The Ultimate Keto Cookbook for Beginners

1001 Easy, Affordable Keto Recipes for Low-Carb High-Fat Meals Lovers and Smart People On a Budget

Marie Johnson

Copyright© 2021 By Marie Johnson
All Rights Reserved

This book is copyright protected. It is only for personal use. You cannot amend, distribute, sell, use, quote or paraphrase any part of the content within this book, without the consent of the author or publisher.

Under no circumstances will any blame or legal responsibility be held against the publisher, or author, for any damages, reparation, or monetary loss due to the information contained within this book, either directly or indirectly.

Disclaimer Notice:

Please note the information contained within this document is for educational and entertainment purposes only. All effort has been executed to present accurate, up to date, reliable, complete information. No warranties of any kind are declared or implied. Readers acknowledge that the author is not engaged in the rendering of legal, financial, medical or professional advice. The content within this book has been derived from various sources. Please consult a licensed professional before attempting any techniques outlined in this book.

By reading this document, the reader agrees that under no circumstances is the author responsible for any losses, direct or indirect, that are incurred as a result of the use of the information contained within this document, including, but not limited to, errors, omissions, or inaccuracies.

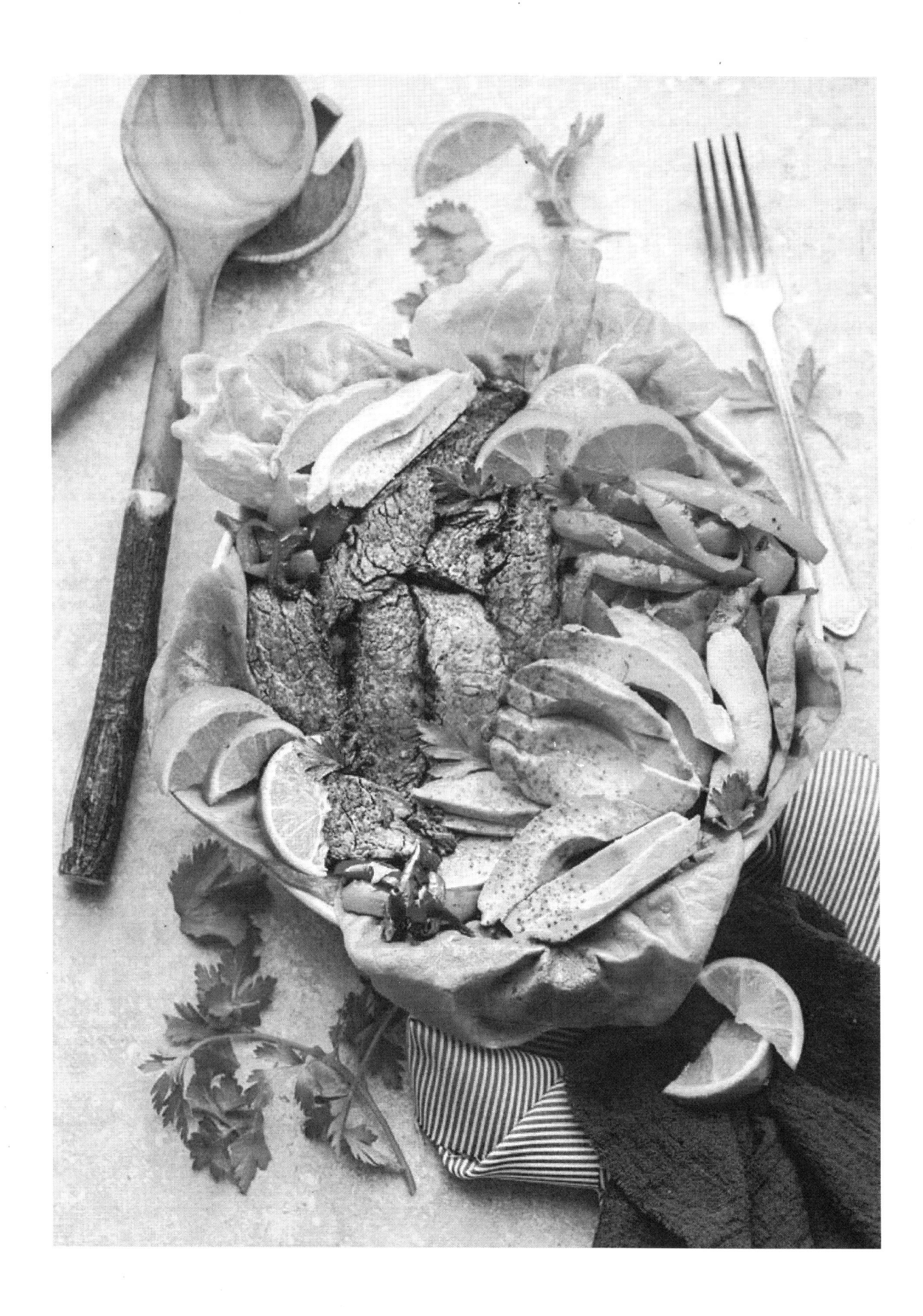

Table of Content

Chapter 1 Breakfast

Coconut and Seed Bagels	1	Pancetta Veg Salad with Kale Frittata	5
Creamy Cashew Lemon Smoothie	1	Cinnamon-Cream-Cheese Almond Waffles	6
Avocado and Berry Smoothie	1	Zucchini and Carrot Coconut Bread	6
Dill-Cream-Cheese Salmon Rolls	1	Mushroom and Broccoli Quiche	6
Bacon and Jalapeño Egg Muffins	2	Cheesy Egg and Bacon Quesadillas	7
Italian Bacon Omelet	2	Swiss Chard, Sausage, and Squash Omelet	7
French Scrambled Eggs	2	Ham, Cheese and Egg Cups	7
Tomato and Bacon Cups	2	Mushroom and Kale Tofu Scramble	8
Chorizo, Kale, and Avocado Eggs	3	Lemony Ginger Pancakes	8
Easy Peanut Butter Smoothie	3	Cheese and Egg Spinach Nests	8
Cheddar Bacon and Egg Frittata	3	Cream Cheese Almond Muffins	9
Spinach-Cucumber Smoothie	3	Jalapeño Pepper Cream Cheese Omelet	9
Broccoli and Ham Egg Bake	4	Pesto Bacon and Avocado Mug Cakes	9
Raspberry and Kale Smoothie	4	Egg and Ham Muffins	10
Sausage Quiche	4	Caramel-Cream Chocolate Crepes	10
Mediterranean Aïoli	4	Creamy Ricotta Almond Cloud Pancakes	11
Avocado Sausage Stacks	5	Gruyere and Mushroom Lettuce Wraps	11
Vanilla Mascarpone Cups	5		

Chapter 2 Snacks and Appetizers

Romano Cheese Meatballs	13	Cocktail Meatballs	18
Caribbean Baked Wings	13	Avocado and Ham Stuffed Eggs	18
Chicken Wings in Spicy Tomato Sauce	13	Sardine Pepper Boats	18
Zucchini Chips	13	Anchovy Fat Bombs	18
Turkey Stuffed Mini Peppers	14	Cauliflower Bites	19
Baked Cocktail Franks	14	Herbed Provolone Cheese Chips	19
Cheese Bites with Pickle	14	Paprika Veggie Bites	19
Cheese and Shrimp Stuffed Celery	14	Crispy Five Seed Crackers	19
Romano and Asiago Cheese Crisps	15	Cheesy Ham and Chicken Bites	20
Traditional Walnut Fat Bombs	15	Avocado-Bacon Sushi	20
Caprese Sticks	15	Cheesy Prosciutto Balls	20
Cheesy Ham-Egg Cups	15	Spicy Chicken Drumettes	20
Bacon-Wrapped Poblano Poppers	16	Beef-Stuffed Peppers	21
Whiskey-Glazed Chicken Wings	16	Cheddar Anchovies Fat Bombs	21
BLT Cups	16	Bacon-Wrapped Enoki Mushrooms	21
Kale Chips	16	Turkey and Avocado Roll-Ups	21
Chicken and Spinach Meatballs	17	Pork Skewers with Greek Dipping Sauce	22
Fajita Spareribs	17	Hot Spare Ribs	22
Cream Cheese Stuffed Mushrooms	17	Meaty Jalapeños	23
Wrapped Asparagus with Prosciutto	17	Mini Bacon and Kale Muffins	23

Chapter 3 Salads

Greek Caper Salad	25	Shrimp Salad with Lemony Mayonnaise	28
Arugula and Avocado Salad	25	Mediterranean Tomato and Avocado Salad	28
Tuna Cheese Caprese Salad	25	Caesar Salad with Salmon and Egg	29
Bacon, Avocado, and Veggies Salad	25	Salmon Fillet and Spinach Cobb Salad	29
Beef and Spinach Salad	26	Kale and Smoked Salmon Salad	29
Marinated Pork and Veg Salad	26	Egg and Chicken Salad in Lettuce Cups	30
Spanish Chicken and Pepper Salad	26	Skirt Steak, Veggies, and Pecan Salad	30
Chicken Thigh Green Salad	27	Yellow Cheddar Pork Patties Salad	30
Tuna Salad with Olives and Lettuce	27	Mackerel and Green Bean Salad	31
Caprese Salad	27	Lemony Prawn and Arugula Salad	31
Classic Greek Salad	27	Garlicky Chicken Salad	32
Feta Cucumber Salad	28	Balsamic Brussels Sprouts Cheese Salad	32
Spinach and Bacon Salad	28		

Chapter 4 Soups

Cauliflower and Lamb Soup	34	Salsa Verde Chicken Soup	39
Turkey Taco Soup	34	Hearty Chicken Soup	39
Lemony Chicken and Chive Soup	34	Pork and Vegetable Soup	40
Green Minestrone Soup	34	Cioppino	40
Chicken and Cabbage Soup	35	Coconut Pumpkin Soup	40
Beef Hamburger Soup	35	Bacon Green Soup	41
Pork Soup	35	Italian Tomato Soup	41
Herbed Beef and Zucchini Soup	35	Cream of Broccoli Soup	41
Lamb and Cheddar Taco Soup	36	Tomato Soup	42
Coconut Carrot Soup	36	Power Green Soup	42
Garlicky Coconut Milk and Tomato Soup	36	Broccoli Soup	42
Easy Chicken and Onion Soup	36	Reuben Beef Soup	42
Coconut Milk and Pumpkin Soup	37	Beef and Mushroom Soup	43
Slow Cooked Faux Lasagna Soup	37	Nacho Soup	43
Super Cheesy Bacon-Cauliflower Soup	37	Leek and Turkey Soup	43
Herbed Beef Soup	37	Cauliflower Soup	44
Zucchini and Celery Soup	38	Rich Taco Soup	44
Cheddar Cauliflower Soup	38	Colden Gazpacho Soup	44
Pork and Mustard Green Soup	38	Cauliflower Soup with Sausage	45
Saffron Coconut Shrimp Soup	39	Curry Green Beans and Shrimp Soup	45

Chapter 5

Grilled Prosciutto-Chicken Wraps	47	Cauliflower Egg Bake	49
Almond and Rind Crusted Zucchini Fritters	47	Bell Pepper and Tomato Sataraš	49
Boiled Stuffed Eggs	47	Balsamic Glazed Brussels Sprouts	50
Paprika Riced Cauliflower	47	Cheddar Buffalo Chicken Bake	50
Chinese Cauliflower Rice with Eggs	48	Mushroom Stroganoff	50
Cottage Kale Stir-Fry	48	Classic Devilled Eggs with Sriracha Mayo	50
Romano Zucchini Cups	48	Broccoli and Cauliflower Mash	51
Indian White Cabbage Stew	48	Zucchini Fritters	51
Pumpkin and Cauliflower Curry	49	Spinach Cheese Balls	51
Creamy Spinach	49	Braised Cream Kale	51

Vegetables and Sides

Colby Bacon-Wrapped Jalapeño Peppers	52	Italian Tomato and Cheese Stuffed Peppers	56
Roasted Cauliflower with Serrano Ham	52	Broccoli Cheese	56
Crispy Chorizo with Parsley	52	Duo-Cheese Broccoli Croquettes	57
Mashed Cauliflower with Bacon and Chives	52	Mascarpone Turkey Pastrami Pinwheels	57
Chicken-Stuffed Cucumber Bites	53	Duo-Cheese Lettuce Rolls	57
Herbed Eggplant	53	Pecorino Cauli Bake with Mayo	57
Tuna-Mayo Topped Dill Pickles	53	Roasted Asparagus	58
Cheese Stuffed Spaghetti Squash	53	Chicken Breast Fritters with Dill Dip	58
Spiced Cauliflower Cheese Bake	54	Mozzarella Prosciutto Wraps with Basil	58
Zucchini Casserole	54	Buttered Broccoli	58
Cumin Green Cabbage Stir-Fry	54	Feta Zucchini and Pepper Gratin	59
Riced Cauliflower Stuffed Bell Peppers	55	Pecorino Mushroom Burgers	59
Herbed Eggplant and Kale Bake	55	Parmesan Cauliflower Fritters	59
Vegetable Mix	55	Prosciutto-Wrapped Piquillo Peppers	60
Zucchini Sticks with Garlic Aioli	56	Avocado Crostini Nori with Walnuts	60

Chapter 6 Vegan and Vegetarian

Cauliflower and Celery Soup	62	Cauliflower Chowder with Fresh Dill	64
Mushroom and Zucchini Stew	62	Parmesan Veggie Fritters	65
Lemony Cucumber-Avocado Salad	62	Italian Broccoli and Spinach Soup	65
Swiss Cheese Broccoli	62	Mexican-Flavored Stuffed Peppers	65
Creamy Cabbage and Cauliflower	63	Peppery Omelet with Cheddar Cheese	66
Mushroom and Bell Pepper Omelet	63	Greek Aubergine-Egg Casserole	66
Egg-Stuffed Avocados	63	Halloumi Asparagus Frittata	66
Summer Stew with Chives	63	Swiss Zucchini Gratin	67
Citrus Asparagus and Cherry Tomato Salad	64	Colby Broccoli Bake	67
Shirataki Mushroom Ramen	64	Double Cheese Kale Bake	67

Chapter 7

Pistachio Nut Salmon with Shallot Sauce	69	Italian Haddock Fillet	73
Greek Tilapia with Tomatoes and Olives	69	Dijon-Tarragon Salmon	73
Tuna Fillet Salade Niçoise	69	Chive-Sauced Chili Cod	73
Anchovies with Caesar Dressing	69	Lobster and Cauliflower Salad Rolls	74
Coconut Shrimp Stew	70	Salmon with Radish and Arugula Salad	74
Dijon Crab Cakes	70	Tuna Omelet Wraps	74
Smoked Salmon and Avocado Omelet	70	Gambas al Ajillo	74
Haddock with Mediterranean Sauce	70	Swedish Herring and Spinach Salad	75
Tilapia Tacos with Cabbage Slaw	71	Baked Tilapia with Black Olives	75
Tilapia and Riced Cauliflower Cabbage Tortillas	71	Garlicky Mackerel Fillet	75
Catalan Shrimp	71	Seared Scallops with Sausage	75
Halibut Tacos with Cabbage Slaw	71	Tuna, Ham and Avocado Wraps	76
Tuna Shirataki Pad Thai	72	Anchovies and Veggies Wraps	76
Sardines with Zoodles	72	Grilled Salmon Steak	76
White Chowder	72	Tiger Shrimp with Chimichurri	76
Cajun Tilapia Fish Burgers	72	Mediterranean Halibut Fillet	77
Salmon Fillets with Broccoli	73	Goan Sole Fillet Stew	77
		Parsley-Lemon Salmon	77

Fish and Seafood

Spanish Cod à La Nage	77	Sardine Burgers	82
Asian Scallop and Vegetable	78	Coconut Mussel Curry	82
Shrimp and Vegetable Bowl	78	Old Bay Sea Bass Fillet	82
Shrimp and Pork Rind Stuffed Zucchini	78	Cheesy Shrimp Stuffed Mushrooms	83
Red Snapper Fillet and Salad	79	Fennel and Trout Parcels	83
Hazelnut Haddock Bake	79	Salmon and Cucumber Panzanella	83
Provençal Lemony Fish Stew	79	Shrimp Jambalaya	84
Shirataki Noodles with Grilled Tuna	80	Thai Tuna Fillet	84
Almond Breaded Hoki	80	Alaskan Cod Fillet	84
Asparagus and Trout Foil Packets	80	Catfish Flakes and Cauliflower Casserole	85
Coconut and Pecorino Fried Shrimp	81	Smoked Haddock Burgers	85
Seafood Chowder	81	Cod Patties with Creamed Horseradish	85
Curry White Fish Fillet	81		

Chapter 8 Poultry

Tikka Masala	87	Mediterranean Roasted Chicken Drumettes	96
Italian Turkey Meatballs with Leeks	87	Classic Jerk Chicken	96
Grilled Lemony Chicken Wings	87	Marinated Chicken with Peanut Sauce	96
Simple White Wine Drumettes	87	Cheddar Bacon Stuffed Chicken Fillets	97
Asian Turkey and Bird's Eye Soup	88	Tuscan Chicken Breast Sauté	97
Turkey and Canadian Bacon Pizza	88	Herbed Balsamic Turkey	97
Grilled Rosemary Wings with Leeks	88	Turkish Chicken Thigh Kebabs	98
Thyme Roasted Drumsticks	88	Turkey Wing Curry	98
Herbed Turkey with Cucumber Salsa	89	Chicken Paella and Chorizo	98
Lemony Rosemary Chicken Thighs	89	Chinese Flavor Chicken Legs	99
Asiago Drumsticks with Spinach	89	Itanlian Chicken Cacciatore	99
Greek Drumettes with Olives	89	Roasted Chicken Breasts with Capers	99
Chipotle Tomato and Pumpkin Chicken Chili	90	Parma Ham-Wrapped Stuffed Chicken	100
Chicken Thigh and Kale Stew	90	Ritzy Baked Chicken with Vegetable	100
Bell Pepper Turkey Casserole	90	Double-Cheese Ranch Chicken	100
Chicken and Bell Pepper Kabobs	91	Baked Chicken in Tomato Purée	101
Chicken Mélange	91	Parmesan Spinach Stuffed Chicken	101
Rind and Cheese Crusted Chicken	91	Homemade Poulet en Papillote	101
Leek and Pumpkin Turkey Stew	92	Hungarian Chicken Thighs	102
Teriyaki Turkey with Peppers	92	Stir-Fried Chicken, Broccoli and Cashew	102
Chicken Drumsticks in Capocollo	92	Chicken with Mayo-Avocado Sauce	102
Olla Tapada	93	Chicken with Cream of Mushroom Soup	103
Chicken and Tomato Packets	93	Garlicky Sweet Chicken Skewers	103
Creamy-Lemony Chicken Thighs	93	Braised Chicken and Veggies	103
Slow Cooked Chicken Cacciatore	94	Bacon-Wrapped Chicken with Asparagus	104
Coconut Turkey Breast	94	Parmesan Chicken Wings with Yogurt Sauce	104
Turkey and Pumpkin Ragout	94	Baked Cheesy Chicken and Spinach	104
Spiced Duck Goulash	95	Lemony Chicken Skewers	105
Italian Asiago and Pepper Stuffed Turkey	95	Paprika Chicken Wings	105
Chicken, Pepper, and Tomato Bake	95	Oregano Chicken Breast	105

Chapter 9 Pork

Pork Paprikash	107	Chili Con Carne	113
Cream of Onion Pork Cutlets	107	Tangy-Garlicky Pork Chops	114
Lemony Mustard Pork Roast	107	Paprika Pork Loin Shoulder	114
Mediterranean Spiced Pork Roast	107	Pork and Yellow Squash Traybake	114
Pork Cutlets with Juniper Berries	108	Creamy Pepper Loin Steaks	115
Bolognese Pork Zoodles	108	Pork Ragout	115
Seared Pork Medallions	108	Roasted Pork Shoulder	115
White Wine Pork with Cabbage	108	Pork Chops and Brussel Sprouts	116
Pork Lettuce Wraps	109	Pork Chops with Greek Salsa	116
Mustard Pork Meatballs	109	Hearty Pork Stew Meat	116
BBQ Grilled Pork Spare Ribs	109	Spicy Pork Meatballs with Seeds	117
Spicy Pork and Capers with Olives	109	Tangy Pork Rib Roast	117
Pork Chops and Bacon	110	Pulled Boston Butt	117
Pork with Raspberry Sauce	110	Pork and Butternut Squash Stew	118
Pork and Beef Meatballs	110	Herbed Pork Chops with Cranberry Sauce	118
Spicy Pork and Spanish Onion	110	Pork Medallions	118
Creamy Dijon Pork Filet Mignon	111	Roasted Stuffed Pork Loin Steak	119
Bacon and Pork Omelet	111	Parmesan Bacon-Stuffed Pork Roll	119
Duo-Cheese Pork and Turkey Patties	111	Pork Chops with Veggies	119
Pork Steaks with Chimichurri Sauce	111	Pork and Veggies Burgers	120
Herbed Pork and Turkey Meatloaf	112	Pork Kofte with Cauliflower Mash	120
Olla Podrida	112	Tomato purée Pork Chops	120
St. Louis Ribs	112	Baked Cheesy Pork and Veggies	121
Pickle and Ham Stuffed Pork	113	Pork and Mashed Cauliflower Crust	121
BBQ Pork Ribs	113	Texas Pulled Boston Butt	121

Chapter 10

King Size Beef Burgers	123	Spicy Beef Brisket Roast	129
Zoodles with Beef Bolognese Sauce	123	Thai Beef Steak with Mushrooms	129
Ground Beef and Cauliflower Curry	123	Juicy Beef with Thyme and Rosemary	129
Simple Beef Burgers	123	Pinwheel Beef and Spinach Steaks	130
Texas Chili	124	Beef and Mushroom Cheeseburgers	130
Chipotle Beef Spare Ribs	124	Beef Meatloaf with Balsamic Glaze	130
Zucchini and Beef Lasagna	124	Lamb Chops with Fennel and Zucchini	131
Beef and Broccoli Casserole	125	Balsamic Glazed Meatloaf	131
Balsamic Mushroom Beef Meatloaf	125	Beef Steaks with Mushrooms and Bacon	131
Beef and Veggie Stuffed Butternut Squash	125	Beef Ragout with Green Beans	132
Lemony Beef Rib Roast	126	Beef Chuck Roast with Mushrooms	132
Mexican Beef and Tomato Chili	126	Veal, Mushroom, and Green Bean Stew	132
Lamb Curry	126	Bacon and Beef Stew	133
Italian Sausage and Okra Stew	127	Pork Rind Crusted Beef Meatballs	133
Beef, Pancetta, and Mushroom Bourguignon	127	Asian-Flavored Beef and Broccoli	133
Beef and Onion Stuffed Zucchinis	127	Creole Beef Tripe Stew with Onions	134
Veggie Cauliflower Rice with Beef Steak	128	Cauliflower and Tomato Beef Curry	134
Beef and Pimiento in Zucchini Boats	128	Grilled Ribeye Steaks with Green Beans	134
Mascarpone Beef Balls with Cilantro	128	Mozzarella Beef Gratin	134

Beef and Lamb

Beef Sausage Casserole with Okra	135	Beef Lasagna with Zucchinis	138
Caribbean Beef with Peppers	135	Juicy Beef Meatballs with Parsley	139
Beef Stew with Black Olives	135	Beef and Cauliflower Rice Casserole	139
Onion Sauced Beef Meatballs	136	Russian Beef and Dill Pickle Gratin	140
Butternut Squash and Beef Stew	136	Beef Tripe with Onions and Tomatoes	140
Flank Steak and Kale Roll	136	Skirt Steak with Green Beans	140
Creamy Reuben Soup with Sauerkraut	137	Herbed Veggie and Beef Stew	141
Beef Brisket with Red Wine	137	Beef and Fennel Provençal	141
Basil Feta Flank Steak Pinwheels	137	Italian Veal Cutlets with Pecorino	142
Beef Chuck Roast with Veggies	138	Grilled Beef Skewers with Fresh Salad	142
Beef Casserole with Cauliflower	138		

Chapter 11 Desserts

Creamy Strawberry Shake	144	Coffee-Coconut Ice Pops	151
Chocolate-Coconut Shake	144	Cheesy Lemonade Fat Bomb	151
Vanilla Chocolate Pudding	144	Baked Cheesecake Bites	152
Chocolate Almond Bark	145	Pumpkin Cheesecake Bites	152
Fresh Strawberry Cheesecake Mousse	145	Chocolate Pecan-Berry Mascarpone Bowl	152
Chocolate Truffles	145	Blackberry Cobbler with Almonds	152
Salted Vanilla Caramels	146	Crispy Strawberry Chocolate Bark	153
Chocolate Fudge	146	Almond-Sour Cream Cheesecake	153
Cheesecake Fat Bomb with Berries	146	Keto Peanut Butter Cookies	153
Bacon Fudge	147	Slow Cooker Chocolate Pot De Crème	154
Classic Flan	147	Lemon Custard	154
Almond Fat Bombs with Chocolate Chips	148	Almond-Peanut Butter Cheesecake	154
Pecan Pralines	148	Strawberry Mousse	155
Panna Cotta	148	Creamy Chocolate Mousse	155
Cinnamon Crusted Almonds	149	Chocolate Chip Ice Cream with Mint	155
Strawberries Coated with Chocolate Chips	149	Avocado-Chocolate Pudding	156
Meringues	149	Pumpkin Compote with Mix Berries	156
Cream Cheese Fat Bombs	150	Ginger-Pumpkin Pudding	156
Lime and Coconut Panna Cotta	150	Blueberry-Pecan Crisp	156
Posset	150	Flaxseed Coconut Bread Pudding	157
Peanut Butter and Chocolate Fat Bombs	151	Blueberry, Strawberry, and Raspberry Parfaits	158
Simple Peanut Butter Fat Bomb	151		

Chapter 12 Sauces and Dressings

Sriracha Sauce	160	Tzatziki Sauce	162
Fettuccine Alfredo	160	Garlic Aioli Sauce	162
BBQ Sauce	160	Tomato and Bacon Dressing	162
Orange Chili Sauce	160	Creamy Caesar Dressing	162
Cheesy Hot Crab Sauce	161	Blue Cheese Dressing	163
Scallion Ginger Dressing	161	Asian Peanut Sauce	163
Marinara	161	Ketchup	163
Parmesan Basil Vinaigrette	161	Strawberry Vinaigrette	163

Appendix 1 Measurement Conversion Chart	164	Appendix 2 Recipe Index	165

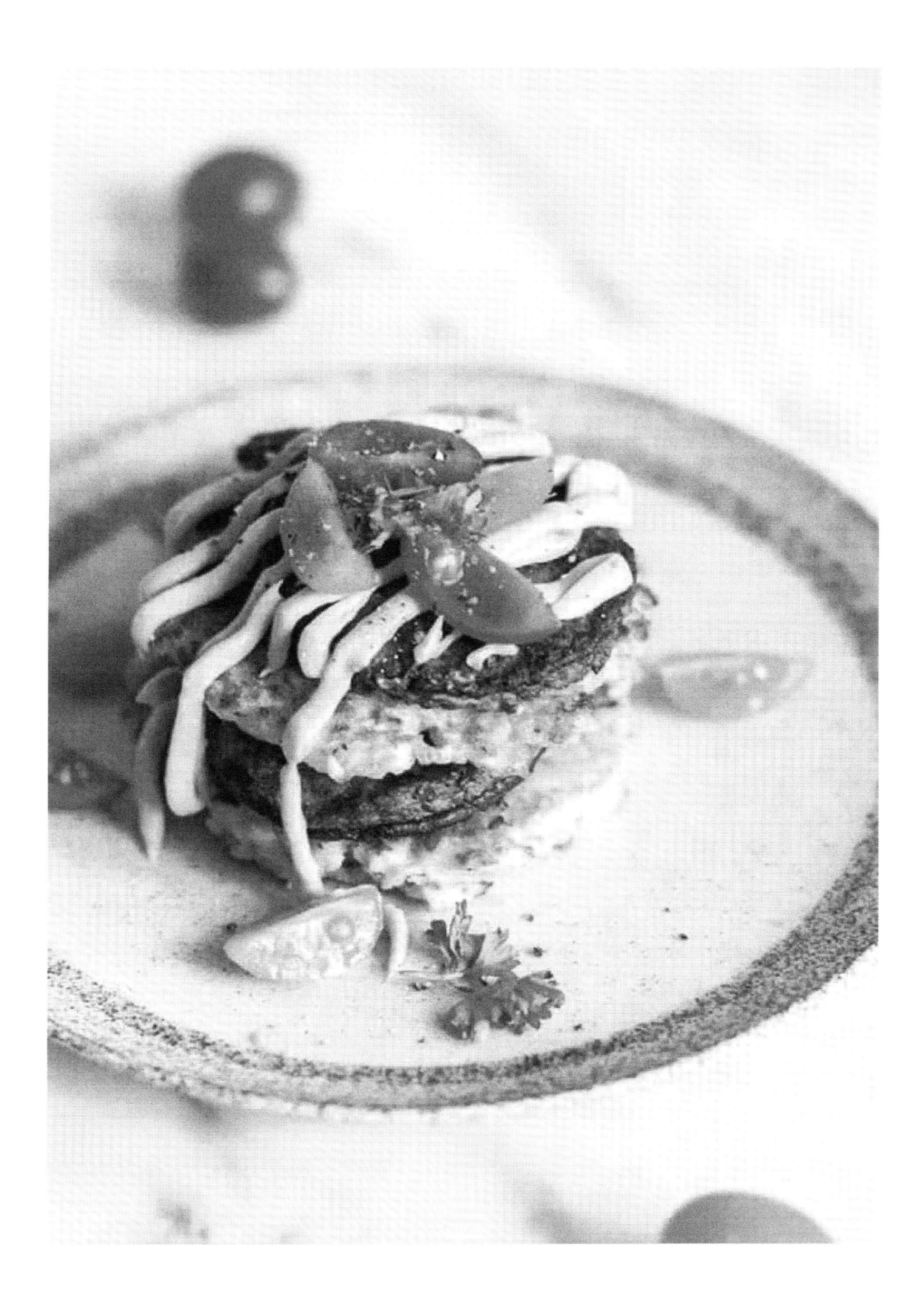

Chapter 1 Breakfast

Coconut and Seed Bagels

Prep time: 5 minutes | Cook time: 20 minutes | Serves 4

½ cup coconut flour
6 eggs, beaten in a bowl
½ cup vegetable broth
¼ cup flax seed meal
¼ cup chia seed meal
1 teaspoon onion powder
1 teaspoon garlic powder
1 teaspoon dried parsley
1 teaspoon chia seeds
1 teaspoon sesame seeds
1 chopped onion

1. Preheat the oven to 350ºF (180ºC).
2. Mix the coconut flour, eggs, broth, flax seed meal, chia seed meal, onion powder, garlic powder, and parsley. Spoon the mixture into a donut tray.
3. In a small bowl, mix the chia seeds, sesame seeds, and onion, and sprinkle on the batter.
4. Bake the bagels for 20 minutes. Serve the bagels with creamy pumpkin soup.

Per Serving
calories: 425 | fat: 19.0g | protein: 33.2g
carbs: 3.3g | net carbs: 0.5g | fiber: 2.8g

Creamy Cashew Lemon Smoothie

Prep time: 5 minutes | Cook time: 0 minutes | Serves 1

1 cup unsweetened cashew milk
¼ cup heavy (whipping) cream
¼ cup freshly squeezed lemon juice
1 scoop plain protein powder
1 tablespoon coconut oil
1 teaspoon Swerve

1. Put the cashew milk, heavy cream, lemon juice, protein powder, coconut oil, and sweetener in a blender and blend until smooth.
2. Pour into a glass and serve immediately.

Per Serving
calories: 503 | fat: 45g | protein: 29g
carbs: 15g | net carbs: 11g | fiber: 4g

Avocado and Berry Smoothie

Prep time: 5 minutes | Cook time: 0 minutes | Serves 2

1 cup unsweetened full-fat coconut milk
1 scoop Perfect Keto Exogenous Ketone Powder in chocolate sea salt
½ avocado
2 tablespoons almond butter
½ cup berries, fresh or frozen (no sugar added if frozen)
½ cup ice cubes
¼ teaspoon liquid stevia (optional)

1. In a blender, combine the coconut milk, protein powder, avocado, almond butter, berries, ice, and stevia (if using).
2. Blend until thoroughly mixed and frothy.
3. Pour into two glasses and enjoy.

Per Serving
calories: 446 | fat: 43g | protein: 7g
carbs: 16g | net carbs: 9g | fiber: 7g

Dill-Cream-Cheese Salmon Rolls

Prep time: 10 minutes | Cook time: 0 minutes | Serves 3

3 tablespoons cream cheese, softened
1 small lemon, zested and juiced
3 teaspoons chopped fresh dill
Salt and black pepper to taste
3 (7-inch) low carb tortillas
6 slices smoked salmon

1. In a bowl, mix the cream cheese, lemon juice, zest, dill, salt, and black pepper.
2. Lay each tortilla on a plastic wrap (just wide enough to cover the tortilla), spread with cream cheese mixture, and top each (one) with two salmon slices. Roll up the tortillas and secure both ends by twisting.
3. Refrigerate for 2 hours, remove plastic, cut off both ends of each wrap, and cut wraps into wheels.

Per Serving
calories: 251 | fat: 16.1g | protein: 17.8g
carbs: 8.7g | net carbs: 7.0g | fiber: 1.7g

Bacon and Jalapeño Egg Muffins

Prep time: 10 minutes | Cook time: 20 minutes | Serves 6

12 eggs
¼ cup coconut milk
Salt and black pepper to taste
1 cup grated Cheddar cheese
12 slices bacon
4 jalapeño peppers, seeded and minced

1. Preheat oven to 370ºF (188ºC).
2. Crack the eggs into a bowl and whisk with coconut milk until combined. Season with salt and pepper, and evenly stir in the Cheddar cheese.
3. Line each hole of a muffin tin with a slice of bacon and fill each with the egg mixture twothirds way up. Top with the jalapeño peppers and bake in the oven for 18 to 20 minutes or until puffed and golden. Remove, allow cooling for a few minutes, and serve with arugula salad.

Per Serving
calories: 301 | fat: 23.8g | protein: 19.8g
carbs: 3.8g | net carbs: 3.3g | fiber: 0.5g

Italian Bacon Omelet

Prep time: 10 minutes | Cook time: 5 minutes | Serves 3

3 ounces (85 g) bacon, diced
2 garlic cloves, minced
1 Italian pepper, chopped
6 eggs, whisked
1 teaspoon Italian seasoning blend
Sea salt and ground black pepper, to season
½ cup goat cheese, shredded

1. Preheat a nonstick skillet over a medium-high flame. Now, cook the bacon until crisp or about 4 minutes; reserve.
2. Add in the garlic and Italian pepper; continue to sauté for a minute or so until aromatic. Pour the eggs into the skillet.
3. Sprinkle with the Italian seasoning blend, salt, and black pepper. Cook until the eggs are golden brown on top. Add the reserved bacon and goat cheese.
4. Fold your omelet in half and serve immediately. Bon appétit!

Per Serving
calories: 481 | fat: 43g | protein: 17g
carbs: 5g | net carbs: 4g | fiber: 1g

French Scrambled Eggs

Prep time: 5 minutes | Cook time: 8 minutes | Serves 3

6 large eggs
1 tablespoon butter, at room temperature
¼ teaspoon ground black pepper
Sea salt, to taste
4 tablespoons crème fraîche

1. Crack the eggs into a bowl and beat them with a wire whisk until the yolks and whites are fully incorporated into each other.
2. Then, melt the butter in a nonstick skillet over a moderate flame. Once hot, add the egg mixture to the skillet.
3. The eggs will start to form curds. Stir until just set but still slightly wet or 8 to 10 minutes. Add in the black pepper, salt, and crème fraiche. Remove from the heat. Enjoy!

Per Serving
calories: 257 | fat: 21g | protein: 13g
carbs: 1g | net carbs: 1g | fiber: 0g

Tomato and Bacon Cups

Prep time: 10 minutes | Cook time: 23 minutes | Serves 6

12 bacon slices
2 tomatoes, diced
1 onion, diced
1 cup shredded Cheddar cheese
1 cup mayonnaise
12 low carb crepes/pancakes
1 teaspoon dried basil
Chopped chives to garnish

1. Fry the bacon in a skillet over medium heat for 5 minutes. Remove and chop with a knife. Transfer to a bowl. Add in Cheddar cheese, tomatoes, onion, mayonnaise, and basil. Mix well set aside.
2. Place the crepes on a flat surface and use egg rings to cut a circle out of each crepe. Grease the muffin cups with cooking spray and fit the circled crepes into them to make a cup.
3. Now, fill the cups with 3 tablespoons of bacon-tomato mixture. Place the muffin cups on a baking sheet, and bake for 18 minutes. Garnish with the chives, and serve with a tomato or cheese sauce.

Per Serving
calories: 426 | fat: 45.1g | protein: 16.1g
carbs: 5.5g | net carbs: 4.2g | fiber: 1.3g

Chorizo, Kale, and Avocado Eggs

Prep time: 7 minutes | Cook time: 13 minutes | Serves 4

1 teaspoon butter
1 red onion, sliced
4 ounces (113 g) chorizo, sliced into thin rounds
1 cup chopped kale
1 ripe avocado, pitted, peeled, chopped
4 eggs
Salt and black pepper to season

1. Preheat oven to 370ºF (188ºC).
2. Melt butter in a cast iron pan over medium heat and sauté the onion for 2 minutes. Add the chorizo and cook for 2 minutes more, flipping once.
3. Introduce the kale in batches with a splash of water to wilt, season lightly with salt, stir and cook for 3 minutes. Mix in the avocado and turn the heat off.
4. Create four holes in the mixture, crack the eggs into each hole, sprinkle with salt and black pepper, and slide the pan into the preheated oven to bake for 6 minutes until the egg whites are set or firm and yolks still runny. Season to taste with salt and pepper, and serve right away with low carb toasts.

Per Serving
calories: 275 | fat: 23.1g | protein: 12.9g
carbs: 7.7g | net carbs: 4.1g | fiber: 3.6g

Easy Peanut Butter Smoothie

Prep time: 5 minutes | Cook time: 0 minutes | Serves 2

1 cup water
¾ cup coconut cream
1 scoop chocolate protein powder
2 tablespoons natural peanut butter
3 ice cubes

1. Put the water, coconut cream, protein powder, peanut butter, and ice in a blender and blend until smooth.
2. Pour into 2 glasses and serve immediately.

Per Serving
calories: 486 | fat: 40g | protein: 30g
carbs: 11g | net carbs: 6g | fiber: 5g

Cheddar Bacon and Egg Frittata

Prep time: 9 minutes | Cook time: 16 minutes | Serves 4

10 slices bacon
10 fresh eggs
3 tablespoons butter, melted
½ cup almond milk
Salt and black pepper to taste
1½ cups Cheddar cheese, shredded
¼ cup chopped green onions

1. Preheat the oven to 400ºF (205ºC) and grease a baking dish with cooking spray. Cook the bacon in a skillet over medium heat for 6 minutes. Once crispy, remove from the skillet to paper towels and discard grease. Chop into small pieces. Whisk the eggs, butter, milk, salt, and black pepper. Mix in the bacon and pour the mixture into the baking dish.
2. Sprinkle with Cheddar cheese and green onions, and bake in the oven for 10 minutes or until the eggs are thoroughly cooked. Remove and cool the frittata for 3 minutes, slice into wedges, and serve warm with a dollop of Greek yogurt.

Per Serving
calories: 326 | fat: 28.1g | protein: 14.9g
carbs: 2.5g | net carbs: 2.1g | fiber: 0.4g

Spinach-Cucumber Smoothie

Prep time: 5 minutes | Cook time: 0 minutes | Serves 2

1 cup coconut milk
1 cup spinach
½ English cucumber, chopped
½ cup blueberries
1 scoop plain protein powder
2 tablespoons coconut oil
4 ice cubes
Mint sprigs, for garnish

1. Put the coconut milk, spinach, cucumber, blueberries, protein powder, coconut oil, and ice in a blender and blend until smooth.
2. Pour into 2 glasses, garnish each with the mint, and serve immediately.

Per Serving
calories: 353 | fat: 32g | protein: 15g
carbs: 9g | net carbs: 6g | fiber: 3g

Broccoli and Ham Egg Bake

Prep time: 5 minutes | Cook time: 20 minutes | Serves 4

2 heads broccoli, cut into small florets
2 red bell peppers, seeded and chopped
¼ cup chopped ham
2 teaspoons butter
1 teaspoon dried oregano plus extra to garnish
Salt and black pepper to taste
8 fresh eggs

1. Preheat oven to 425ºF (220ºC).
2. Melt the butter in a frying pan over medium heat; brown the ham, stirring frequently, about 3 minutes.
3. Arrange the broccoli, bell peppers, and ham on a foil-lined baking sheet in a single layer, toss to combine; season with salt, oregano, and black pepper. Bake for 10 minutes until the vegetables have softened.
4. Remove, create eight indentations with a spoon, and crack an egg into each. Return to the oven and continue to bake for an additional 5 to 7 minutes until the egg whites are firm.
5. Season with salt, black pepper, and extra oregano, share the bake into four plates and serve with strawberry lemonade (optional).

Per Serving
calories: 345 | fat: 27.9g | protein: 11.0g
carbs: 8.9g | net carbs: 4.2g | fiber: 4.7g

Raspberry and Kale Smoothie

Prep time: 10 minutes | Cook time: 0 minutes | Serves 2

1 cup water
½ cup raspberries
½ cup shredded kale
¾ cup cream cheese
1 tablespoon coconut oil
1 scoop vanilla protein powder

1. Put the water, raspberries, kale, cream cheese, coconut oil, and protein powder in a blender and blend until smooth.
2. Pour into 2 glasses and serve immediately.

Per Serving
calories: 436 | fat: 36g | protein: 28g
carbs: 11g | net carbs: 6g | fiber: 5g

Sausage Quiche

Prep time: 15 minutes | Cook time: 40 minutes | Serves 6

6 eggs
12 ounces (340 g) raw sausage roll
10 cherry tomatoes, halved
2 tablespoons heavy cream
2 tablespoons Parmesan cheese
¼ teaspoon salt
A pinch of black pepper
2 tablespoons chopped parsley
5 eggplant slices

1. Preheat your oven to 370ºF (188ºC).
2. Grease a pie dish with cooking spray. Press the sausage roll at the bottom of a pie dish. Arrange the eggplant slices on top of the sausage. Top with cherry tomatoes.
3. Whisk the eggs along with the heavy cream, salt, Parmesan cheese, and black pepper. Spoon the mixture over the sausage. Bake for about 40 minutes until browned around the edges. Serve warm, sprinkled with parsley.

Per Serving
calories: 341 | fat: 28.1g | protein: 16.9g
carbs: 6.2g | net carbs: 2.9g | fiber: 3.3g

Mediterranean Aïoli

Prep time: 10 minutes | Cook time: 0 minutes | Serves 6

2 egg yolks
1 teaspoon stone-ground mustard
½ teaspoon sea salt
A pinch of ground black pepper
1 teaspoon garlic, crushed
1 tablespoon lemon juice
½ cup extra-virgin olive oil
1 tablespoon fresh chives

1. Whisk the egg yolks and add them to your food processor.
2. Add in the mustard, salt, black pepper, garlic, and lemon juice; continue mixing until everything is well incorporated.
3. Now, with the machine running, add the oil to the egg yolk mixture in a steady stream. Mix until you reach your desired thickness.
4. Garnish with chives. Keep for about 1 week in the refrigerator. Bon appétit!

Per Serving
calories: 94 | fat: 9g | protein: 2g
carbs: 1g | net carbs: 1g | fiber: 0g

Avocado Sausage Stacks

Prep time: 5 minutes | Cook time: 15 minutes | Serves 6

6 Italian sausage patties
4 tablespoons olive oil
2 ripe avocados, pitted
2 teaspoons fresh lime juice
Salt and black pepper to taste
6 fresh eggs
Red pepper flakes to garnish

1. In a skillet, warm the oil over medium heat and fry the sausage patties about 8 minutes until lightly browned and firm. Remove the patties to a plate.
2. Spoon the avocado into a bowl, mash with the lime juice, and season with salt and black pepper. Spread the mash on the sausages.
3. Boil 3 cups of water in a wide pan over high heat, and reduce to simmer (don't boil).
4. Crack each egg into a small bowl and gently put the egg into the simmering water; poach for 2 to 3 minutes. Use a perforated spoon to remove from the water on a paper towel to dry. Repeat with the other 5 eggs. Top each stack with a poached egg, sprinkle with chili flakes, salt, black pepper, and chives. Serve with turnip wedges.

Per Serving
calories: 388 | fat: 22.9g | protein: 16.1g carbs: 9.6g | net carbs: 5.1g | fiber: 4.5g

Vanilla Mascarpone Cups

Prep time: 5 minutes | Cook time: 15 minutes | Serves 6

¾ cup mascarpone cheese
¼ cup natural yogurt
3 eggs, beaten
1 tablespoon walnuts, ground
4 tablespoons erythritol
½ teaspoon vanilla essence
⅓ teaspoon ground cinnamon

1. Set oven to 360°F (182°C) and grease a muffin pan. Mix all ingredients in a bowl. Split the batter into the muffin cups. Bake for 12 to 15 minutes. Remove and set on a wire rack to cool slightly before serving.

Per Serving
calories: 182 | fat: 13.6g | protein: 10.4g carbs: 3.8g | net carbs: 3.6g | fiber: 0.2g

Pancetta Veg Salad with Kale Frittata

Prep time: 7 minutes | Cook time: 15 minutes | Serves 4

6 slices pancetta
4 tomatoes, cut into 1-inch chunks
1 large cucumber, seeded and sliced
1 small red onion, sliced
¼ cup balsamic vinegar
Salt and black pepper to taste
8 eggs
1 bunch kale, chopped
Salt and black pepper to taste
6 tablespoons grated Parmesan cheese
4 tablespoons olive oil
1 large white onion, sliced
3 ounces (85 g) beef salami, thinly sliced
1 clove garlic, minced

1. Place the pancetta in a skillet and fry over medium heat until crispy, about 4 minutes. Remove to a cutting board and chop.
2. Then, in a small bowl, whisk the vinegar, 2 tablespoons of olive oil, salt, and pepper to make the dressing.
3. Next, combine the tomatoes, red onion, and cucumber in a salad bowl, drizzle with the dressing and toss the veggies. Sprinkle with the pancetta and set aside.
4. Reheat the broiler to 400°F (205°C).
5. Crack the eggs into a bowl and whisk together with half of the Parmesan, salt, and pepper. Set aside.
6. Next, heat the remaining olive oil in the cast iron pan over medium heat. Sauté the onion and garlic for 3 minutes. Add the kale to the skillet, season with salt and pepper, and cook for 2 minutes. Top with the salami, stir and cook further for 1 minute. Pour the egg mixture all over the kale, reduce the heat to medium-low, cover, and cook the ingredients for 4 minutes.
7. Sprinkle the remaining cheese on top and transfer the pan to the oven. Broil to brown on top for 1 minute. When ready, remove the pan and run a spatula around the edges of the frittata; slide it onto a warm platter. Cut the frittata into wedges and serve.

Per Serving
calories: 454 | fat: 30.1g | protein: 26.5g carbs: 8.7g | net carbs: 4.5g | fiber: 4.2g

Cinnamon-Cream-Cheese Almond Waffles

Prep time: 15 minutes | Cook time: 10 minutes | Serves 6

Spread:
8 ounces (227 g) cream cheese, at room temperature
1 teaspoon cinnamon powder
3 tablespoons Swerve brown sugar
Cinnamon powder for garnishing

Waffles:
5 tablespoons melted butter
1½ cups unsweetened almond milk
7 large eggs
¼ teaspoon liquid stevia
½ teaspoon baking powder
1½ cups almond flour

1. Combine the cream cheese, cinnamon, and Swerve with a hand mixer until smooth. Cover and chill until ready to use.
2. To make the waffles, whisk the butter, milk, and eggs in a medium bowl. Add the stevia and baking powder and mix. Stir in the almond flour and combine until no lumps exist. Let the batter sit for 5 minutes to thicken. Spritz a waffle iron with a non-stick cooking spray. Ladle a ¼ cup of the batter into the waffle iron and cook according to the manufacturer's instructions until golden, about 10 minutes in total. Repeat with the remaining batter.
3. Slice the waffles into quarters; apply the cinnamon spread in between each of two waffles and snap. Sprinkle with cinnamon powder and serve.

Per Serving
calories: 308 | fat: 24.1g | protein: 11.9g
carbs: 9.6g | net carbs: 7.8g | fiber: 1.8g

Zucchini and Carrot Coconut Bread

Prep time: 15 minutes | Cook time: 55 minutes | Serves 4

1 cup shredded carrots
1 cup shredded zucchini, squeezed
⅓ cup coconut flour
1 teaspoon vanilla extract
6 eggs
1 tablespoon coconut oil
¾ teaspoon baking soda
1 tablespoon cinnamon powder
½ teaspoon salt
½ cup Greek yogurt
1 teaspoon apple cider vinegar
½ teaspoon nutmeg powder

1. Preheat the oven to 350ºF (180ºC) and grease the loaf pan with cooking spray. Set aside.
2. Mix the carrots, zucchini, coconut flour, vanilla extract, eggs, coconut oil, baking soda, cinnamon powder, salt, Greek yogurt, vinegar, and nutmeg. Pour the batter into the loaf pan and bake for 55 minutes.
3. Remove the bread after and let cool for 5 minutes. Preserve the bread and use it for toasts, sandwiches, or served with soups and salads.

Per Serving
calories: 176 | fat: 10.6g | protein: 11.5g
carbs: 4.5g | net carbs: 1.7g | fiber: 2.8g

Mushroom and Broccoli Quiche

Prep time: 15 minutes | Cook time: 55 to 60 minutes | Serves 6

12 eggs
1½ cups shredded Cheddar cheese
1½ cups almond milk
½ teaspoon dried thyme
Salt to taste
¼ cup sliced mushrooms
½ cup chopped broccoli
1 clove garlic, minced

Quiche Pastry:
¾ cup almond flour
A pinch of salt
2 ounces (57 g) cold butter
½ teaspoon baking powder
1 tablespoon cold water
2 eggs
Cooking spray

1. Preheat the oven to 370ºF (188ºC).
2. In a large bowl, mix all the crust ingredients until dough is formed. Press it into a greased baking dish and bake for 20-25 minutes until lightly golden.
3. Spread the Cheddar cheese in the pie crust. Beat the eggs with the almond milk, thyme, and salt, then, stir in the mushrooms, broccoli, and garlic.
4. Pour the ingredients into the pie crust and bake in the oven for 35 minutes until the quiche is set.
5. Remove and serve sliced with a tomato and avocado salad.

Per Serving
calories: 486 | fat: 39.6g | protein: 24.6g
carbs: 7.1g | net carbs: 6.2g | fiber: 0.9g

Cheesy Egg and Bacon Quesadillas

Prep time: 14 minutes | Cook time: 16 minutes | Serves 4

8 low carb tortilla shells	1½ cups grated Swiss cheese
6 eggs	5 bacon slices
1 cup water	1 medium onion, thinly sliced
3 tablespoons butter	1 tablespoon chopped parsley
1½ cups grated Cheddar cheese	

1. Bring the eggs to a boil in water over medium heat for 10 minutes. Transfer the eggs to an ice water bath, peel the shells, and chop them; set aside.
2. Meanwhile, as the eggs cook, fry the bacon in a skillet over medium heat for 4 minutes until crispy. Remove and chop. Plate and set aside too.
3. Fetch out ⅔ of the bacon fat and sauté the onions in the remaining grease over medium heat for 2 minutes; set aside. Melt 1 tablespoon of butter in a skillet over medium heat.
4. Lay one tortilla in a skillet; sprinkle with some Swiss cheese. Add some chopped eggs and bacon over the cheese, top with onion, and sprinkle with some Cheddar cheese. Cover with another tortilla shell. Cook for 45 seconds, then carefully flip the quesadilla, and cook the other side too for 45 seconds. Remove to a plate and repeat the cooking process using the remaining tortilla shells.
5. Garnish with parsley and serve warm.

Per Serving
calories: 450 | fat: 48.6g | protein: 29.2g
carbs: 9.3g | net carbs: 6.9g | fiber: 2.4g

Swiss Chard, Sausage, and Squash Omelet

Prep time: 6 minutes | Cook time: 4 minutes | Serves 1

2 eggs	4 ounces (113 g) roasted squash
1 cup Swiss chard, chopped	1 tablespoon olive oil
4 ounces (113 g) sausage, chopped	Salt and black pepper, to taste
2 tablespoons ricotta cheese	Fresh parsley to garnish

1. Beat the eggs in a bowl, season with salt and pepper; stir in the swiss chard and the ricotta cheese.
2. In another bowl, mash the squash and add to the egg mixture. Heat ¼ tablespoon of olive oil in a pan over medium heat. Add sausage and cook until browned on all sides, turning occasionally.
3. Drizzle the remaining olive oil. Pour the egg mixture over. Cook for about 2 minutes per side until the eggs are thoroughly cooked and lightly browned. Remove the pan and run a spatula around the edges of the omelet; slide it onto a warm platter. Fold in half, and serve sprinkled with fresh parsley.

Per Serving
calories: 557 | fat: 51.6g | protein: 32.2g
carbs: 12.9g | net carbs: 7.4g | fiber: 5.5g

Ham, Cheese and Egg Cups

Prep time: 10 minutes | Cook time: 5 minutes | Serves 6

6 thin slices ham	Garlic salt and ground black pepper, to taste
1 teaspoon mustard	6 ounces (170 g) Colby cheese, shredded
6 eggs	
4 ounces (113 g) cream cheese	
½ teaspoon red pepper flakes, crushed	2 tablespoons green onions, chopped

1. Spritz a muffin tin with nonstick cooking spray. Place the ham slices over each muffin cup and gently press down until a cup shape forms.
2. In a mixing dish, whisk the mustard, eggs, cream cheese, red pepper, garlic salt, and black pepper.
3. Divide the egg mixture between the cups. Top with the shredded Colby cheese. Bake in the preheated oven at 360ºF (182ºC) approximately 25 minutes.
4. Transfer the muffin tin to a wire rack before serving. Garnish with green onions and serve. Bon appétit!

Per Serving
calories: 258 | fat: 19g | protein: 18g
carbs: 3g | net carbs: 3g | fiber: 0g

Mushroom and Kale Tofu Scramble

Prep time: 5 minutes | Cook time: 26 minutes | Serves 4

2 tablespoons butter	crumbled
1 cup sliced white mushrooms	Salt and black pepper to taste
2 cloves garlic, minced	½ cup thinly sliced kale
16 ounces (454 g) firm tofu, pressed and	6 fresh eggs

1. Melt the butter in a non-stick skillet over medium heat, and sauté the mushrooms for 5 minutes until they lose their liquid. Add the garlic and cook for 1 minute.
2. Crumble the tofu into the skillet, season with salt and black pepper. Cook with continuous stirring for 6 minutes. Introduce the kale in batches and cook to soften for about 7 minutes. Crack the eggs into a bowl, whisk until well combined and creamy in color, and pour all over the kale. Use a spatula to immediately stir the eggs while cooking until scrambled and no more runny, about 5 minutes. Plate, and serve with low carb crusted bread.

Per Serving

calories: 470 | fat: 38.7g | protein: 24.9g carbs: 7.6g | net carbs: 4.9g | fiber: 2.7g

Lemony Ginger Pancakes

Prep time: 14 minutes | Cook time: 1 minutes | Serves 4

2 cups almond flour	powder
1 teaspoon baking powder	⅓ teaspoon salt
1½ teaspoons cinnamon powder	2 eggs
⅓ cup Swerve brown sugar	1¼ cups almond milk
¼ teaspoon baking soda	½ cup lemon juice
1 teaspoon ginger	½ teaspoon lemon zest
	3½ tablespoon olive oil

Lemon Sauce:

½ cup Swerve	2 tablespoons lemon juice
1 teaspoon arrowroot starch	2½ tablespoons butter
1¼ cup hot water	Lemon zest to taste

1. In a bowl, mix the almond flour, baking powder, cinnamon powder, Swerve brown sugar, baking soda, ginger powder, salt, eggs, almond milk, lemon juice, lemon zest, and olive oil.
2. Heat oil in a skillet over medium heat and spoon 4 to 5 tablespoons of the mixture into the skillet. Cook the batter for 1 minute, flip it and cook the other side for another minute. Remove the pancake onto a plate after and repeat the cooking process until the batter is exhausted.
3. Mix the Swerve and arrowroot starch in a medium saucepan. Set the pan over medium heat and gradually stir the water until it thickens, about 1 minute.
4. Turn the heat off and add the butter, lemon juice, and lemon zest. Stir the mixture until the butter melts. After, drizzle the sauce on the pancakes immediately and serve them warm.

Per Serving

calories: 325 | fat: 24.1g | protein: 7.2g carbs: 8.9g | net carbs: 5.6g | fiber: 3.3g

Cheese and Egg Spinach Nests

Prep time: 13 minutes | Cook time: 22 minutes | Serves 4

2 tablespoons olive oil	shredded Parmesan cheese
1 clove garlic, grated	2 tablespoons shredded gouda cheese
½ pound (227 g) spinach, chopped	
Salt and black pepper to taste	4 eggs
2 tablespoons	

1. Preheat oven to 350ºF (180ºC). Warm the oil in a non-stick skillet over medium heat; add the garlic and sauté until softened for 2 minutes. Add the spinach to wilt for about 5 minutes, and season with salt and black pepper. Allow cooling.
2. Grease a baking sheet with cooking spray, mold 4 (firm and separate) spinach nests on the sheet, and crack an egg into each nest. Sprinkle with Parmesan and gouda cheese. Bake for 15 minutes just until the egg whites have set and the yolks are still runny. Plate the nests and serve right away with low carb toasts and coffee.

Per Serving

calories: 231 | fat: 17.6g | protein: 12.2g carbs: 5.4g | net carbs: 4.1g | fiber: 1.3g

Cream Cheese Almond Muffins

Prep time: 10 minutes | Cook time: 20 minutes | Serves 4

2 drops liquid stevia
2 cups almond flour
2 teaspoons baking powder
½ teaspoon salt
8 ounces (227 g) cream cheese, softened
¼ cup melted butter
1 egg
1 cup unsweetened almond milk

1. Preheat oven to 400ºF (205ºC) and grease a 12-cup muffin tray with cooking spray. Mix the flour, baking powder, and salt in a large bowl.
2. In a separate bowl, beat the cream cheese, stevia, and butter using a hand mixer and whisk in the egg and milk. Fold in the flour, and spoon the batter into the muffin cups two-thirds way up.
3. Bake for 20 minutes until puffy at the top and golden brown, remove to a wire rack to cool slightly for 5 minutes before serving. Serve with tea.

Per Serving
calories: 321 | fat: 30.5g | protein: 4.1g carbs: 8.1g | net carbs: 5.9g | fiber: 2.2g

Jalapeño Pepper Cream Cheese Omelet

Prep time: 15 minutes | Cook time: 5 minutes | Serves 1

2 tablespoons cream cheese, softened at room temperature
4 tablespoons shredded cheddar cheese, divided into 2 tablespoons and 2 tablespoons
2 tablespoons cooked bacon bits
1½ teaspoons thinly sliced green onions
1½ teaspoons finely diced seeded jalapeño pepper (about ⅛ medium)
2 large eggs
2 tablespoons heavy cream
¼ teaspoon sea salt
⅛ teaspoon black pepper
1 tablespoon butter

1. In a medium bowl, mash together the cream cheese, 2 tablespoons of the cheddar, and the bacon bits. Stir in the green onions and jalapeño. Set the cream cheese mixture aside.
2. In another medium bowl, whisk together the eggs, heavy cream, sea salt, and black pepper.
3. In a medium skillet, melt the butter over medium heat. Pour in the egg mixture. Cover and cook for 1 to 2 minutes, until mostly cooked through. You can lift with a spatula to get more of the egg underneath if needed, but don't stir or scramble.
4. Drop dollops of the cream cheese mixture onto half of the omelet, distributing as evenly as possible. Use a spatula to fold the omelet over. Sprinkle the remaining 2 tablespoons cheddar cheese on top.
5. Reduce the heat to medium-low. Cover and cook for a couple of minutes, until the cheese melts on top and inside.

Per Serving
calories: 416 | fat: 35g | protein: 22g carbs: 3g | net carbs: 3g | fiber: 0g

Pesto Bacon and Avocado Mug Cakes

Prep time: 6 minutes | Cook time: 2 minutes | Serves 2

¼ cup flax meal
1 egg
2 tablespoons heavy cream
2 tablespoons pesto
Filling:
2 tablespoons cream cheese
4 slices bacon
¼ cup almond flour
¼ teaspoon baking soda
Salt and black pepper, to taste
½ medium avocado, sliced

1. Mix together the dry muffin ingredients in a bowl. Add egg, heavy cream, and pesto, and whisk well with a fork. Season with salt and pepper. Divide the mixture between two ramekins.
2. Place in the microwave and cook for 60-90 seconds. Leave to cool slightly before filling.
3. Meanwhile, in a skillet, over medium heat, cook the bacon slices until crispy. Transfer to paper towels to soak up excess fat; set aside. Invert the muffins onto a plate and cut in half, crosswise. To assemble the sandwiches: spread cream cheese and top with bacon and avocado slices.

Per Serving
calories: 512 | fat: 38.3g | protein: 16.3g carbs: 10.3g | net carbs: 4.4g | fiber: 5.9g

Egg and Ham Muffins

Prep time: 15 minutes | Cook time: 25 minutes | Serves 9

2 cups chopped smoked ham
⅓ cup grated Parmesan cheese
¼ cup almond flour
9 eggs
⅓ cup mayonnaise, sugar-free
¼ teaspoon garlic powder
¼ cup chopped onion
Sea salt to taste

1. Preheat your oven to 370ºF (188ºC).
2. Lightly grease nine muffin pans with cooking spray and set aside. Place the onion, ham, garlic powder, and salt, in a food processor, and pulse until ground. Stir in the mayonnaise, almond flour, and Parmesan cheese. Press this mixture into the muffin cups.
3. Make sure it goes all the way up the muffin sides so that there will be room for the egg. Bake for 5 minutes. Crack an egg into each muffin cup. Return to the oven and bake for 20 more minutes or until the tops are firm to the touch and eggs are cooked. Leave to cool slightly before serving.

Per Serving
calories: 366 | fat: 28.1g | protein: 13.6g | carbs: 1.3g | net carbs: 1.0g | fiber: 0.3g

Caramel-Cream Chocolate Crepes

Prep time: 20 minutes | Cook time: 15 minutes | Serves 4

4 tablespoons coconut flour
4 tablespoons unsweetened cocoa powder
½ teaspoon baking powder
4 egg whites
Caramel Cream:
½ cup salted butter
4 tablespoons Swerve brown sugar
½ cup plus 4 tablespoons flax milk
2 tablespoons erythritol
2 tablespoons olive oil

1 teaspoon vanilla extract
1 cup heavy cream

1. In a bowl, mix the coconut flour, cocoa powder, and baking powder together. Set aside.
2. Then, in another bowl, whisk the egg whites, ½ cup flax milk, erythritol, and the olive oil. Pour the wet ingredients into the dry ingredients, and whisk until smooth.
3. Set a skillet over medium heat, grease with cooking spray, and pour in a ladleful of the batter. Swirl the pan quickly to spread the dough all around the skillet and cook the crepe for 2-3 minutes.
4. When it is firm enough to touch and cooked through, slide the crepe into a flat plate. Wipe the pan with a napkin and continue cooking until the remaining batter has finished. Put the butter and brown sugar in a pot and melt the butter over medium heat while stirring continually. Keep cooking for 4 minutes after the butter has melted; be careful not to burn.
5. Stir in the cream, reduce the heat to low, and let the sauce simmer for 10 minutes while stirring continually. Turn the heat off and stir in the vanilla extract. Once the crepes are ready, drizzle the caramel sauce over them, and serve with a cup of coffee.

Per Serving
calories: 331 | fat: 21.1g | protein: 10.9g | carbs: 6.9g | net carbs: 5.0g | fiber: 1.9g

Creamy Ricotta Almond Cloud Pancakes

Prep time: 5 minutes | Cook time: 5 minutes | Serves 4

1 cup almond flour
1 teaspoon baking powder
2½ tablespoons Swerve
⅓ teaspoon salt

1¼ cups ricotta cheese
⅓ cup coconut milk
2 large eggs
1 cup heavy whipping cream

1. In a medium bowl, whisk the almond flour, baking powder, Swerve, and salt. Set aside.
2. Crack the eggs into the blender and process on medium speed for 30 seconds. Add the ricotta cheese, continue processing it, and gradually pour the coconut milk in while you keep on blending. In about 90 seconds, the mixture will be creamy and smooth. Pour it into the dry ingredients and whisk to combine.
3. Set a skillet over medium heat and let it heat for a minute. Then, fetch a soup spoonful of mixture into the skillet and cook it for 1 minute.
4. Flip the pancake and cook further for 1 minute. Remove onto a plate and repeat the cooking process until the batter is exhausted. Serve the pancakes with whipping cream.

Per Serving
calories: 406 | fat: 30.5g | protein: 11.4g | carbs: 8.8g | net carbs: 6.4g | fiber: 2.4g

Gruyere and Mushroom Lettuce Wraps

Prep time: 10 minutes | Cook time: 10 minutes | Serves 4

Wraps:
6 eggs
2 tablespoons almond milk
Filling:
1 teaspoon olive oil
1 cup mushrooms, chopped
Salt and black pepper, to taste
½ teaspoon cayenne pepper

1 tablespoon olive oil
Sea salt, to taste

8 fresh lettuce leaves
4 slices Gruyere cheese
2 tomatoes, sliced

1. Mix all the ingredients for the wraps thoroughly.
2. Set a frying pan over medium heat. Add in ¼ of the mixture and cook for 4 minutes on both sides. Do the same thrice and set the wraps aside, they should be kept warm.
3. In a separate pan over medium heat, warm 1 teaspoon of olive oil. Cook the mushrooms for 5 minutes until soft; add cayenne pepper, black pepper, and salt. Set 1-2 lettuce leaves onto every wrap, split the mushrooms among the wraps and top with tomatoes and cheese.

Per Serving
calories: 471 | fat: 43.9g | protein: 19.4g | carbs: 6.5g | net carbs: 5.3g | fiber: 1.2g

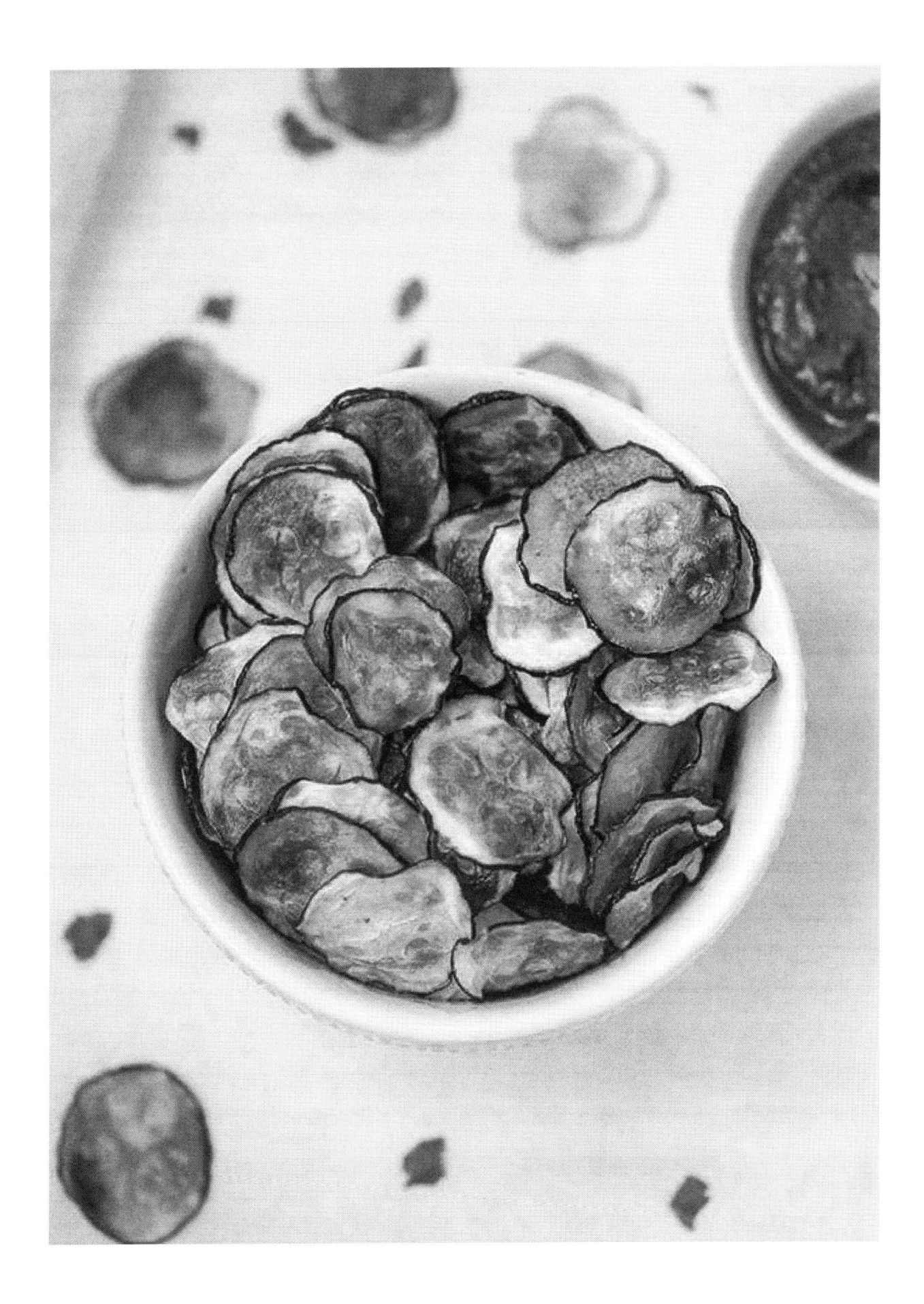

Chapter 2 Snacks and Appetizers

Romano Cheese Meatballs

Prep time: 5 minutes | Cook time: 20 minutes | Serves 10

½ ground turkey
1 pound (454 g) ground beef
4 ounces (113 g) pork rinds
¼ cup coconut milk
1 shallot, chopped
2 garlic cloves, minced
Sea salt and ground black pepper, to taste
½ cup Romano cheese, grated

1. Thoroughly combine all ingredients in a mixing bowl; shape the mixture into bite-sized meatballs.
2. Place your meatballs on a parchment-lined baking sheet; brush your meatballs with olive oil.
3. Bake for 10 minutes; rotate the pan and bake for a further 10 minutes. Serve with cocktail sticks and enjoy!

Per Serving
calories: 247 | fat: 18g | protein: 19g
carbs: 1g | net carbs: 1g | fiber: 0g

Caribbean Baked Wings

Prep time: 15 minutes | Cook time: 45 minutes | Serves 2

4 chicken wings
1 tablespoon coconut aminos
2 tablespoons rum
2 tablespoons butter
1 tablespoon onion powder
1 tablespoon garlic powder
½ teaspoon salt
¼ teaspoon freshly ground black pepper
½ teaspoon red pepper flakes
¼ teaspoon dried dill
2 tablespoons sesame seeds

1. Pat dry the chicken wings. Toss the chicken wings with the remaining ingredients until well coated. Arrange the chicken wings on a parchment-lined baking sheet.
2. Bake in the preheated oven at 420ºF (216ºC) for 45 minutes until golden brown.
3. Serve with your favorite sauce for dipping. Bon appétit!

Per Serving
calories: 287 | fat: 18.6g | protein: 15.5g
carbs: 5.1g | net carbs: 3.3g | fiber: 1.8g

Chicken Wings in Spicy Tomato Sauce

Prep time: 10 minutes | Cook time: 45 minutes | Serves 6

3 pounds (1.4 kg) chicken wings
Sea salt and ground black pepper, to taste
Sauce:
2 vine-ripe tomatoes
1 onion
2 garlic cloves
½ teaspoon paprika
½ teaspoon cayenne pepper
1 teaspoon chili pepper

1. Start by preheating your oven to 400ºF (205ºC). Set a wire rack inside a rimmed baking sheet.
2. Season the chicken wings with salt, black pepper, paprika, and cayenne pepper. Bake the wings approximately 45 minutes or until the skin is crispy.
3. To make the sauce, purée all ingredients in your food processor. Bon appétit!

Per Serving
calories: 309 | fat: 8g | protein: 50g
carbs: 5g | net carbs: 4g | fiber: 1g

Zucchini Chips

Prep time: 10 minutes | Cook time: 20 minutes | Serves 2

1 tablespoon extra-virgin olive oil
¼ teaspoon sea salt
1 teaspoon hot paprika
½ pound (227 g) zucchini, sliced into rounds
2 tablespoons Parmesan cheese, grated

1. Gently toss the sliced zucchini with the olive oil, salt, and paprika. Place them on a tinfoil-lined baking sheet.
2. Sprinkle the Parmesan cheese evenly over each zucchini round.
3. Bake in the preheated oven at 400ºF (205ºC) for 15 to 20 minutes or until your chips turns a golden-brown color.

Per Serving
calories: 53 | fat: 4.5g | protein: 1.6g
carbs: 1.5g | net carbs: 0.9g | fiber: 0.6g

Turkey Stuffed Mini Peppers

Prep time: 10 minutes | Cook time: 10 minutes | Serves 5

2 teaspoons olive oil
1 teaspoon mustard seeds
5 ounces (142 g) ground turkey
Salt and ground black pepper, to taste
10 mini bell peppers, cut in half lengthwise, stems and seeds removed
2 ounces (57 g) garlic and herb seasoned chevre goat cheese, crumbled

1. Heat the oil in a skillet over medium-high heat. Once hot, cook mustard seeds with ground turkey until the turkey is no longer pink. Crumble with a fork. Season with salt and black pepper.
2. Lay the pepper halves cut-side-up on a parchment-lined baking sheet. Spoon the meat mixture into the center of each pepper half.
3. Top each pepper with cheese. Bake in the preheated oven at 400ºF (205ºC) for 10 minutes. Bon appétit!

Per Serving
calories: 200 | fat: 17.1g | protein: 7.8g
carbs: 2.9g | net carbs: 2.0g | fiber: 0.9g

Baked Cocktail Franks

Prep time: 5 minutes | Cook time: 12 minutes | Serves 10

2 tablespoons olive oil
18 ounces (510 g) cocktail franks
Sea salt and red pepper flakes, to taste
2 tablespoons wholegrain mustard

1. Start by preheating your oven to 360ºF (182ºC). Then, brush a baking pan with olive oil. Place the cocktail franks on the baking pan.
2. Sprinkle them with the salt and red pepper; add in the mustard and toss to combine.
3. Bake approximately 12 minutes until they are golden brown. Serve warm and enjoy!

Per Serving
calories: 155 | fat: 12g | protein: 9g
carbs: 5g | net carbs: 4g | fiber: 1g

Cheese Bites with Pickle

Prep time: 15 minutes | Cook time: 0 minutes | Serves 10

10 ounces (283 g) Swiss cheese, shredded
10 ounces (283 g) cottage cheese
¼ cup sour cream
1 tablespoon pickle, minced
Sea salt and ground black pepper, to season
1 teaspoon granulated garlic
¾ cup pecans, finely chopped

1. Beat the Swiss cheese, cottage cheese, sour cream, minced pickles, and seasonings until everything is well incorporated.
2. Place the mixture for 2 hours in your refrigerator. Form the mixture into bite-sized balls using your hands and a spoon.
3. Roll the cheese balls over the chopped pecans to coat them evenly. Bon appétit!

Per Serving
calories: 200 | fat: 15.6g | protein: 11.4g
carbs: 4.8g | net carbs: 3.8g | fiber: 1.0g

Cheese and Shrimp Stuffed Celery

Prep time: 10 minutes | Cook time: 5 minutes | Serves 6

5 ounces (142 g) shrimp
10 ounces (283 g) cottage cheese, at room temperature
4 ounces (113 g) Coby cheese, shredded
2 scallions, chopped
1 teaspoon yellow mustard
Sea salt, to taste
½ teaspoon oregano
6 stalks celery, cut into halves

1. Gently pat the shrimp dry with a paper towel.
2. Cook the shrimp in a lightly greased skillet over medium-high heat for 2 minutes; turn them over and cook for a further 2 minutes.
3. Chop the shrimp and transfer to a mixing bowl. Add in the cheese, scallions, mustard, and spices. Mix to combine well.
4. Divide the shrimp mixture between the celery stalks and serve. Bon appétit!

Per Serving
calories: 127 | fat: 6.1g | protein: 13.4g
carbs: 4.2g | net carbs: 3.7g | fiber: 0.5g

Romano and Asiago Cheese Crisps

Prep time: 15 minutes | Cook time: 30 minutes | Serves 8

1¼ cups Romano cheese, grated
½ cup Asiago cheese, grated
2 ripe tomatoes, peeled
½ teaspoon sea salt
½ teaspoon chili powder
1 teaspoon dried oregano
1 teaspoon dried basil
1 teaspoon dried parsley flakes
1 teaspoon garlic powder

1. Mix the cheese in a bowl. Place tablespoon-sized heaps of the mixture onto parchmentlined baking pans.
2. Bake in the preheated oven at 380°F (193°C) approximately 7 minutes until beginning to brown around the edges.
3. Let them stand for about 15 minutes until crisp.
4. Meanwhile, purée the tomatoes in your food processor. Bring the puréed tomatoes to a simmer, add the remaining ingredients and cook for 30 minutes or until it has thickened and cooked through.
5. Serve the cheese crisps with the spicy tomato sauce on the side. Bon appétit!

Per Serving
calories: 110 | fat: 7.5g | protein: 8.4g
carbs: 2.0g | net carbs: 1.6g | fiber: 0.4g

Traditional Walnut Fat Bombs

Prep time: 5 minutes | Cook time: 1 minute | Serves 10

2 tablespoons keto chocolate protein powder
¼ cup erythritol
5 ounces (142 g) butter
3 ounces (85 g) walnut butter
10 whole walnuts, halved

1. In a sauté pan, melt the butter, protein powder, and Erythritol over a low flame, for 1 minute. Stir until smooth and well mixed.
2. Spoon the mixture into a piping bag and pipe into mini cupcake liners. Add the walnut halves to each mini cupcake.
3. Place in your refrigerator for at least 2 hours. Bon appétit!

Per Serving
calories: 260 | fat: 27g | protein: 5g
carbs: 3g | net carbs: 1g | fiber: 2g

Caprese Sticks

Prep time: 10 minutes | Cook time: 0 minutes | Serves 8

2 tablespoons extra-virgin olive oil
2 tablespoons red wine vinegar
1 tablespoon Italian seasoning blend
8 pieces Prosciutto
8 pieces Soppressata
16 grape tomatoes
8 black olives, pitted
8 ounces (227 g) Mozzarella, cubed
2 tablespoons fresh basil leaves, chopped
1 red bell pepper, sliced
1 yellow bell pepper, sliced
Coarse sea salt, to taste

1. In a small mixing bowl, make the vinaigrette by whisking the oil, vinegar, and Italian seasoning blend. Set aside.
2. Slide the ingredients on the prepared skewers.
3. Arrange the sticks on serving platter. Season with salt to taste. Serve the vinaigrette on the side and enjoy!

Per Serving
calories: 142 | fat: 8.3g | protein: 12.8g
carbs: 3.2g | net carbs: 2.2g | fiber: 1.0g

Cheesy Ham-Egg Cups

Prep time: 5 minutes | Cook time: 13 minutes | Serves 9

9 slices ham
Coarse salt and ground black pepper, to season
1 teaspoon jalapeño pepper, seeded and minced
½ cup Swiss cheese, shredded
9 eggs

1. Begin by preheating your oven to 390°F (199°C). Lightly grease a muffin pan with cooking spray.
2. Line each cup with a slice of ham; add salt, black pepper, jalapeño, and cheese. Crack an egg into each ham cup.
3. Bake in the preheated oven about 13 minutes or until the eggs are cooked through. Bon appétit!

Per Serving
calories: 137 | fat: 9g | protein: 12g
carbs: 2g | net carbs: 1g | fiber: 1g

Bacon-Wrapped Poblano Poppers

Prep time: 15 minutes | Cook time: 30 minutes | Serves 16

10 ounces (283 g) cottage cheese, at room temperature
6 ounces (170 g) Swiss cheese, shredded
Sea salt and ground black pepper, to taste
½ teaspoon shallot powder
½ teaspoon cumin powder
⅓ teaspoon mustard seeds
16 poblano peppers, deveined and halved
16 thin slices bacon, sliced lengthwise

1. Mix the cheese, salt, black pepper, shallot powder, cumin, and mustard seeds until well combined.
2. Divide the mixture between the pepper halves. Wrap each pepper with 2 slices of bacon; secure with toothpicks.
3. Arrange the stuffed peppers on the rack in the baking sheet.
4. Bake in the preheated oven at 390°F (199°C) for about 30 minutes until the bacon is sizzling and browned. Bon appétit!

Per Serving
calories: 184 | fat: 14.1g | protein: 8.9g
carbs: 5.8g | net carbs: 5.0g | fiber: 0.8g

Whiskey-Glazed Chicken Wings

Prep time: 5 minutes | Cook time: 50 to 55 minutes | Serves 5

2 tablespoons extra-virgin olive oil
2 pounds (907 g) chicken wings
1 tablespoon whiskey
1 tablespoon Taco seasoning mix
1 cup tomato purée

1. Start by preheating your oven to 410°F (210°C). Toss the chicken wings with the other ingredients until well coated.
2. Place the wings onto a rack in the baking pan. Bake in the preheated oven for 50 to 55 minutes until a meat thermometer reads 165°F (74°C).
3. Serve with dipping sauce, if desired. Enjoy!

Per Serving
calories: 293 | fat: 12g | protein: 41g
carbs: 4g | net carbs: 3g | fiber: 1g

BLT Cups

Prep time: 10 minutes | Cook time: 10 minutes | Serves 10

5 ounces (142 g) bacon, chopped
5 tablespoons Parmigiano-Reggiano cheese, grated
1 teaspoon adobo sauce
2 tablespoons mayonnaise
Sea salt and ground black pepper, to taste
2 tablespoons green onions, minced
10 pieces lettuce
10 tomatoes cherry tomatoes, discard the insides

1. Preheat a frying pan over moderate heat. Cook the bacon in the frying pan until crisp, about 7 minutes; reserve.
2. In a mixing bowl, thoroughly combine the cheese, adobo sauce, mayo, salt, black pepper, and green onions. Divide the mayo mixture between the cherry tomatoes.
3. Divide the cooked bacon between the cherry tomatoes. Top with the lettuce and serve immediately. Bon appétit!

Per Serving
calories: 93 | fat: 8.2g | protein: 2.6g
carbs: 1.5g | net carbs: 1.1g | fiber: 0.4g

Kale Chips

Prep time: 15 minutes | Cook time: 15 minutes | Serves 2

2 cups kale, torn into pieces
1 tablespoons olive oil
Sea salt, to taste
¼ teaspoon pepper
½ teaspoon onion powder
½ teaspoon garlic powder
½ teaspoon fresh dill, minced
½ tablespoon fresh parsley, minced

1. Start by preheating your oven to 320°F (160°C).
2. Toss the kale leaves with all other ingredients until well coated. Bake for 10 to 14 minutes, depending on how crisp you like them.
3. Store the kale chips in an airtight container for up to a week. Bon appétit!

Per Serving
calories: 69 | fat: 6.5g | protein: 0.5g
carbs: 1.5g | net carbs: 1.0g | fiber: 0.5g

Chicken and Spinach Meatballs

Prep time: 15 minutes | Cook time: 25 minutes | Serves 10

1½ pounds (680 g) ground chicken
8 ounces (227 g) Parmigiano-Reggiano cheese, grated
1 teaspoon garlic, minced
1 tablespoon Italian seasoning mix
1 egg, whisked
8 ounces (227 g) spinach, chopped
½ teaspoon mustard seeds
Sea salt and ground black pepper, to taste
½ teaspoon paprika

1. Mix the ingredients until everything is well incorporated.
2. Now, shape the meat mixture into 20 meatballs. Transfer your meatballs to a baking sheet and brush them with a nonstick cooking oil.
3. Bake in the preheated oven at 390°F (199°C) for about 25 minutes or until golden brown. Serve with cocktail sticks and enjoy!

Per Serving
calories: 210 | fat: 12.4g | protein: 19.4g
carbs: 4.5g | net carbs: 4.0g | fiber: 0.5g

Fajita Spareribs

Prep time: 5 minutes | Cook time: 2 hours 30 minutes | Serves 4

2 pounds (907 g) St. Louis-style spareribs
1 tablespoon Fajita seasoning mix
2 cloves garlic, pressed
½ cup chicken bone broth
1 cup tomato purée

1. Toss the spareribs with the Fajita seasoning mix, garlic, chicken bone broth, and tomato purée until well coated.
2. Arrange the spare ribs on a tinfoil-lined baking sheet.
3. Bake in the preheated oven at 260°F (127°C) for 2 hours and 30 minutes.
4. Place under the preheated broiler for about 8 minutes until the sauce is lightly caramelized. Bon appétit!

Per Serving
calories: 344 | fat: 14g | protein: 50g
carbs: 5g | net carbs: 4g | fiber: 1g

Cream Cheese Stuffed Mushrooms

Prep time: 15 minutes | Cook time: 40 minutes | Serves 10

20 button mushrooms, stalks removed
6 ounces (170 g) cream cheese
¼ cup mayonnaise
¼ teaspoon mustard seeds
½ teaspoon celery seeds
Sea salt and black pepper, to taste

1. Adjust an oven rack to the center position. Brush your mushrooms with nonstick cooking spray and arrange them on a baking sheet.
2. Roast your mushrooms in the preheated oven at 375°F (190°C) for 40 minutes until the mushrooms release liquid.
3. In the meantime, mix the remaining ingredients until well combined. Spoon the mixture into the roasted mushroom caps. Bon appétit!

Per Serving
calories: 104 | fat: 9.8g | protein: 2.6g
carbs: 2.0g | net carbs: 1.5g | fiber: 0.5g

Wrapped Asparagus with Prosciutto

Prep time: 15 minutes | Cook time: 20 minutes | Serves 6

1½ pounds (680 g) asparagus spears, trimmed
1 teaspoon shallot powder
½ teaspoon granulated garlic
½ teaspoon paprika
Kosher salt and ground black pepper, to taste
1 tablespoon sesame oil
10 slices prosciutto

1. Toss the asparagus spears with the shallot powder, garlic, paprika, salt, and black pepper. Drizzle sesame oil all over the asparagus spears.
2. Working one at a time, wrap a prosciutto slice on each asparagus spear; try to cover the entire length of the asparagus spear.
3. Place the wrapped asparagus spears on a parchment-lined roasting pan. Bake in the preheated oven at 390°F (199°C) for about 18 minutes or until thoroughly cooked. Bon appétit!

Per Serving
calories: 120 | fat: 6.5g | protein: 10.1g
carbs: 6.2g | net carbs: 3.2g | fiber: 3.0g

Cocktail Meatballs

Prep time: 15 minutes | Cook time: 20 minutes | Serves 2

¼ pound (113 g) ground turkey
¼ pound (113 g) ground pork
1 ounce (28 g) bacon, chopped
¼ cup flaxseed meal
½ teaspoon garlic, pressed
1 egg, beaten
½ cup Cheddar cheese, shredded
Sea salt, to season
¼ teaspoon ground black pepper
¼ teaspoon cayenne pepper
¼ teaspoon marjoram

1. Start by preheating your oven to 400ºF (205ºC).
2. Thoroughly combine all ingredients in a mixing bowl. Now, form the mixture into meatballs.
3. Place your meatballs in a parchment-lined baking sheet. Bake in the preheated oven for about 18 minutes, rotating the pan halfway through.
4. Serve with toothpicks and enjoy!

Per Serving
calories: 570 | fat: 42.3g | protein: 40.2g
carbs: 6.4g | net carbs: 0.8g | fiber: 5.6g

Avocado and Ham Stuffed Eggs

Prep time: 5 minutes | Cook time: 12 minutes | Serves 4

4 large eggs
½ avocado, mashed
½ teaspoon yellow mustard
1 garlic clove, minced
2 ounces (57 g) cooked ham, chopped

1. Place the eggs in a saucepan and fill with enough water. Bring the water to a rolling boil; heat off. Cover and allow the eggs to sit for about 12 minutes; let them cool.
2. Slice the eggs into halves; mix the yolks with the avocado, mustard and garlic.
3. Divide the avocado filling among the egg whites. Top with the chopped ham. Bon appétit!

Per Serving
calories: 128 | fat: 9g | protein: 9g
carbs: 3g | net carbs: 1g | fiber: 2g

Sardine Pepper Boats

Prep time: 10 minutes | Cook time: 10 minutes | Serves 3

2 eggs
½ red onion, chopped
½ teaspoon garlic clove, minced
2 ounces (57 g) canned boneless sardines, drained and chopped
¼ freshly ground
black pepper
½ cup tomatoes, chopped
¼ cup mayonnaise
3 tablespoons Ricotta cheese
3 bell peppers, deveined and halved

1. Place the eggs and water in a saucepan; bring to a rapid boil; immediately remove from the heat.
2. Allow it to sit, covered, for 10 minutes. Then, discard the shells, rinse the eggs under cold water, and chop them.
3. Thoroughly combine the onion, garlic, sardines, black pepper, tomatoes, mayonnaise, and cheese.
4. Stuff the pepper halves and serve well chilled. Bon appétit!

Per Serving
calories: 372 | fat: 31.2g | protein: 16.1g
carbs: 5.9g | net carbs: 4.5g | fiber: 1.4g

Anchovy Fat Bombs

Prep time: 15 minutes | Cook time: 0 minutes | Serves 10

8 ounces (227 g) Cheddar cheese, shredded
6 ounces (170 g) cream cheese, at room temperature
4 ounces (113 g) canned anchovies,
chopped
½ yellow onion, minced
1 teaspoon fresh garlic, minced
Sea salt and ground black pepper, to taste

1. Mix all of the above ingredients in a bowl. Place the mixture in your refrigerator for 1 hour.
2. Then, shape the mixture into bite-sized balls.
3. Serve immediately.

Per Serving
calories: 123 | fat: 8.8g | protein: 7.4g
carbs: 3.3g | net carbs: 3.3g | fiber: 0g

Cauliflower Bites

Prep time: 10 minutes | Cook time: 30 minutes | Serves 2

1½ cups cauliflower florets
1 tablespoon butter, softened
1 egg, whisked
Sea salt and ground black pepper, to taste
1 teaspoon Italian seasoning mix
½ cup Asiago cheese, grated

1. Pulse the cauliflower in your food processor; now, heat the butter in a nonstick skillet and cook the cauliflower until golden.
2. Add the remaining ingredients and blend together until well incorporated.
3. Form the mixture into balls and flatten them with the palm of your hand. Arrange on a tinfoil-lined baking pan.
4. Bake in the preheated oven at 400°F (205°C) for 25 to 30 minutes. Serve with homemade ketchup. Bon appétit!

Per Serving
calories: 235 | fat: 19.1g | protein: 12.4g carbs: 4.4g | net carbs: 2.9g | fiber: 1.5g

Herbed Provolone Cheese Chips

Prep time: 5 minutes | Cook time: 9 minutes | Serves 5

6 ounces (170 g) (170 g) provolone cheese, grated
½ teaspoon garlic powder
½ teaspoon shallot powder
¼ teaspoon ground black pepper
1 teaspoon dried dill
½ teaspoon dried oregano
1 teaspoon paprika

1. Place the grated provolone cheese in small heaps on a roasting pan lined with Silpat mat. Make sure to leave enough room in between them.
2. Sprinkle the herbs and spices over them.
3. Bake in the preheated oven at 395°F (202°C) for about 9 minutes, Transfer to a cooling rack and let it sit for 20 minutes before serving. Serve with a homemade salsa sauce if desired.

Per Serving
calories: 119 | fat: 9g | protein: 9g carbs: 1g | net carbs: 1g | fiber: 0g

Paprika Veggie Bites

Prep time: 5 minutes | Cook time: 0 minutes | Serves 3

1 teaspoon Dijon mustard
½ cup cream cheese
¼ cup mayonnaise
1 cucumber, cut into rounds
1 bell pepper, seeded and cut into 4 pieces lengthwise
1 teaspoon paprika

1. Mix the Dijon mustard, cream cheese, and mayonnaise in a bowl; stir to combine.
2. Place the cucumber and bell peppers on a serving platter. Divide the cheese mixture between the vegetables.
3. Sprinkle paprika over the vegetable bites. Serve well chilled.

Per Serving
calories: 164 | fat: 17g | protein: 2g carbs: 3g | net carbs: 2g | fiber: 1g

Crispy Five Seed Crackers

Prep time: 5 minutes | Cook time: 1 hour | Serves 12

¼ cup chia seeds
¼ cup sesame seeds
¼ cup flax seeds
¼ cup sunflower seeds
¼ cup pumpkin seeds
¼ cup almond meal
1 teaspoon psyllium husk powder
Coarse sea salt, to taste
¼ teaspoon ground cumin
¾ cup boiling water
4 tablespoons coconut oil, melted

1. Thoroughly combine the seeds, almond meal, psyllium husk powder, salt, and ground cumin until well mixed.
2. Pour the boiling water over the seed mixture; add in the melted coconut oil.
3. Spread out the batter thinly on a tinfoil-lined baking pan. Bake in the preheated oven at 310°F (154°C) for 30 minutes.
4. Rotate the pan and continue to bake an additional 25 to 30 minutes. Heat off. Allow your crackers to dry in the warm oven for 50 to 60 minutes longer. Bon appétit!

Per Serving
calories: 128 | fat: 13g | protein: 4g carbs: 3g | net carbs: 1g | fiber: 2g

Cheesy Ham and Chicken Bites

Prep time: 5 minutes | Cook time: 22 to 24 minutes | Serves 5

5 slices ham
5 chicken fillets, about ¼-inch thin
3 ounces (85 g)
Ricotta cheese
⅓ cup Colby cheese, grated
½ cup tomato purée

1. Place a slice of ham on each chicken fillet.
2. Thoroughly combine the Ricotta cheese and Colby cheese until everything is well incorporated.
3. Then, divide the cheese mixture between the chicken fillets. Roll them up and secure with toothpicks.
4. Transfer them to a lightly oiled baking tray. Bake in the preheated oven at 390ºF (199ºC) for 18 minutes, flipping them once or twice.
5. Pour the spicy tomato purée over the chicken roll-ups and bake another 4 to 6 minutes or until everything is thoroughly cooked. Bon appétit!

Per Serving
calories: 289 | fat: 11g | protein:37 g carbs: 7g | net carbs: 5g | fiber: 2g

Avocado-Bacon Sushi

Prep time: 5 minutes | Cook time: 0 minutes | Serves 8

1 teaspoon garlic paste
2 scallions, finely chopped
4 ounces (113 g) cream cheese, softened
1 teaspoon adobo
sauce
1 avocado, mashed
2 tablespoons fresh lemon juice
8 bacon slices
1 tablespoon toasted sesame seeds

1. In a mixing bowl, thoroughly combine the garlic paste, scallions, cream cheese, adobo sauce, avocado, and fresh lemon juice.
2. Divide the mixture evenly between the bacon slices. Roll up tightly and garnish with toasted sesame seeds. Enjoy!

Per Serving
calories: 350 | fat: 37g | protein: 2g carbs: 4g | net carbs: 2g | fiber: 2g

Cheesy Prosciutto Balls

Prep time: 5 minutes | Cook time: 0 minutes | Serves 4

2 ounces (57 g) goat cheese, crumbled
2 ounces (57 g) feta cheese crumbled
3 ounces (85 g) prosciutto, chopped
1 red bell pepper, seeded and finely chopped
2 tablespoons sesame seeds, toasted

1. Thoroughly combine the cheese, prosciutto and pepper until everything is well incorporated. Shape the mixture into balls.
2. Arrange these keto balls on a platter and place them in the refrigerator until ready to serve.
3. Roll the keto balls in toasted sesame seeds before serving. Bon appétit!

Per Serving
calories: 176 | fat: 13g | protein: 13g carbs: 2g | net carbs: 1g | fiber: 1g

Spicy Chicken Drumettes

Prep time: 5 minutes | Cook time: 23 minutes | Serves 6

2 pounds (907 g) chicken drumettes
Sea salt and ground black pepper, to taste
½ teaspoon paprika
1 teaspoon cayenne pepper
1 teaspoon dried oregano
⅓ cup hot sauce
1 tablespoon stone-ground mustard
1 teaspoon garlic powder

1. Pat dry the chicken drumettes with paper towels. Season them with salt, black pepper, paprika, cayenne pepper, and oregano.
2. Brush the drumettes with cooking oil and transfer to a roasting pan. Bake at 420ºF (216ºC) for 18 minutes.
3. Toss with the hot sauce, mustard and garlic powder; broil for 5 minutes more or until the chicken drumettes are golden brown and thoroughly cooked. Bon appétit!

Per Serving
calories: 179 | fat: 3g | protein: 34g carbs: 2g | net carbs: 1g | fiber: 1g

Beef-Stuffed Peppers

Prep time: 5 minutes | Cook time: 30 minutes | Serves 6

¾ pound (340 g) ground beef
½ cup onion, chopped
2 garlic cloves, minced
12 mini peppers, seeded
½ cup Cheddar cheese, shredded

1. Heat up a lightly oiled sauté pan over a moderate flame. Brown the ground beef for 3 to 4 minutes, crumbling with a fork.
2. Stir in the onions and garlic; continue to sauté an additional 2 minutes or until tender and aromatic.
3. Cook the peppers in boiling water until just tender or approximately 7 minutes.
4. Arrange the stuffed peppers on a tinfoil-lined baking pan. Divide the beef mixture among the peppers. Top with the shredded Cheddar cheese.
5. Bake in the preheated oven at 360ºF (182ºC) approximately 17 minutes. Serve at room temperature. Bon appétit!

Per Serving
calories: 207 | fat: 10g | protein: 20g
carbs: 7g | net carbs: 5g | fiber: 2g

Cheddar Anchovies Fat Bombs

Prep time: 5 minutes | Cook time: 0 minutes | Serves 2

2 (2-ounce / 57-g) cans anchovies, drained
⅓ cup cream cheese, chilled
⅓ cup Cheddar cheese, shredded
1 tablespoon Dijon mustard
2 scallions, chopped

1. Mix all of the above ingredients until everything is well incorporated. Shape the mixture into bite-sized balls.
2. Serve well chilled and enjoy!

Per Serving
calories: 391 | fat: 27g | protein: 34g
carbs: 3g | net carbs: 2g | fiber: 1g

Bacon-Wrapped Enoki Mushrooms

Prep time: 10 minutes | Cook time: 40 minutes | Serves 5

½ pound (227 g) enoki mushrooms
5 slices bacon, cut into halves

Dipping Sauce:
½ cup water
2 tablespoons sesame oil
2 tablespoons coconut aminos
1 teaspoon monk fruit powder
1 large clove garlic, minced
½ teaspoon ground ginger
1 teaspoon Chinese five-spice powder
Kosher salt and ground black pepper, to taste

1. Wrap the mushrooms with the bacon and secure with toothpicks. Arrange on a parchment-lined baking tray and bake at 380ºF (193ºC) for 40 minutes, flipping once halfway through cooking.
2. In the meantime, make the sauce by whisking all ingredients in a wok or deep saucepan. Cook over medium heat until thickened and reduced.
3. Serve the bacon dippers with the sauce on the side.

Per Serving
calories: 323 | fat: 33g | protein: 2g
carbs: 5g | net carbs: 3g | fiber: 2g

Turkey and Avocado Roll-Ups

Prep time: 5 minutes | Cook time: 0 minutes | Serves 8

½ fresh lemon, juiced
2 avocados, pitted, peeled and diced
16 slices cooked turkey breasts, deli-sliced
Salt and black pepper, to taste
16 slices Swiss cheese

1. Drizzle fresh lemon juice over your avocados. Place 1-2 avocado pieces on the turkey breast slice.
2. Season with salt and black pepper to taste.
3. Add the slice of Swiss cheese; repeat with the remaining ingredients. Roll them up and arrange on a nice serving platter. Bon appétit!

Per Serving
calories: 332 | fat: 24g | protein: 23g
carbs: 7g | net carbs: 3g | fiber: 4g

Pork Skewers with Greek Dipping Sauce

Prep time: 15 minutes | Cook time: 10 minutes | Serves 2

½ pound (227 g) pork loin, cut into bite-sized pieces
2 garlic cloves, pressed
1 scallion stalk, chopped
¼ cup dry red wine
Dipping Sauce:
½ cup Greek yogurt
½ teaspoon dill, ground
½ Lebanese cucumber, grated
1 teaspoon garlic, minced

1 thyme sprig
1 rosemary sprig
1 tablespoon lemon juice
1 teaspoon stone ground mustard
1 tablespoon olive oil

Sea salt, to taste
½ teaspoon ground black pepper
2 tablespoons cilantro leaves, roughly chopped

1. Place the pork loin in a ceramic dish; add in the garlic, scallions, wine, thyme, rosemary, lemon juice, mustard, and olive oil. Let them marinate in your refrigerator for 2 to 3 hours Thread the pork pieces onto bamboo skewers. Grill them for 5 to 6 minutes per side.
2. Meanwhile, whisk the remaining ingredients until well mixed. Serve the pork skewers with the sauce for dipping and enjoy!

Per Serving

calories: 313 | fat: 20.0g | protein: 29.2g | carbs: 2.2g | net carbs: 1.6g | fiber: 0.6g

Hot Spare Ribs

Prep time: 20 minutes | Cook time: 2 hours | Serves 2

1 pound (454 g) spare ribs
1 teaspoon Dijon mustard
1 tablespoon rice wine
Salt and ground black pepper, to season
1 teaspoon garlic, pressed
Hot Sauce:
1 teaspoon Sriracha sauce
1 tablespoon olive oil
1 cup tomato sauce, sugar-free

½ shallot powder
1 teaspoon cayenne pepper
½ teaspoon ground allspice
1 tablespoon avocado oil

1 teaspoon garlic, minced
Salt, to season

1. Arrange the spare ribs on a parchment-lined baking pan. Add the remaining ingredients for the ribs and toss until well coated.
2. Bake in the preheated oven at 360ºF (182ºC) for 1 hour. Rotate the pan and roast an additional 50 to 60 minutes. Baste the ribs with the cooking liquid periodically.
3. In the meantime, whisk the sauce ingredients until well mixed. Pour the hot sauce over the ribs. Place under the broiler and broil for 7 to 9 minutes or until an internal temperature reaches 145ºF (63ºC).
4. Brush the sauce onto each rib and serve warm. Bon appétit!

Per Serving

calories: 471 | fat: 27.1g | protein: 48.6g | carbs: 6.6g | net carbs: 4.6g | fiber: 2.0g

Meaty Jalapeños

Prep time: 15 minutes | Cook time: 40 minutes | Serves 10

2 ounces (57 g) bacon, chopped
½ pound (227 g) ground pork
½ pound (227 g) ground beef
½ cup red onion, chopped
2 garlic cloves, minced
1 teaspoon taco seasoning mix
Sea salt and ground black pepper, to season
½ cup tomato purée
1 teaspoon stone-ground mustard
20 jalapeño peppers, deveined and halved lengthwise
4 ounces (113 g) Parmesan cheese, preferably freshly grated

1. Preheat a nonstick skillet over medium-high heat. Now, cook the bacon, pork, and beef for about 4 minutes until no longer pink.
2. Add in the onion and garlic and cook an additional 3 minutes until they are tender. Sprinkle with the taco seasoning mix, salt, and black pepper. Fold in the tomato purée and mustard.
3. Continue to cook over medium-low heat for 4 minutes more. Spoon the mixture into jalapeño peppers.
4. Bake in the preheated oven at 390ºF (199ºC) for about 20 minutes. Top with Parmesan cheese and bake an additional 6 minutes or until cheese is golden on the top. Bon appétit!

Per Serving
calories: 190 | fat: 13.3g | protein: 12.6g | carbs: 4.8g | net carbs: 3.6g | fiber: 1.2g

Mini Bacon and Kale Muffins

Prep time: 5 minutes | Cook time: 30 minutes | Serves 6

2 slices cooked bacon, chopped
½ cup scallions, chopped
1 garlic clove, minced
1 cup kale, torn into small pieces
4 eggs, well whisked
4 tablespoons Greek yogurt
Kosher salt and ground white pepper, to season

1. Add cupcake liners to a mini muffin tin. Mix the bacon with the scallions, garlic, and kale. Fold in the eggs and yogurt. Mix to combine well.
2. Season with salt and ground white pepper; divide the mixture between the cupcake liners.
3. Bake in the preheated oven at 360ºF (182ºC) for 30 minutes or until your muffins are thoroughly cooked and firm.
4. Let cool for about 5 minutes; lastly, run a butter knife around the edges of each muffin to loosen it. Serve warm or at room temperature. Enjoy!

Per Serving
calories: 88 | fat: 7g | protein: 6g | carbs: 2g | net carbs: 1g | fiber: 1g

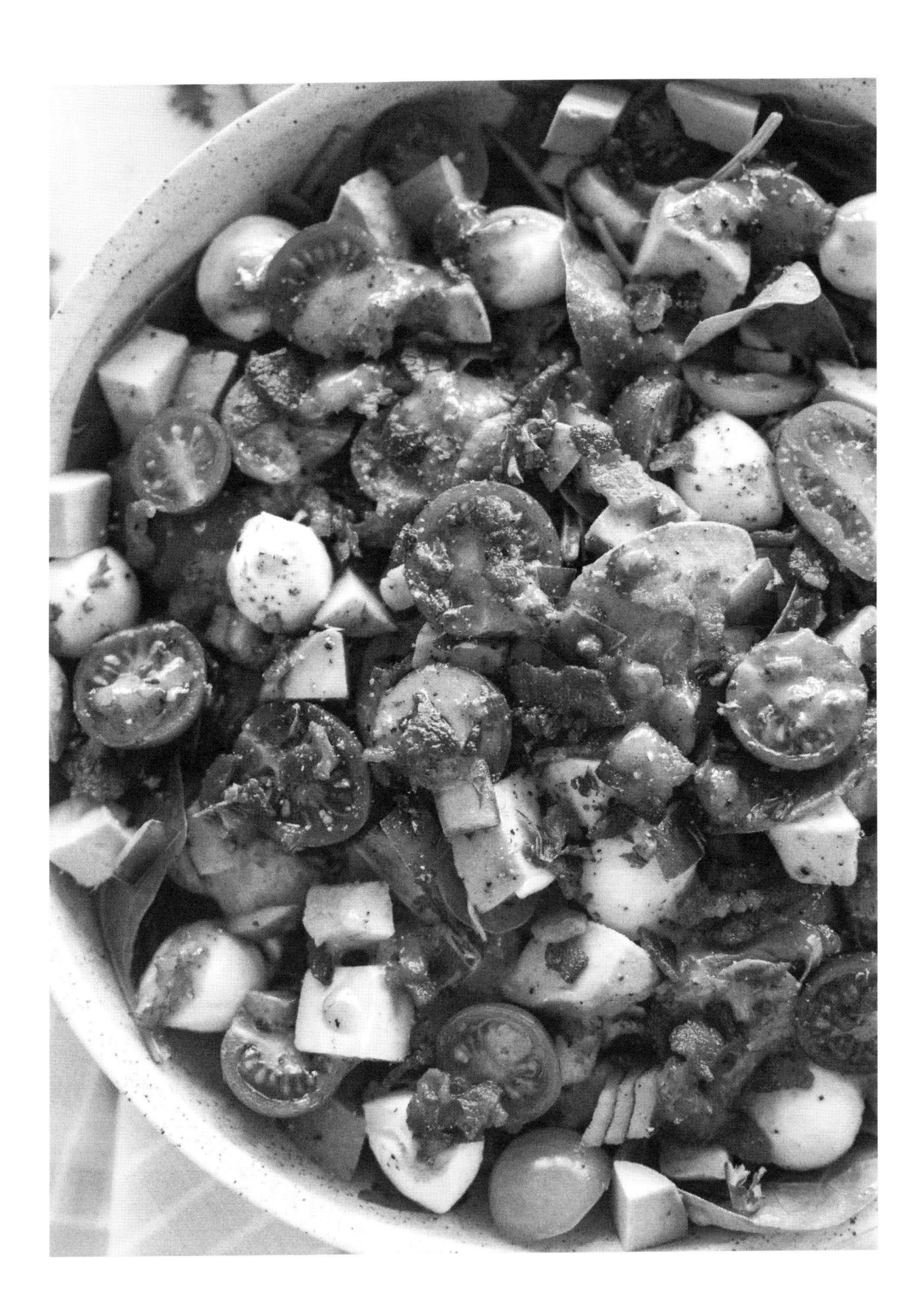

Chapter 3 Salads

Greek Caper Salad

Prep time: 10 minutes | Cook time: 0 minutes | Serves 4

5 tomatoes, chopped
1 large cucumber, chopped
1 green bell pepper, chopped
1 small red onion, chopped
16 Kalamata olives, chopped
4 tablespoons capers
7 ounces (198 g) Feta cheese, chopped
1 teaspoon oregano, dried
4 tablespoons olive oil
Salt to taste

1. Place tomatoes, pepper, cucumber, onion, Feta and olives in a bowl. Mix to combine. Season with salt. Combine the capers, olive oil and oregano in a small bowl. Drizzle the dressing over the salad.

Per Serving
calories: 324 | fat: 27.8g | protein: 9.4g
carbs: 11.9g | net carbs: 8.0g | fiber: 3.9g

Arugula and Avocado Salad

Prep time: 15 minutes | Cook time: 0 minutes | Serves 4

Salad:
6 cups baby arugula
1 avocado, diced
½ cup cherry tomatoes, halved
⅓ cup shaved Parmesan cheese
¼ cup thinly sliced red onions
¼ cup pili nuts or pine nuts

Dressing:
3 tablespoons extra-virgin olive oil
1 tablespoon red wine vinegar
1 small clove garlic, pressed or minced
Salt and pepper, to taste

1. Place all the salad ingredients in a large bowl and gently toss.
2. In a small bowl, stir together the dressing ingredients. Toss the salad with the dressing right before serving.

Per Serving
calories: 274 | fat: 23.9g | protein: 8.7g
carbs: 9.0g | net carbs: 4.0g | fiber: 5.0g

Tuna Cheese Caprese Salad

Prep time: 10 minutes | Cook time: 0 minutes | Serves 4

2 (10 ounce / 283-g) cans tuna chunks in water, drained
2 tomatoes, sliced
8 ounces (283 g) fresh mozzarella cheese, sliced
6 basil leaves
½ cup black olives, pitted and sliced
1 tablespoon extra virgin olive oil
½ lemon, juiced

1. Place the tuna in the center of a serving platter. Arrange the cheese and tomato slices around the tuna. Alternate a slice of tomato, cheese, and a basil leaf.
2. To finish, scatter the black olives over the top, drizzle with olive oil and lemon juice and serve.

Per Serving
calories: 360 | fat: 31g | protein: 21g
carbs: 3g | net carbs: 1g | fiber: 2g

Bacon, Avocado, and Veggies Salad

Prep time: 10 minutes | Cook time: 0 minutes | Serves 4

2 large avocados, 1 chopped and 1 sliced
1 spring onion, sliced
4 cooked bacon slices, crumbled
2 cups spinach
2 small lettuce heads, chopped
2 hard-boiled eggs, chopped

Vinaigrette:
1 tablespoon olive oil
1 teaspoon Dijon mustard
1 tablespoon apple cider vinegar

1. Combine the spinach, lettuce, eggs, chopped avocado, and spring onion, in a large bowl. Whisk together the vinaigrette ingredients in another bowl. Pour the dressing over, toss to combine and top with the sliced avocado and bacon.

Per Serving
calories: 350 | fat: 33g | protein: 7g
carbs: 11g | net carbs: 3g | fiber: 8g

Beef and Spinach Salad

Prep time: 15 minutes | Cook time: 20 minutes | Serves 4

3 tablespoons olive oil
½ pound (227 g) beef rump steak, cut into strips
Salt and black pepper, to taste
1 teaspoon cumin
A pinch of dried thyme
2 garlic cloves, minced
4 ounces (113 g) Feta cheese, crumbled
½ cup pecans, toasted
2 cups spinach
1½ tablespoons lemon juice
¼ cup fresh mint, chopped

1. Season the beef with salt, 1 tablespoon of olive oil, garlic, thyme, pepper, and cumin. Place on a preheated to medium heat grill, and cook for 10 minutes, flip once. Remove the grilled beef to a cutting board, leave to cool, and slice into strips.
2. Sprinkle the pecans on a lined baking sheet, place in the oven at 350ºF (180ºC), and toast for 10 minutes. In a salad bowl, combine the spinach with black pepper, mint, remaining olive oil, salt, lemon juice, Feta cheese, and pecans, and toss well to coat. Top with the beef slices and enjoy.

Per Serving
calories: 435 | fat: 43.1g | protein: 17.1g
carbs: 5.3g | net carbs: 3.4g | fiber: 1.9g

Marinated Pork and Veg Salad

Prep time: 15 minutes | Cook time: 15 minutes | Serves 6

¼ cup rice vinegar
¼ cup rice wine
¼ cup coconut aminos
1 tablespoon brown mustard
1 jalapeño pepper, chopped
2 garlic cloves, pressed
2 tablespoons olive oil
2 pounds (907 g) pork rib chops
Flaky sea salt and ground black pepper, to taste
½ teaspoon celery seeds
6 cups lettuce, torn into small pieces
1 bell pepper, deseeded and sliced
1 cucumber, sliced
1 tomato, sliced
4 scallions, chopped
½ lemon, juiced
½ cup sour cream, for garnish

1. Place the vinegar, wine, coconut aminos, mustard, jalapeño pepper, garlic, and pork in a ceramic dish. Cover and let it marinate for 2 hours in your refrigerator.
2. Heat the olive oil in an oven-safe pan over a medium-high flame.
3. Discard the marinade and cook the pork rib chops for 3 to 5 minutes. Flip them over using a pair of tongs. Cook an additional 4 minutes or until a good crust is formed.
4. Sprinkle with salt, black pepper, and celery seeds. Then, bake the pork rib chops in the preheated oven for 10 minutes until an instant-read thermometer reads 145ºF (63ºC).
5. Shred the pork rib chops and reserve. Add the lettuce, bell pepper, cucumber, tomato, and scallions to a salad bowl. Top with the shredded pork, drizzle lemon juice over everything and garnish with sour cream. Enjoy!

Per Serving
calories: 297 | fat: 14.1g | protein: 35.2g
carbs: 6.0g | net carbs: 4.5g | fiber: 1.5g

Spanish Chicken and Pepper Salad

Prep time: 10 minutes | Cook time: 15 minutes | Serves 6

1½ pounds (680 g) chicken breasts
½ cup dry white wine
1 onion, chopped
2 Spanish peppers, deveined and chopped
1 Spanish naga chili pepper, chopped
2 garlic cloves, minced
2 cups arugula
¼ cup mayonnaise
1 tablespoon balsamic vinegar
1 tablespoon stone-ground mustard
Sea salt and freshly ground black pepper, to season

1. Place the chicken breasts in a saucepan. Add the wine to the saucepan and cover the chicken with water. Bring to a boil over medium-high heat.
2. Reduce to a simmer and cook partially covered for 10 to 14 minutes (an instant-read thermometer should register 165ºF (74ºC)).
3. Transfer the chicken from the poaching liquid to a cutting board; cut into bite-sized pieces and transfer to a salad bowl.
4. Add the remaining ingredients to the salad bowl and gently stir to combine. Serve well chilled.

Per Serving
calories: 280 | fat: 16.2g | protein: 27.2g
carbs: 4.9g | net carbs: 4.0g | fiber: 0.9g

Chicken Thigh Green Salad

Prep time: 10 minutes | Cook time: 15 minutes | Serves 2

2 chicken thighs, skinless
Sea salt and cayenne pepper, to season
½ teaspoon Dijon mustard
1 tablespoon red wine vinegar
¼ cup mayonnaise
1 small-sized celery stalk, chopped
2 spring onion stalks, chopped
½ head Romaine lettuce, torn into pieces
½ cucumber, sliced

1. Fry the chicken thighs until thoroughly heated and crunchy on the outside; an instant-read thermometer should read about 165ºF (74ºC).
2. Discard the bones and chop the meat.
3. Place the other ingredients in a serving bowl and stir until everything is well incorporated. Layer the chopped chicken thighs over the salad.
4. Serve well chilled and enjoy!

Per Serving
calories: 455 | fat: 29.1g | protein: 40.2g
carbs: 6.6g | net carbs: 2.8g | fiber: 3.8g

Tuna Salad with Olives and Lettuce

Prep time: 5 minutes | Cook time: 0 minutes | Serves 2

1 cup canned tuna, drained
1 teaspoon onion flakes
1 tablespoon mayonnaise
1 cup shredded romaine lettuce
1 tablespoon lime juice
Sea salt, to taste
6 black olives, pitted and sliced

1. Combine the tuna, mayonnaise, lime juice, and salt in a small bowl; mix to combine well. In a salad platter, arrange the shredded lettuce and onion flakes. Spread the tuna mixture over; top with black olives to serve.

Per Serving
calories: 248 | fat: 20g | protein: 19g
carbs: 3g | net carbs: 2g | fiber: 1g

Caprese Salad

Prep time: 15 minutes | Cook time: 0 minutes | Serves 5

2 medium tomatoes, each cut into 5 slices
Coarse salt to taste
6 ounces (170 g) fresh Mozzarella, cut into 10 slices
2 avocados, cut into 30 thin slices
3 to 4 large basil leaves, chopped, plus additional leaves for garnish
¼ cup extra-virgin olive oil or avocado oil
1 lime, halved
Ground black pepper
Italian seasoning (optional)

1. Lay the tomato slices on a serving plate and sprinkle with salt. On top of each tomato, stack a Mozzarella slice, 3 avocado slices, and some chopped basil.
2. Drizzle with the oil and squeeze some lime juice over the top.
3. Sprinkle with pepper and Italian seasoning, if using. Garnish each stack with a basil leaf, if desired.

Per Serving
calories: 284 | fat: 25.7g | protein: 7.5g
carbs: 8.0g | net carbs: 3.5g | fiber: 4.5g

Classic Greek Salad

Prep time: 10 minutes | Cook time: 0 minutes | Serves 4

5 tomatoes, chopped
1 large cucumber, chopped
1 green bell pepper, chopped
1 small red onion, chopped
16 kalamata olives, chopped
1 tablespoon capers
1 cup feta cheese, chopped
1 teaspoon oregano, dried
1 tablespoon olive oil
Salt to taste

1. Place tomatoes, bell pepper, cucumber, onion, feta cheese and olives in a bowl; mix to combine well. Season with salt. Combine capers, olive oil, and oregano, in a bowl. Drizzle with the dressing to serve.

Per Serving
calories: 323 | fat: 28g | protein: 9g
carbs: 12g | net carbs: 8g | fiber: 4g

Feta Cucumber Salad

Prep time: 10 minutes | Cook time: 0 minutes | Serves 5

2 medium-large cucumbers
½ cup thinly sliced red onions
Dressing:
¼ cup extra-virgin olive oil
1 tablespoon red wine vinegar
1 tablespoon Swerve
4 ounces (113 g) Feta cheese, crumbled
Salt and pepper to taste
confectioners'-style sweetener
½ teaspoon dried ground oregano

1. Peel the cucumbers as desired and cut in half lengthwise, then slice.
2. In a medium-sized bowl, toss the cucumbers with the onions. Add the Feta and gently toss to combine.
3. Make the dressing: Place all the ingredients in a small bowl and whisk to combine.
4. Serve right away or place in the refrigerator to chill before serving. To serve, gently toss the salad with the dressing and season to taste with salt and pepper.

Per Serving
calories: 172 | fat: 15.2g | protein: 4.5g
carbs: 6.5g | net carbs: 3.7g | fiber: 2.8g

Spinach and Bacon Salad

Prep time: 15 minutes | Cook time: 0 minutes | Serves 4

8 cups baby spinach
4 slices bacon, pan-fried and chopped
3 large eggs, hard-boiled and sliced
10 grape tomatoes, halved
2 avocados, sliced or cubed
½ medium red onion, thinly sliced
½ cup sliced white mushrooms
⅓ cup chopped pecans
Ground black pepper
¾ cup ranch or blue cheese dressing

1. In a large bowl, gently toss the spinach, bacon, hard-boiled eggs, tomatoes, avocados, onion, mushrooms, and pecans. Season with pepper to taste.
2. Top with the dressing just before serving.

Per Serving
calories: 402 | fat: 34.6g | protein: 12.9g
carbs: 11.1g | net carbs: 7.4g | fiber: 3.7g

Shrimp Salad with Lemony Mayonnaise

Prep time: 10 minutes | Cook time: 0 minutes | Serves 4

1 small head cauliflower, cut into florets
⅓ cup diced celery
½ cup sliced black
Dressing:
½ cup mayonnaise
1 teaspoon apple cider vinegar
¼ teaspoon celery seeds
A pinch of black
olives
2 cups cooked large shrimp
1 tablespoon dill, chopped
pepper
1 tablespoon lemon juice
1 teaspoon Swerve
Salt to taste

1. Combine the cauliflower, celery, shrimp, and dill in a large bowl.
2. Whisk together the mayonnaise, vinegar, celery seeds, black pepper, sweetener, and lemon juice in another bowl. Season with salt to taste. Pour the dressing over and gently toss to combine; refrigerate for 1 hour. Top with olives to serve.

Per Serving
calories: 182 | fat: 15g | protein: 12g
carbs: 4g | net carbs: 2g | fiber: 2g

Mediterranean Tomato and Avocado Salad

Prep time: 5 minutes | Cook time: 0 minutes | Serves 4

3 tomatoes, sliced
1 large avocado, sliced
8 kalamata olives
¼ pound (113 g) buffalo mozzarella
cheese, sliced
1 tablespoon pesto sauce
1 tablespoon olive oil

1. Arrange the tomato slices on a serving platter and place the avocado slices in the middle.
2. Arrange the olives around the avocado slices and drop pieces of mozzarella on the platter.
3. Drizzle the pesto sauce all over, and drizzle olive oil as well.

Per Serving
calories: 290 | fat: 25g | protein: 9g
carbs: 9g | net carbs: 4g | fiber: 5g

Caesar Salad with Salmon and Egg

Prep time: 5 minutes | Cook time: 27 minutes | Serves 4

2 cups water
8 eggs
2 cups torn romaine lettuce
½ cup smoked salmon, chopped
6 slices bacon
1 tablespoon Heinz low carb Caesar dressing

1. Boil the water in a pot over medium heat for 5 minutes and bring to simmer. Crack each egg into a small bowl and gently slide into the water. Poach for 2 to 3 minutes, remove with a perforated spoon, transfer to a paper towel to dry, and plate. Poach the remaining 7 eggs.
2. Put the bacon in a skillet and fry over medium heat until browned and crispy, about 6 minutes, turning once. Remove, allow cooling, and chop in small pieces.
3. Toss the lettuce, smoked salmon, bacon, and Caesar dressing in a salad bowl. Divide the salad into 4 plates, top with two eggs each, and serve immediately or chilled.

Per Serving
calories: 260 | fat: 21g | protein: 8g
carbs: 6g | net carbs: 5g | fiber: 1g

Salmon Fillet and Spinach Cobb Salad

Prep time: 5 minutes | Cook time: 25 minutes | Serves 2

4 bacon slices
2 large eggs
2 (6-ounce / 170-g) salmon fillets
Pink Himalayan salt, to taste
Freshly ground black pepper, to taste
1 tablespoon butter, if needed
1 avocado, sliced
6 ounces (170-g) organic baby spinach
¼ cup crumbled blue cheese
1 tablespoon olive oil

1. In a medium skillet over medium-high heat, cook the bacon on both sides until crispy, about 8 minutes. Transfer the bacon to a paper towel–lined plate.
2. Bring a small saucepan filled with water to a boil over high heat. Put the eggs on to softboil, turn the heat down to medium-high, and cook for about 6 minutes.
3. Meanwhile, pat the salmon fillets on both sides with a paper towel to remove excess moisture. Season both sides with pink Himalayan salt and pepper.
4. With the bacon grease still in the skillet, add the salmon. If you need more grease in the pan, add some butter to the bacon grease.
5. Cook the salmon on medium-high heat for 5 minutes on each side, or until it reaches your preferred degree of doneness. (I like it medium-rare.)
6. Meanwhile, transfer the bacon to a cutting board and chop it. Peel the softboiled eggs. Season the avocado with pink Himalayan salt and pepper.
7. Divide the spinach, bacon, and avocado between two plates.
8. Carefully halve the softboiled eggs and place them on the salads. Sprinkle the blue cheese crumbles over the salads.
9. Top with the salmon, drizzle the salads with the olive oil, and serve.

Per Serving
calories: 623 | fat: 43g | protein: 54g
carbs: 12g | net carbs: 5g | fiber: 7g

Kale and Smoked Salmon Salad

Prep time: 15 minutes | Cook time: 0 minutes | Serves 4

¼ cup extra virgin olive oil
1 tablespoon lemon juice
½ teaspoon garlic powder
½ teaspoon sea salt
¼ teaspoon black pepper
6 ounces (170 g) chopped and deribbed kale (from 8 to 10 ounces / 227 to 283 g untrimmed)
¼ cup salted roasted sunflower seeds
8 ounces (227 g) smoked salmon, cut into pieces

1. In a large bowl, whisk together the olive oil, lemon juice, garlic powder, sea salt, and black pepper.
2. Add the chopped kale. Use your hands to massage the kale with the dressing mixture. Grab a bunch, squeeze with the dressing, release, and repeat. Do this for a couple of minutes, until the kale starts to soften.
3. Add the sunflower seeds and smoked salmon. Toss together.

Per Serving
calories: 258 | fat: 20.0g | protein: 14.0g
carbs: 6.0g | net carbs: 6.0g | fiber: 0g

Egg and Chicken Salad in Lettuce Cups

Prep time: 10 minutes | Cook time: 18 minutes | Serves 4

2 chicken breasts, cut into pieces
1 tablespoon olive oil
Salt and black pepper to season
6 large eggs
1½ cups water
2 tomatoes, seeded, chopped
6 tablespoon Greek yogurt
1 head green lettuce, firm leaves removed for cups

1. Preheat oven to 400ºF (205ºC). Put the chicken pieces in a bowl, drizzle with olive oil, and sprinkle with salt and black pepper. Mix the ingredients until the chicken is well coated with the seasoning.
2. Put the chicken on a prepared baking sheet and spread out evenly. Slide the baking sheet in the oven and bake the chicken until cooked through and golden brown for 8 minutes, turning once.
3. Bring the eggs to boil in salted water in a pot over medium heat for 10 minutes. Run the eggs in cold water, peel, and chop into small pieces. Transfer to a salad bowl.
4. Remove the chicken from the oven when ready and add to the salad bowl. Include the tomatoes and Greek yogurt; mix evenly with a spoon. Layer two lettuce leaves each as cups and fill with two tablespoons of egg salad each. Serve with chilled blueberry juice.

Per Serving
calories: 325 | fat: 25g | protein: 21g
carbs: 7g | net carbs: 4g | fiber: 3g

Skirt Steak, Veggies, and Pecan Salad

Prep time: 15 minutes | Cook time: 10 minutes | Serves 2

8 ounces (227 g) skirt steak
Pink Himalayan salt
Freshly ground black pepper
1 tablespoon butter
2 romaine hearts or 2 cups chopped romaine
½ cup halved grape tomatoes
¼ cup crumbled blue cheese
¼ cup pecans
1 tablespoon olive oil

1. Heat a large skillet over high heat.
2. Pat the steak dry with a paper towel, and season both sides with pink Himalayan salt and pepper.
3. Add the butter to the skillet. When it melts, put the steak in the skillet.
4. Sear the steak for about 3 minutes on each side, for medium-rare.
5. Transfer the steak to a cutting board and let it rest for at least 5 minutes.
6. Meanwhile, divide the romaine between two plates, and top with the grape tomato halves, blue cheese, and pecans. Drizzle with the olive oil.
7. Slice the skirt steak across the grain, top the salads with it, and serve.

Per Serving
calories: 451 | fat: 36g | protein: 30g
carbs: 7g | net carbs: 5g | fiber: 2g

Yellow Cheddar Pork Patties Salad

Prep time: 5 minutes | Cook time: 20 minutes | Serves 4

1 pound (454 g) ground pork
Salt and black pepper to season
1 tablespoon olive oil
2 hearts romaine lettuce, torn into pieces
2 firm tomatoes, sliced
¼ red onion, sliced
3 ounces (85 g) yellow cheddar cheese, shredded

1. Season the pork with salt and black pepper, mix and make medium-sized patties out of them.
2. Heat the oil in a skillet over medium heat and fry the patties on both sides for 10 minutes until browned and cook within. Transfer to a wire rack to drain oil. When cooled, cut into quarters.
3. Mix the lettuce, tomatoes, and red onion in a salad bowl, season with a little oil, salt, and black pepper. Toss and add the pork on top.
4. Melt the cheese in the microwave for about 90 seconds. Drizzle the cheese over the salad and serve.

Per Serving
calories: 310 | fat: 23g | protein: 22g
carbs: 9g | net carbs: 2g | fiber: 7g

Mackerel and Green Bean Salad

Prep time: 10 minutes | Cook time: 11 minutes | Serves 2

2 mackerel fillets
2 hard-boiled eggs, sliced
1 tablespoon coconut oil
2 cups green beans
1 avocado, sliced
4 cups mixed salad greens
1 tablespoon olive oil
1 tablespoon lemon juice
1 teaspoon Dijon mustard
Salt and black pepper, to taste

1. Fill a saucepan with water and add the green beans and salt. Cook over medium heat for about 3 minutes. Drain and set aside.
2. Melt the coconut oil in a pan over medium heat. Add the mackerel fillets and cook for about 4 minutes per side, or until opaque and crispy. Divide the green beans between two salad bowls. Top with mackerel, eggs, and avocado slices.
3. In a bowl, whisk together the lemon juice, olive oil, mustard, salt, and pepper, and drizzle over the salad.

Per Serving

calories: 525 | fat: 42g | protein: 27g | carbs: 22g | net carbs: 8g | fiber: 14g

Lemony Prawn and Arugula Salad

Prep time: 10 minutes | Cook time: 3 minute | Serves 4

4 cups baby arugula
½ cup garlic mayonnaise
1 tablespoon olive oil
1 pound (454 g) tiger prawns, peeled and
deveined
1 teaspoon Dijon mustard
Salt and chili pepper to season
2 tablespoons lemon juice

1. First, make the dressing: add the mayonnaise, lemon juice and mustard in a small bowl. Mix until smooth and creamy. Set aside until ready to use.
2. Heat 1 tablespoon of olive oil in a skillet over medium heat, add the prawns, season with salt, and chili pepper, and fry for 3 minutes on each side until prawns are pink. Set aside to a plate.
3. Place the arugula in a serving bowl and pour half of the dressing on the salad. Toss with 2 spoons until mixed, and add the remaining dressing. Divide salad onto 4 plates and top with prawns.

Per Serving

calories: 215 | fat: 20g | protein: 8g | carbs: 3g | net carbs: 2g | fiber: 1g

Garlicky Chicken Salad

Prep time: 10 minutes | Cook time: 8 minutes | Serves 4

2 chicken breasts, boneless, skinless, flattened
Salt and black pepper, to taste
1 tablespoon garlic powder
1 teaspoon olive oil
1½ cups mixed salad greens
1 tablespoon red wine vinegar
1 cup crumbled blue cheese

1. Season the chicken with salt, black pepper, and garlic powder. Heat oil in a pan over high heat and fry the chicken for 4 minutes on both sides until golden brown. Remove chicken to a cutting board and let cool before slicing.
2. Toss salad greens with red wine vinegar and share the salads into 4 plates. Divide chicken slices on top and sprinkle with blue cheese. Serve.

Per Serving
calories: 286 | fat: 23g | protein: 14g | carbs: 5g | net carbs: 4g | fiber: 1g

Balsamic Brussels Sprouts Cheese Salad

Prep time: 10 minutes | Cook time: 20 minutes | Serves 6

2 pound (907 g) Brussels sprouts, halved
1 tablespoon olive oil
Salt and black pepper to taste
2½ tablespoon balsamic vinegar
¼ head red cabbage, shredded
1 tablespoon Dijon mustard
1 cup Pecorino Romano cheese, grated

1. Preheat oven to 400ºF (205ºC) and line a baking sheet with foil. Toss the brussels sprouts with olive oil, a little salt, black pepper, and balsamic vinegar, in a bowl, and spread on the baking sheet in an even layer. Bake until tender on the inside and crispy on the outside, about 20 to 25 minutes.
2. Transfer to a salad bowl and add the red cabbage, Dijon mustard and half of the cheese. Mix until well combined. Sprinkle with the remaining cheese, share the salad onto serving plates, and serve with the salmon.

Per Serving
calories: 210 | fat: 18g | protein: 4g | carbs: 12g | net carbs: 6g | fiber: 6g

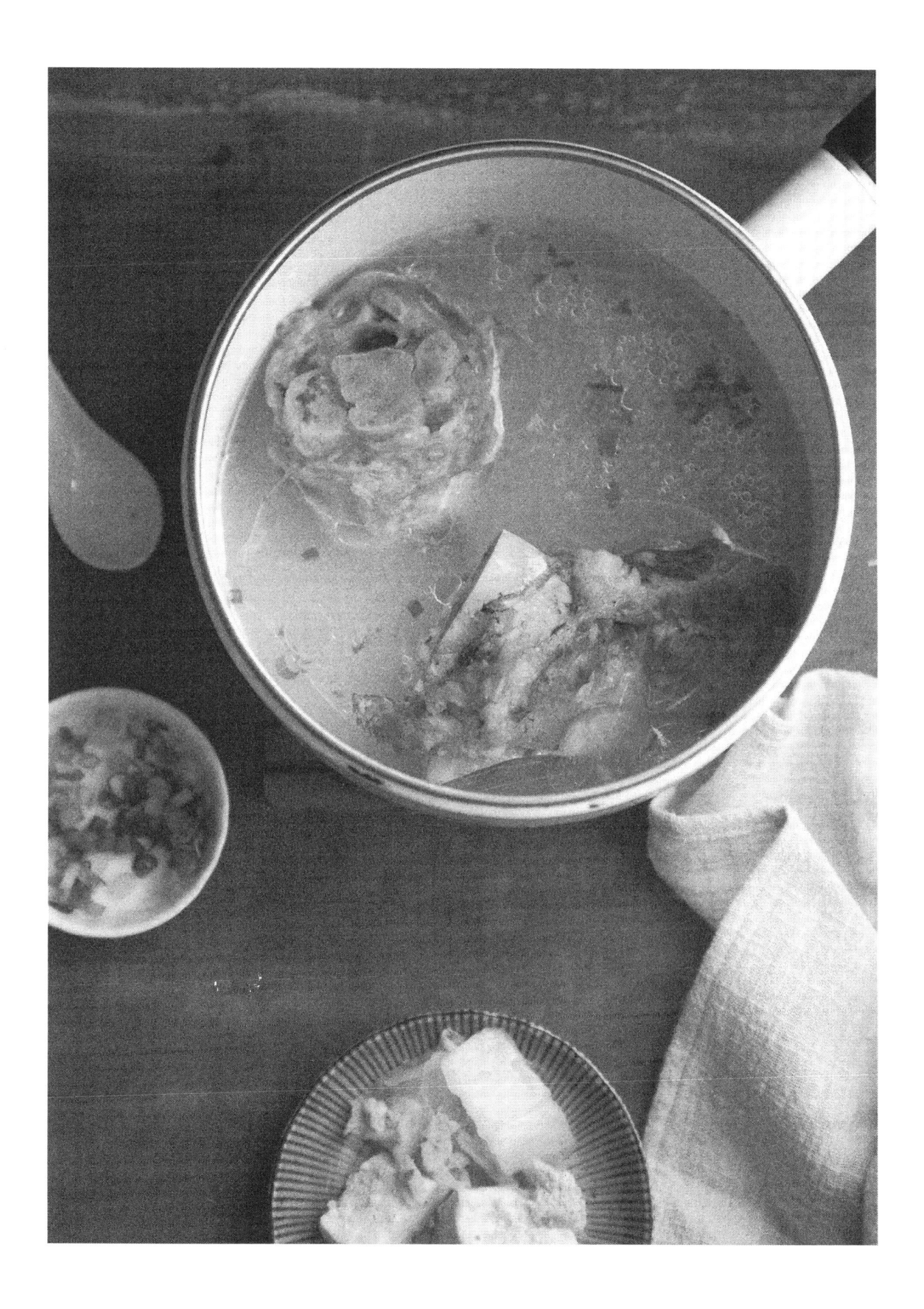

Chapter 4 Soups

Cauliflower and Lamb Soup

Prep time: 10 minutes | Cook time: 4 hours | Serves 6

1 pound (454 g) ground lamb
5 cups beef broth
1 cauliflower head, cut into florets
1 cup heavy cream
1 yellow onion, chopped
2 cloves garlic, chopped
1 tablespoon freshly chopped thyme
½ teaspoon cracked black pepper
½ teaspoon salt

1. Add the ground lamb and cauliflower to the base of a stockpot.
2. Add in the remaining ingredients minus the heavy cream, and cook on high for 4 hours.
3. Warm the heavy cream before adding to the soup. Use an immersion blender to blend the soup until creamy.

Per Serving
calories: 264 | fat: 14.0g | protein: 26.9g
carbs: 5.9g | net carbs: 3.9g | fiber: 2.0g

Turkey Taco Soup

Prep time: 10 minutes | Cook time: 4 hours | Serves 6

1 pound (454 g) ground turkey
5 cups chicken bone broth (you can also use regular chicken broth)
1 cup canned diced tomatoes (no sugar added)
1 cup whipped cream
cheese
1 yellow onion, chopped
1 tablespoon chili powder
1 teaspoon cumin
1 teaspoon garlic powder
1 teaspoon onion powder

1. Add all the ingredients to the base of a Crock-Pot minus the cream cheese and cover with the chicken broth.
2. Set on high and cook for 4 hours adding in the cream cheese at the 3.5 hour mark.
3. Stir well before serving.

Per Serving
calories: 336 | fat: 22.9g | protein: 27.9g
carbs: 5.9g | net carbs: 4.8g | fiber: 1.1g

Lemony Chicken and Chive Soup

Prep time: 10 minutes | Cook time: 4 hours | Serves 4

2 boneless, skinless chicken breasts
6 cups chicken broth
¼ cup freshly squeezed lemon juice
2 tablespoons chives, chopped
1 yellow onion, chopped
2 cloves garlic, chopped
Salt and pepper, to taste

1. Add all the ingredients to a slow cooker and cook on high for 4 hours.
2. Once cooked, shred the chicken and stir back into the soup.

Per Serving
calories: 172 | fat: 5.9g | protein: 22.1g
carbs: 6.0g | net carbs: 5.0g | fiber: 1.0g

Green Minestrone Soup

Prep time: 10 minutes | Cook time: 12 minutes | Serves 4

1 tablespoon butter
1 tablespoon onion-garlic puree
2 heads broccoli, cut in florets
2 stalks celery, chopped
5 cups vegetable broth
1 cup baby spinach
Salt and black pepper to taste
1 tablespoon Gruyere cheese, grated

1. Melt the butter in a saucepan over medium heat and sauté the onion-garlic puree for 3 minutes until softened. Mix in the broccoli and celery, and cook for 4 minutes until slightly tender. Pour in the broth, bring to a boil, then reduce the heat to medium-low and simmer covered for about 5 minutes.
2. Drop in the spinach to wilt, adjust the seasonings, and cook for 4 minutes. Ladle soup into serving bowls. Serve with a sprinkle of grated Gruyere cheese.

Per Serving
calories: 227 | fat: 20g | protein: 8g
carbs: 9g | net carbs: 2g | fiber: 7g

Chicken and Cabbage Soup

Prep time: 15 minutes | Cook time: 40 minutes | Serves 6

1 rotisserie chicken, shredded
6 cups water
2 tablespoons butter
2 celery stalks, chopped
½ onion, chopped
1 bay leaf
Sea salt and ground black pepper, to taste
1 tablespoon fresh cilantro, chopped
2 cups green cabbage, sliced into strips

1. Cook the bones and carcass from a leftover chicken with water over medium-high heat for 15 minutes. Then, reduce to a simmer and cook an additional 15 minutes. Reserve the chicken along with the broth.
2. Let it cool enough to handle, shred the meat into bite-size pieces.
3. Melt the butter in a large stockpot over medium heat. Sauté the celery and onion until tender and fragrant.
4. Add bay leaf, salt, pepper, and broth, and let it simmer for 10 minutes.
5. Add the reserved chicken, cilantro, and cabbage. Simmer for an additional 10 to 11 minutes, until the cabbage is tender. Bon appétit!

Per Serving
calories: 266 | fat: 23.6g | protein: 9.4g carbs: 4.2g | net carbs: 2.6g | fiber: 1.6g

Beef Hamburger Soup

Prep time: 10 minutes | Cook time: 4 hours | Serves 6

1 pound (454 g) lean ground beef
½ cup no-sugar added marinara sauce
½ cup beef broth
½ cup shredded Cheddar cheese
1 yellow onion, chopped
2 cloves garlic, chopped
Salt and pepper, to taste

1. Add all the ingredients to a slow cooker minus the shredded cheese and cook on high for 4 hours.
2. Stir in the cheese and serve.

Per Serving
calories: 210 | fat: 9.1g | protein: 25.8g carbs: 5.0g | net carbs: 4.0g | fiber: 1.0g

Pork Soup

Prep time: 10 minutes | Cook time: 25 minutes | Serves 5

2 teaspoons olive oil
1 pound (454 g) ground pork
2 shallots, chopped
1 celery stalk, chopped
1 fresh Italian pepper, deveined and chopped
5 cups beef bone broth
2 tablespoons fresh cilantro, roughly chopped

1. Heat 1 teaspoon of the olive oil in a soup pot over a medium-high flame. Brown the ground pork until no longer pink or about 4 minutes, crumbling with a spatula; reserve.
2. In the same pot, heat the remaining teaspoon of olive oil. Sauté the shallot until just tender and fragrant.
3. Add in the chopped celery and Italian pepper along with the reserved cooked pork.
4. Pour in the beef bone broth. When it comes to a boil, turn the heat to simmer. Let it simmer, partially covered, for 25 minutes until everything is cooked through.
5. Season with salt to taste, ladle into soup bowls, and garnish each serving with fresh cilantro. Bon appétit!

Per Serving
calories: 293 | fat: 20.5g | protein: 23.5g carbs: 1.5g | net carbs: 1.3g | fiber: 0.2g

Herbed Beef and Zucchini Soup

Prep time: 10 minutes | Cook time: 4 to 6 hours | Serves 6

1 pound (454 g) lean ground beef
4 cups beef broth
1 zucchini, diced
2 stalks celery, chopped
½ cup diced tomatoes
1 yellow onion, chopped
2 cloves garlic, chopped
1 teaspoon freshly chopped thyme
1 teaspoon freshly chopped rosemary
Salt and pepper, to taste

1. Add all the ingredients to a slow cooker and cook on high for 4 to 6 hours.
2. Stir well before serving.

Per Serving
calories: 186 | fat: 6.0g | protein: 7.1g carbs: 5.0g | net carbs: 4.0g | fiber: 1.0g

Lamb and Cheddar Taco Soup

Prep time: 10 minutes | Cook time: 4 to 6 hours | Serves 6

1 pound (454 g) ground lamb
4 cups beef broth
1 cup shredded Cheddar cheese
1 cup diced tomatoes
1 green bell pepper, chopped
1 yellow onion, chopped
2 cloves garlic, chopped
1 teaspoon ground cumin
1 teaspoon ground coriander
1 teaspoon paprika
½ teaspoon cayenne pepper
Salt and pepper, to taste

1. Add all the ingredients to a slow cooker minus the shredded cheese and cook on high for 4 to 6 hours.
2. Stir in the shredded cheese and serve.

Per Serving
calories: 266 | fat: 12.9g | protein: 30.1g
carbs: 5.9g | net carbs: 4.8g | fiber: 1.1g

Coconut Carrot Soup

Prep time: 15 minutes | Cook time: 40 minutes | Serves 8

6 cups vegetable broth
¼ cup full-fat unsweetened coconut milk
¾ pound (340 g) carrots, peeled and chopped
2 teaspoons grated ginger
1 teaspoon ground turmeric
1 sweet yellow onion, chopped
2 cloves garlic, chopped
Pinch of sea salt and pepper, to taste

1. Add all the ingredients minus the coconut milk to a stockpot over medium heat and bring to a boil. Reduce to a simmer and cook for 40 minutes or until the carrots are tender.
2. Use an immersion blender and blend the soup until smooth. Stir in the coconut milk.
3. Enjoy right away and freeze any leftovers.

Per Serving
calories: 74 | fat: 3.0g | protein: 4.1g
carbs: 7.1g | net carbs: 4.9g | fiber: 2.2g

Garlicky Coconut Milk and Tomato Soup

Prep time: 15 minutes | Cook time: 30 minutes | Serves 6

6 cups vegetable broth
½ cup full-fat unsweetened coconut milk
1½ cups canned diced tomatoes
1 yellow onion, chopped
3 cloves garlic, chopped
1 teaspoon Italian seasoning
1 bay leaf
Pinch of salt and pepper, to taste
Fresh basil, for serving

1. Add all the ingredients minus the coconut milk and fresh basil to a stockpot over medium heat and bring to a boil. Reduce to a simmer and cook for 30 minutes.
2. Remove the bay leaf, and then use an immersion blender to blend the soup until smooth. Stir in the coconut milk.
3. Garnish with fresh basil and serve.

Per Serving
calories: 105 | fat: 6.9g | protein: 6.1g
carbs: 5.8g | net carbs: 4.8g | fiber: 1.0g

Easy Chicken and Onion Soup

Prep time: 10 minutes | Cook time: 30 minutes | Serves 2

2 chicken drumsticks, skinless and boneless
½ white onion, chopped
1 stalk celery, chopped
1 teaspoon poultry seasoning mix
1 tablespoon fresh cilantro, chopped

1. Place the chicken in a stockpot. Add enough water to cover by about an inch.
2. Now, add in the chopped onion, celery and poultry seasoning mix. Bring to a boil over medium-high heat. Turn the temperature to medium-low and cook for 35 to 40 minutes.
3. As for the chicken, the meat thermometer should register 165ºF (74ºC). Make sure to add extra water during the cooking as needed to keep the ingredients covered.
4. Season to taste and serve with fresh cilantro. Bon appétit!

Per Serving
calories: 167 | fat: 4.8g | protein: 25.5g
carbs: 3.2g | net carbs: 2.6g | fiber: 0.6g

Coconut Milk and Pumpkin Soup

Prep time: 15 minutes | Cook time: 30 minutes | Serves 6

6 cups vegetable broth
1 cup canned pumpkin
1 cup full-fat coconut milk
1 teaspoon freshly chopped sage
2 cloves garlic, chopped
Pinch of salt and pepper, to taste

1. Add all the ingredients minus the coconut milk to a stockpot over medium heat and bring to a boil. Reduce to a simmer and cook for 30 minutes.
2. Add the coconut milk and stir.

Per Serving
calories: 145 | fat: 10.8g | protein: 6.2g
carbs: 6.9g | net carbs: 5.0g | fiber: 1.9g

Slow Cooked Faux Lasagna Soup

Prep time: 20 minutes | Cook time: 6 hours | Serves 6

3 tablespoons extra-virgin olive oil, divided
1 pound (454 g) ground beef
½ sweet onion, chopped
2 teaspoons minced garlic
4 cups beef broth
1 (28-ounce / 794-g) can diced tomatoes, undrained
1 zucchini, diced
1½ tablespoons dried basil
2 teaspoons dried oregano
4 ounces (113 g) cream cheese
1 cup shredded mozzarella

1. Lightly grease the insert of the slow cooker with 1 tablespoon of the olive oil.
2. In a large skillet over medium-high heat, heat the remaining 2 tablespoons 2. of the olive oil. Add the ground beef and sauté until it is cooked through, about 6 minutes.
3. Add the onion and garlic and sauté for an additional 3 minutes.
4. Transfer the meat mixture to the insert.
5. Stir in the broth, tomatoes, zucchini, basil, and oregano.
6. Cover and cook on low for 6 hours.
7. Stir in the cream cheese and mozzarella and serve.

Per Serving
calories: 472 | fat: 36g | protein: 30g
carbs: 9g | net carbs: 6g | fiber: 3g

Super Cheesy Bacon-Cauliflower Soup

Prep time: 15 minutes | Cook time: 6 hours | Serves 6

1 tablespoon extra-virgin olive oil
4 cups chicken broth
2 cups coconut milk
2 cups chopped cooked chicken
1 cup chopped cooked bacon
2 cups chopped cauliflower
1 sweet onion, chopped
3 teaspoons minced garlic
½ cup cream cheese, cubed
2 cups shredded cheddar cheese

1. Lightly grease the insert of the slow cooker with the olive oil.
2. Place the broth, coconut milk, chicken, bacon, cauliflower, onion, and garlic in the insert.
3. Cover and cook on low for 6 hours.
4. Stir in the cream cheese and Cheddar and serve.

Per Serving
calories: 540 | fat: 44g | protein: 35g
carbs: 7g | net carbs: 6g | fiber: 1g

Herbed Beef Soup

Prep time: 15 minutes | Cook time: 40 minutes | Serves 6

1 pound (454 g) beef chuck roast, cubed
6 cups beef bone broth (you can also use regular beef broth)
1 yellow onion, chopped
2 cloves garlic, chopped
2 carrots, chopped
2 stalks celery, sliced
1 teaspoon fresh thyme, chopped
½ teaspoon dried oregano
1 handful fresh basil, chopped
Salt and pepper, to taste
1 tablespoon coconut oil, for cooking

1. Add the coconut oil to a skillet and brown the beef over medium heat.
2. Add the beef and the remaining ingredients minus the basil to a stockpot and bring to a boil.
3. Reduce to a simmer and cook for about 30 minutes or until the vegetables are tender.
4. Serve with freshly chopped basil.

Per Serving
calories: 220 | fat: 9.0g | protein: 29.0g
carbs: 6.0g | net carbs: 5.0g | fiber: 1.0g

Zucchini and Celery Soup

Prep time: 10 minutes | Cook time: 15 minutes | Serves 3

2 teaspoons extra-virgin olive oil
½ pound (227 g) zucchini, peeled and diced
½ shallot, chopped
½ cup celery, chopped
½ teaspoon garlic powder
¼ teaspoon red pepper flakes
2 cups vegetable broth

1. Heat 1 teaspoon of the olive oil in a soup pot over medium-high heat; cook your zucchini for 1 to 2 minutes or until just tender; reserve.
2. In the same pot, heat the remaining teaspoon of olive oil; sauté the shallot until tender and translucent.
3. Add the remaining ingredients to the sautéed vegetables in the soup pot. Reduce the heat to medium-low, cover and let it cook for 15 minutes or until thoroughly heated.
4. Ladle into serving bowls and serve warm. Bon appétit!

Per Serving
calories: 57 | fat: 3.2g | protein: 2.2g
carbs: 3.6g | net carbs: 2.5g | fiber: 1.1g

Cheddar Cauliflower Soup

Prep time: 5 minutes | Cook time: 20 minutes | Serves 4

1 tablespoon butter
½ onion, chopped
2 cups riced/shredded cauliflower (I buy it pre-riced at Trader Joe's)
1 cup chicken broth
2 ounces (57 g) cream cheese
1 cup heavy (whipping) cream
Pink Himalayan salt
Freshly ground pepper
½ cup shredded Cheddar cheese (I use sharp Cheddar)

1. In a medium saucepan over medium heat, melt the butter. Add the onion and cook, stirring occasionally, until softened, about 5 minutes.
2. Add the cauliflower and chicken broth, and allow the mixture to come to a boil, stirring occasionally.
3. Lower the heat to medium-low and simmer until the cauliflower is soft enough to mash, about 10 minutes.
4. Add the cream cheese, and mash the mixture.
5. Add the cream and purée the mixture with an immersion blender (or you can pour the soup into the blender, blend it, and then pour it back into the pan and reheat it a bit).
6. Season the soup with pink Himalayan salt and pepper.
7. Pour the soup into four bowls, top each with the shredded Cheddar cheese, and serve.

Per Serving
calories: 372 | fat: 35g | protein: 9g
carbs: 9g | net carbs: 6g | fiber: 3g

Pork and Mustard Green Soup

Prep time: 15 minutes | Cook time: 20 minutes | Serves 2

1 tablespoon olive oil
1 bell pepper, deveined and chopped
2 garlic cloves, pressed
½ cup scallions, chopped
½ pound (227 g) ground pork (84% lean)
1 cup beef bone broth
1 cup water
½ teaspoon crushed red pepper flakes
Sea salt and freshly cracked black pepper, to season
1 bay laurel
1 teaspoon fish sauce
2 cups mustard greens, torn into pieces
1 tablespoon fresh parsley, chopped

1. Heat the olive oil in a stockpot over a moderate flame. Coat, once hot, sauté the pepper, garlic, and scallions until tender or about 3 minutes.
2. After that, stir in the ground pork and cook for 5 minutes more or until well browned, stirring periodically.
3. Add in the beef bone broth, water, red pepper, salt, black pepper, and bay laurel. Reduce the temperature to simmer and cook, covered, for 10 minutes. Afterwards, stir in the fish sauce and mustard greens.
4. Remove from the heat; let it stand until the greens are wilted. Ladle into individual bowls and serve garnished with fresh parsley.

Per Serving
calories: 345 | fat: 25.1g | protein: 23.2g
carbs: 6.2g | net carbs: 3.2g | fiber: 3.0g

Saffron Coconut Shrimp Soup

Prep time: 5 minutes | Cook time: 15 minutes | Serves 4

1 tablespoon coconut oil
1 red bell pepper, chopped
2 teaspoons minced garlic
2 teaspoons grated fresh ginger
4 cups chicken stock
1 (15-ounce / 425-g) can coconut milk
1 pound shrimp, peeled, deveined, and chopped
1 cup shredded kale
Juice of 1 lime
½ cup warm water
Pinch saffron threads
Sea salt, for seasoning
2 tablespoons chopped fresh cilantro

1. Sauté the vegetables. In a large saucepan over medium heat, warm the coconut oil. Add the red pepper, garlic, and ginger and sauté until they've softened, about 5 minutes.
2. Simmer the soup. Add the chicken stock and coconut milk and bring the soup to a boil, then reduce the heat to low and stir in the shrimp, kale, and lime juice. Simmer the soup until the shrimp is cooked through, about 5 minutes.
3. Mix in the saffron. While the soup is simmering, stir the saffron and the warm water together in a small bowl and let it sit for 5 minutes. Stir the saffron mixture into the soup when the shrimp is cooked, and simmer the soup for 3 minutes more.
4. Season and serve. Season with salt. Ladle the soup into bowls, garnish it with the cilantro, and serve it hot.

Per Serving
calories: 504 | fat: 36g | protein: 32g
carbs: 15g | net carbs: 12g | fiber: 3g

Salsa Verde Chicken Soup

Prep time: 10 minutes | Cook time: 5 minutes | Serves 4

½ cup salsa verde
2 cups cooked and shredded chicken
2 cups chicken broth
1 cup shredded cheddar cheese
4 ounces (113 g) cream cheese
½ teaspoon chili powder
½ teaspoon ground cumin
½ teaspoon fresh cilantro, chopped
Salt and black pepper, to taste

1. Combine the cream cheese, salsa verde, and broth, in a food processor; pulse until smooth. Transfer the mixture to a pot and place over medium heat. Cook until hot, but do not bring to a boil. Add chicken, chili powder, and cumin and cook for about 3-5 minutes, or until it is heated through.
2. Stir in cheddar cheese and season with salt and pepper to taste. If it is very thick, add a few tablespoons of water and boil for 1-3 more minutes. Serve hot in bowls sprinkled with fresh cilantro.

Per Serving
calories: 346 | fat: 23g | protein: 25g
carbs: 4g | net carbs: 3g | fiber: 1g

Hearty Chicken Soup

Prep time: 10 minutes | Cook time: 30 minutes | Serves 6

½ cup grass-fed butter
½ onion, chopped
2 celery stalks, chopped
2 teaspoons minced garlic
¼ cup arrowroot
5 cups chicken stock
3 cups shredded cooked chicken
Zest and juice of 1 lemon
1 cup heavy (whipping) cream
Sea salt, for seasoning
Freshly ground black pepper, for seasoning
1 tablespoon chopped fresh oregano

1. Sauté the vegetables. In a medium stockpot over medium-high heat, melt the butter. Add the onion, celery, and garlic and sauté until they've softened, about 5 minutes.
2. Make the soup base. Add the arrowroot and whisk until it forms a paste. Whisk in the chicken stock.
3. Thicken the soup. Bring the soup to a boil, then reduce the heat to low and simmer, stirring it from time to time, until the soup thickens, about 15 minutes.
4. Add the remaining ingredients. Stir in the chicken, lemon zest, lemon juice, and cream and simmer until the chicken is heated through, about 10 minutes.
5. Season and serve. Season the soup with salt and pepper. Ladle the soup into bowls, garnish with the oregano, and serve it hot.

Per Serving
calories: 501 | fat: 36g | protein: 28g
carbs: 13g | net carbs: 10g | fiber: 3g

Pork and Vegetable Soup

Prep time: 5 minutes | Cook time: 20 minutes | Serves 5

1½ pounds (680 g) pork stew meat, cubed
5 cups vegetable broth
½ cup scallions, chopped
2 bell peppers, chopped
1 celery stalk, chopped

1. Spritz the bottom of a large soup pot with nonstick cooking spray. Heat up the pot over medium-high heat.
2. Now, brown the meat for 5 minutes, stirring frequently. Deglaze the skillet with a splash of vegetable broth, scraping up any brown bits stuck to the bottom. After that, stir in the remaining ingredients and bring to a rolling boil.
3. Turn the heat to simmer; cover and let it simmer for 15 minutes until everything is thoroughly warmed.
4. Ladle into individual bowls and serve hot. Bon appétit!

Per Serving
calories: 303 | fat: 18g | protein: 29g
carbs: 4g | net carbs: 3g | fiber: 1g

Cioppino

Prep time: 10 minutes | Cook time: 30 minutes | Serves 6

2 tablespoons olive oil
½ onion, chopped
2 celery stalks, sliced
1 red bell pepper, chopped
1 tablespoon minced garlic
2 cups fish stock
1 (15-ounce / 425-g) can coconut milk
1 cup crushed tomatoes
2 tablespoons tomato purée
1 tablespoon chopped fresh basil
2 teaspoons chopped fresh oregano
½ teaspoon sea salt
½ teaspoon freshly ground black pepper
¼ teaspoon red pepper flakes
10 ounces (283 g) salmon, cut into 1-inch pieces
½ pound (227) shrimp, peeled and deveined
12 clams or mussels, cleaned and debearded but in the shell

1. Sauté the vegetables. In a large stockpot over medium-high heat, warm the olive oil. Add the onion, celery, red bell pepper, and garlic and sauté until they've softened, about 4 minutes.
2. Make the soup base. Stir in the fish stock, coconut milk, crushed tomatoes, tomato purée, basil, oregano, salt, pepper, and red pepper flakes. Bring the soup to a boil, then reduce the heat to low and simmer the soup for 10 minutes.
3. Add the seafood. Stir in the salmon and simmer until it goes opaque, about 5 minutes. Add the shrimp and simmer until they're almost cooked through, about 3 minutes. Add the mussels and let them simmer until they open, about 3 minutes. Throw out any mussels that don't open.
4. Serve. Ladle the soup into bowls and serve it hot.

Per Serving
calories: 377 | fat: 29g | protein: 24g
carbs: 9g | net carbs: 7g | fiber: 2g

Coconut Pumpkin Soup

Prep time: 15 minutes | Cook time: 6 hours | Serves 6

1 tablespoon extra-virgin olive oil
4 cups chicken broth
2 cups coconut milk
1 pound pumpkin, diced
½ sweet onion, chopped
1 tablespoon grated fresh ginger
2 teaspoons minced garlic
½ teaspoon ground cinnamon
¼ teaspoon ground nutmeg
¼ teaspoon freshly ground black pepper
¼ teaspoon salt
pinch ground allspice
1 cup heavy (whipping) cream
2 cups chopped cooked chicken

1. Lightly grease the insert of the slow cooker with the olive oil.
2. Place the broth, coconut milk, pumpkin, onion, ginger, garlic, cinnamon, nutmeg, pepper, salt, and allspice in the insert.
3. Cover and cook on low for 6 hours.
4. Using an immersion blender or a regular blender, purée the soup.
5. If you removed the soup from the insert to purée, add it back to the pot, and stir in the cream and chicken.
6. Keep heating the soup on low for 15 minutes to heat the chicken through, and then serve warm.

Per Serving
calories: 389 | fat: 32g | protein: 16g
carbs: 10g | net carbs: 5g | fiber: 5g

Bacon Green Soup

Prep time: 15 minutes | Cook time: 15 minutes | Serves 4

2 slices bacon, chopped
2 tablespoons scallions, chopped
1 carrot, chopped
1 celery, chopped
Salt and ground black pepper, to taste
1 teaspoon garlic, finely chopped
½ teaspoon dried rosemary
1 sprig thyme, stripped and chopped
½ head green cabbage, shredded
½ head broccoli, broken into small florets
3 cups water
1 cup chicken stock
½ cup full-fat yogurt

1. Heat a stockpot over medium heat; now, sear the bacon until crisp. Reserve the bacon and 1 tablespoon of fat.
2. Then, cook scallions, carrots, and celery in 1 tablespoon of reserved fat. Add salt, pepper, and garlic; cook an additional 1 minute or until fragrant.
3. Now, stir in rosemary, thyme, cabbage, and broccoli. Pour in water and stock, bringing to a rapid boil; reduce heat and let it simmer for 10 minutes more.
4. Add yogurt and cook an additional 5 minutes, stirring occasionally. Use an immersion blender, to purée your soup until smooth.
5. Taste and adjust the seasonings. Garnish with the cooked bacon just before serving.

Per Serving
calories: 96 | fat: 7.7g | protein: 3.0g
carbs: 4.2g | net carbs: 3.2g | fiber: 1.0g

Italian Tomato Soup

Prep time: 15 minutes | Cook time: 30 minutes | Serves 4

1½ tablespoons olive oil
½ cup scallions, chopped
1 teaspoon fresh garlic, minced
1 teaspoon dried oregano
½ teaspoon dried rosemary
1½ pounds (680 g) Roma tomatoes, diced
2 cups Brodo di Pollo (Italian broth)
2 tablespoons tomato paste
2 cups mustard greens, torn into pieces
Sea salt and ground black pepper, to taste
2 tablespoons fresh Italian parsley, roughly chopped

1. Heat the olive oil in a soup pot over a moderate flame. Now, sauté the scallions until softened or 3 to 4 minutes.
2. Then, stir in the garlic, oregano, and rosemary, and continue to sauté an additional 30 seconds.
3. Then, stir in the Roma tomatoes, Italian broth, and tomato paste; bring to a boil. Now, reduce the heat to medium-low and let it cook, partially covered, for 20 to 25 minutes.
4. Puree the soup in your blender and return it to the pot. Add in the mustard greens; season with salt and black pepper.
5. Next, cook over a moderate flame until the greens wilt. Garnish with fresh Italian parsley and serve immediately.

Per Serving
calories: 105 | fat: 7.3g | protein: 2.5g
carbs: 6.1g | net carbs: 2.9g | fiber: 3.2g

Cream of Broccoli Soup

Prep time: 15 minutes | Cook time: 20 minutes | Serves 4

3 tablespoons olive oil
1 celery rib, chopped
½ white onion, finely chopped
1 teaspoon ginger-garlic paste
1 (1-pound / 454-g) head broccoli, broken into florets
4 cups vegetable broth
½ cup double cream
1½ cups Monterey Jack cheese, grated

1. Heat the olive oil in a soup pot over moderate heat. Now, sauté the celery rib and onion until they have softened.
2. Fold in the ginger-garlic paste and broccoli; pour in the vegetable broth and bring to boil. Turn the heat to simmer. Continue to cook for a further 13 minutes or until the broccoli is cooked through.
3. Fold in the cream, stir and remove from heat. Divide your soup between four ramekins and top them with the Monterey Jack cheese.
4. Broil for about 5 minutes or until cheese is bubbly and golden. Bon appétit!

Per Serving
calories: 324 | fat: 28.1g | protein: 13.3g
carbs: 4.3g | net carbs: 3.8g | fiber: 0.5g

Tomato Soup

Prep time: 10 minutes | Cook time: 14 minutes | Serves 6

1 tablespoon butter
2 large red onions, diced
½ cup raw cashew nuts, diced
2 (28-ounce / 794-g) cans tomatoes
1 teaspoon fresh thyme leaves, extra to garnish
1½ cups water
Salt and black pepper to taste
1 cup heavy cream

1. Melt butter in a pot over medium heat and sauté the onions for 4 minutes until softened.
2. Stir in the tomatoes, thyme, water, cashews, and season with salt and black pepper. Cover and bring to simmer for 10 minutes until thoroughly cooked.
3. Open, turn the heat off, and puree the ingredients with an immersion blender. Adjust to taste and stir in the heavy cream. Spoon into soup bowls and serve.

Per Serving
calories: 310 | fat: 27g | protein: 11g
carbs: 12g | net carbs: 10g | fiber: 2g

Power Green Soup

Prep time: 10 minutes | Cook time: 14 minutes | Serves 6

1 broccoli head, chopped
1 cup spinach
1 onion, chopped
2 garlic cloves, minced
½ cup watercress
5 cups veggie stock
1 cup coconut milk
1 tablespoon butter
1 bay leaf
Salt and black pepper, to taste

1. Melt the butter in a large pot over medium heat. Add onion and garlic, and cook for 3 minutes. Add broccoli and cook for an additional 5 minutes. Pour the stock over and add the bay leaf. Close the lid, bring to a boil, and reduce the heat. Simmer for about 3 minutes.
2. At the end, add spinach and watercress, and cook for 3 more minutes. Stir in the coconut cream, salt and black pepper. Discard the bay leaf, and blend the soup with a hand blender.

Per Serving
calories: 392 | fat: 37g | protein: 5g
carbs: 11g | net carbs: 6g | fiber: 5g

Broccoli Soup

Prep time: 10 minutes | Cook time: 14 minutes | Serves 4

¾ cup heavy cream
1 onion, diced
1 teaspoon minced garlic
4 cups chopped broccoli
4 cups veggie broth
1 tablespoon butter
3 cups grated cheddar cheese
Salt and black pepper, to taste
½ bunch fresh mint, chopped

1. Melt the butter in a large pot over medium heat. Sauté onion and garlic for 3 minutes or until tender, stirring occasionally. Season with salt and black pepper. Add the broth, broccoli and bring to a boil.
2. Reduce the heat and simmer for 10 minutes. Puree the soup with a hand blender until smooth. Add in 2 ¾ cups of the cheddar cheese and cook about 1 minute. Taste and adjust the seasoning. Stir in the heavy cream. Serve in bowls with the remaining cheddar cheese and sprinkled with fresh mint.

Per Serving
calories: 561 | fat: 52g | protein: 24g
carbs: 11g | net carbs: 7g | fiber: 4g

Reuben Beef Soup

Prep time: 10 minutes | Cook time: 20 minutes | Serves 6

1 onion, diced
6 cups beef stock
1 teaspoon caraway seeds
2 celery stalks, diced
2 garlic cloves, minced
2 cups heavy cream
1 cup sauerkraut, shredded
1 pound (454 g) corned beef, chopped
1 tablespoon butter
1½ cup swiss cheese, shredded
Salt and black pepper, to taste

1. Melt the butter in a large pot. Add onion and celery, and fry for 3 minutes until tender. Add garlic and cook for another minute.
2. Pour the beef stock over and stir in sauerkraut, salt, caraway seeds, and add a pinch of black pepper. Bring to a boil. Reduce the heat to low, and add the corned beef. Cook for about 15 minutes, adjust the seasoning. Stir in heavy cream and cheese and cook for 1 minute.

Per Serving
calories: 450 | fat: 37g | protein: 23g
carbs: 9g | net carbs: 8g | fiber: 1g

Beef and Mushroom Soup

Prep time: 10 minutes | Cook time: 40 minutes | Serves 6

1 pound (454 g) beef chuck, cubed
1½ cups cremini mushrooms
6 cups beef broth
½ cup heavy cream
½ cup whipped cream cheese
1 yellow onion, chopped
2 cloves garlic, chopped
Salt and pepper, to taste
1 tablespoon coconut oil, for cooking

1. Add the coconut oil to a skillet and brown the beef.
2. Once cooked, add the beef to the base of a stockpot with all of the ingredients minus the heavy cream. Mix well.
3. Bring to a simmer and whisk again until the cream cheese is mixed evenly into the soup.
4. Cook for 30 minutes.
5. Warm the heavy cream, and then add to the soup.

Per Serving
calories: 316 | fat: 18.9g | protein: 30.1g
carbs: 5.0g | net carbs: 4.0g | fiber: 1.0g

Nacho Soup

Prep time: 15 minutes | Cook time: 6 hours | Serves 8

3 tablespoons extra-virgin olive oil, divided
1 pound (454 g) ground chicken
1 sweet onion, diced
1 red bell pepper, chopped
2 teaspoons minced garlic
2 tablespoons taco seasoning
4 cups chicken broth
2 cups coconut milk
1 tomato, diced
1 jalapeño pepper, chopped
2 cups shredded cheddar cheese
½ cup sour cream, for garnish
1 scallion, white and green parts, chopped, for garnish

1. Lightly grease the insert of the slow cooker with 1 tablespoon of the olive oil.
2. In a large skillet over medium-high heat, heat the remaining 2 tablespoons of the olive oil. Add the chicken and sauté until it is cooked through, about 6 minutes.
3. Add the onion, red bell pepper, garlic, and taco seasoning, and sauté for an additional 3 minutes.
4. Transfer the chicken mixture to the insert, and stir in the broth, coconut milk, tomato, and jalapeño pepper.
5. Cover and cook on low for 6 hours.
6. Stir in the cheese.
7. Serve topped with the sour cream and scallion.

Per Serving
calories: 434 | fat: 35g | protein: 22g
carbs: 9g | net carbs: 7g | fiber: 2g

Leek and Turkey Soup

Prep time: 15 minutes | Cook time: 1 hour 10 minutes | Serves 2

3 cups water
½ pound (227 g) turkey thighs
1 cup cauliflower, broken into small florets
1 large-sized leek, chopped
1 small-sized stalk celery, chopped
½ head garlic, split horizontally
¼ teaspoon turmeric powder
¼ teaspoon Turkish sumac
¼ teaspoon fennel seeds
½ teaspoon mustard seeds
1 bay laurel
Sea salt and freshly ground black pepper, to season
1 teaspoon coconut aminos
1 whole egg

1. Add the water and turkey thighs to a pot and bring it to a rolling boil. Cook for about 40 minutes; discard the bones and shred the meat using two forks.
2. Stir in the cauliflower, leeks, celery, garlic, and spices. Reduce the heat to simmer and let it cook until everything is heated through, about 30 minutes.
3. Afterwards, add the coconut aminos and egg; whisk until the egg is well incorporated into the soup. Serve hot and enjoy!

Per Serving
calories: 217 | fat: 8.2g | protein: 25.1g
carbs: 6.7g | net carbs: 4.5g | fiber: 2.2g

Cauliflower Soup

Prep time: 10 minutes | Cook time: 17 minutes | Serves 4

1 tablespoon butter
1 onion, chopped
2 head cauliflower, cut into florets
2 cups water
Salt and black pepper to taste
3 cups almond milk
1 cup shredded white cheddar cheese
3 bacon strips

1. Melt the butter in a saucepan over medium heat and sauté the onion for 3 minutes until fragrant.
2. Include the cauli florets, sauté for 3 minutes to slightly soften, add the water, and season with salt and black pepper. Bring to a boil, and then reduce the heat to low. Cover and cook for 10 minutes. Puree cauliflower with an immersion blender until the ingredients are evenly combined and stir in the almond milk and cheese until the cheese melts. Adjust taste with salt and black pepper.
3. In a non-stick skillet over high heat, fry the bacon, until crispy. Divide soup between serving bowls, top with crispy bacon, and serve hot.

Per Serving
calories: 402 | fat: 37g | protein: 8g | carbs: 9g | net carbs: 6g | fiber: 3g

Rich Taco Soup

Prep time: 5 minutes | Cook time: 4¼ hours | Serves 4

1 pound (454 g) ground beef
Pink Himalayan salt, to taste
Freshly ground black pepper, to taste
2 cups beef broth (I use Kettle & Fire Bone Broth)
1 (10-ounce / 283-g) can diced tomatoes (I use Rotel)
1 tablespoon taco seasoning
8 ounces (227 g) cream cheese

1. With the crock insert in place, preheat the slow cooker to low.
2. On the stove top, in a medium skillet over medium-high heat, sauté the ground beef until browned, about 8 minutes, and season with pink Himalayan salt and pepper.
3. Add the ground beef, beef broth, tomatoes, taco seasoning, and cream cheese to the slow cooker.
4. Cover and cook on low for 4 hours, stirring occasionally.
5. Ladle into four bowls and serve.

Per Serving
calories: 422 | fat: 33g | protein: 25g | carbs: 6g | net carbs: 5g | fiber: 1g

Colden Gazpacho Soup

Prep time: 15 minutes | Cook time: 0 minutes | Serves 6

2 small green peppers, roasted
2 large red peppers, roasted
2 medium avocados, flesh scoped out
2 garlic cloves
2 spring onions, chopped
1 cucumber, chopped
1 cup olive oil
1 tablespoon lemon juice
4 tomatoes, chopped
7 ounces (198 g) goat cheese
1 small red onion, chopped
1 tablespoon apple cider vinegar
Salt, to taste

1. Place the peppers, tomatoes, avocados, red onion, garlic, lemon juice, olive oil, vinegar, and salt, in a food processor. Pulse until your desired consistency is reached. Taste and adjust the seasoning.
2. Transfer the mixture to a pot. Stir in cucumber and spring onions. Cover and chill in the fridge at least 2 hours. Divide the soup between 6 bowls. Serve topped with goat cheese and an extra drizzle of olive oil.

Per Serving

calories: 528 | fat: 46g | protein: 8g | carbs: 7g | net carbs: 4g | fiber: 3g

Cauliflower Soup with Sausage

Prep time: 10 minutes | Cook time: 35 minutes | Serves 4

1 cauliflower head, chopped
1 turnip, chopped
1 tablespoon butter
1 chorizo sausage, sliced

2 cups chicken broth
1 small onion, chopped
2 cups water
Salt and black pepper, to taste

1. Melt 1 tablespoon of the butter in a large pot over medium heat. Stir in onion and cook until soft and golden, about 3-4 minutes. Add cauliflower and turnip, and cook for another 5 minutes.
2. Pour the broth and water over. Bring to a boil, simmer covered, and cook for about 20 minutes until the vegetables are tender.
3. Remove from heat. Melt the remaining butter in a skillet. Add the chorizo sausage and cook for 5 minutes until crispy. Puree the soup with a hand blender until smooth.
4. Taste and adjust the seasonings. Serve the soup in deep bowls topped with the chorizo sausage.

Per Serving

calories: 251 | fat: 19g | protein: 10g | carbs: 8g | net carbs: 6g | fiber: 2g

Curry Green Beans and Shrimp Soup

Prep time: 10 minutes | Cook time: 10 minutes | Serves 4

1 tablespoon butter
1 pound (454 g) jumbo shrimp, peeled and deveined
1 teaspoon ginger-garlic puree

1 tablespoon red curry paste
6 ounces (170 g) coconut milk
Salt and chili pepper to taste
1 bunch green beans, halved

1. Melt butter in a medium saucepan over medium heat. Add the shrimp, season with salt and black pepper, and cook until they are opaque, 2 to 3 minutes. Remove shrimp to a plate. Add the ginger-garlic puree and red curry paste to the butter and sauté for 2 minutes until fragrant.
2. Stir in the coconut milk; add the shrimp, salt, chili pepper, and green beans. Cook for 4 minutes. Reduce the heat to a simmer and cook an additional 3 minutes, occasionally stirring. Adjust taste with salt, fetch soup into serving bowls, and serve with cauli rice.

Per Serving

calories: 375 | fat: 35g | protein: 9g | carbs: 4g | net carbs: 2g | fiber: 2g

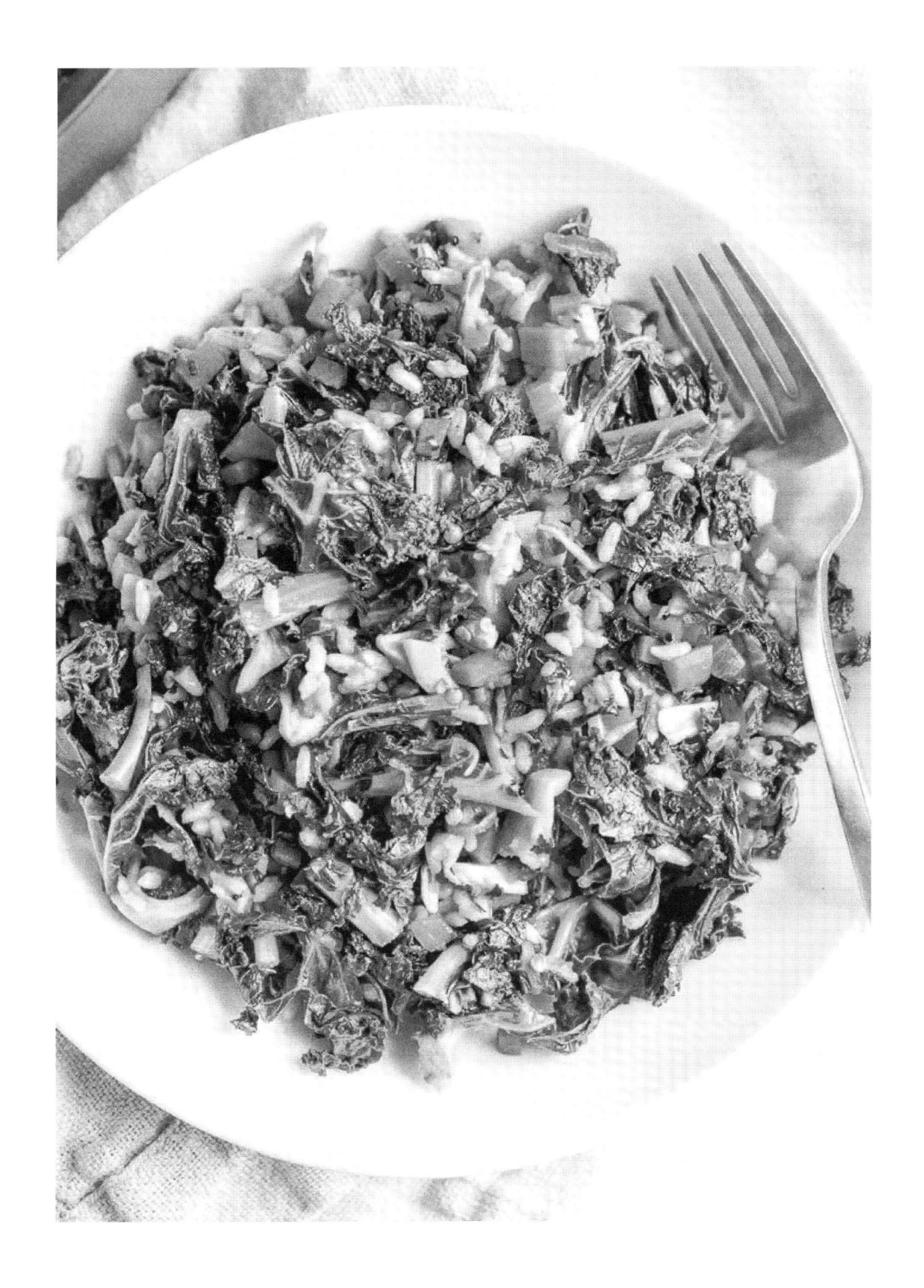

Chapter 5 Vegetables and Sides

Grilled Prosciutto-Chicken Wraps

Prep time: 5 minutes | Cook time: 6 minutes | Serves 8

¼ teaspoon garlic powder
8 ounces (227 g) Provolone cheese
8 raw chicken tenders
Salt and black pepper, to taste
8 prosciutto slices

1. Pound the chicken until half an inch thick. Season with salt, black pepper, and garlic powder. Cut the provolone cheese into 8 strips. Place a slice of prosciutto on a flat surface. Place one chicken tender on top. Top with a provolone strip.
2. Roll the chicken and secure with previously soaked skewers. Grill the wraps for 3 minutes per side.

Per Serving
calories: 271 | fat: 13g | protein: 35g
carbs: 2g | net carbs: 1g | fiber: 1g

Almond and Rind Crusted Zucchini Fritters

Prep time: 13 minutes | Cook time: 2 minutes | Serves 2

2 tablespoons olive oil
3 eggs, whisked
1 teaspoon garlic, pressed
½ pound (227 g) zucchini, grated
⅓ cup almond meal
2 tablespoons pork rinds
¼ teaspoon paprika
Sea salt and ground black pepper, to taste
½ cup Swiss cheese, shredded

1. Add the grated zucchini to a colander. Add ½ teaspoon of salt, toss and let it sit for 10 minutes. After that, drain the zucchini completely using a cheese cloth.
2. Heat the olive oil in a skillet over medium-high flame. In a mixing bowl, combine the zucchini with the remaining ingredients until everything is well incorporated.
3. Make the fritters, flattening them with a spatula; cook for 2 minutes on both sides. Bon appétit!

Per Serving
calories: 462 | fat: 36.0g | protein: 27.5g
carbs: 7.6g | net carbs: 4.8g | fiber: 2.8g

Boiled Stuffed Eggs

Prep time: 5 minutes | Cook time: 10 minutes | Serves 6

6 eggs
1 tablespoon Sriracha
⅓ cup mayonnaise
Salt, to taste

1. Place the eggs in a saucepan and cover with salted water. Bring to a boil over medium heat. Boil for 10 minutes. Place the eggs in an ice bath and let cool for 10 minutes.
2. Peel and slice in half lengthwise. Scoop out the yolks to a bowl; mash with a fork. Whisk together the Sriracha, mayonnaise, mashed yolks, and salt, in a bowl. Spoon this mixture into egg whites.

Per Serving
calories: 92 | fat: 6g | protein: 6g
carbs: 3g | net carbs: 3g | fiber: 0g

Paprika Riced Cauliflower

Prep time: 4 minutes | Cook time: 6 minutes | Serves 4

1 tablespoon butter
1 pound (454 g) cauliflower florets
2 cloves garlic, minced
1 tablespoon smoked paprika
Flaky salt, to taste

1. Melt the butter in a frying pan over a moderate flame.
2. Pulse the cauliflower in your food processor until your cauliflower has broken down into rice-sized chunks approximately 6 seconds.
3. Add the cauliflower rice to the frying pan and cook, covered, for 5 minutes. Stir in the garlic and smoked paprika. Continue to sauté an additional minute or so.
4. Season with salt to taste and serve immediately. Bon appétit!

Per Serving
calories: 57 | fat: 3.2g | protein: 2.3g
carbs: 6.1g | net carbs: 3.8g | fiber: 2.3g

Chinese Cauliflower Rice with Eggs

Prep time: 7 minutes | Cook time: 8 minutes | Serves 3

½ pound (227 g) fresh cauliflower
1 tablespoon sesame oil
½ cup leeks, chopped
1 garlic, pressed
Sea salt and freshly ground black pepper, to taste
½ teaspoon Chinese five-spice powder
1 teaspoon oyster sauce
½ teaspoon light soy sauce
1 tablespoon Shaoxing wine
3 eggs

1. Pulse the cauliflower in a food processor until it resembles rice.
2. Heat the sesame oil in a pan over medium-high heat; sauté the leeks and garlic for 2 to 3 minutes. Add the prepared cauliflower rice to the pan, along with salt, black pepper, and Chinese five-spice powder.
3. Next, add oyster sauce, soy sauce, and wine. Let it cook, stirring occasionally, until the cauliflower is crisp-tender, about 5 minutes.
4. Then, add the eggs to the pan; stir until everything is well combined. Serve warm and enjoy!

Per Serving
calories: 132 | fat: 8.8g | protein: 7.2g
carbs: 6.2g | net carbs: 4.4g | fiber: 1.8g

Cottage Kale Stir-Fry

Prep time: 10 minutes | Cook time: 10 minutes | Serves 3

½ tablespoon olive oil
1 teaspoon fresh garlic, chopped
9 ounces (255 g) kale, torn into pieces
½ cup Cottage cheese, creamed
½ teaspoon sea salt

1. Heat the olive oil in a saucepan over a moderate flame. Now, cook the garlic until just tender and aromatic.
2. Then, stir in the kale and continue to cook for about 10 minutes until all liquid evaporates.
3. Fold in the Cottage cheese and salt; stir until everything is heated through. Enjoy!

Per Serving
calories: 94 | fat: 4.5g | protein: 7.0g
carbs: 6.2g | net carbs: 3.5g | fiber: 2.7g

Romano Zucchini Cups

Prep time: 10 minutes | Cook time: 15 minutes | Serves 4

1 teaspoon sea salt
1 (½-pound / 227-g) zucchini, grated
½ cup almond flour
2 eggs, beaten
1 cup Romano cheese, grated

1. Place the salt and grated zucchini in a bowl; let it sit for 15 minutes, squeeze using a cheesecloth and discard the liquid.
2. Now, stir in the almond flour, eggs, and Romano cheese. Spritz a 12-cup mini-muffin pan with cooking spray.
3. Bake in the preheated oven for 15 minutes until the surface is no longer wet to the touch. Let them cool about 5 minutes to set up. Bon appétit!

Per Serving
calories: 225 | fat: 18.0g | protein: 13.4g
carbs: 3.0g | net carbs: 1.5g | fiber: 1.5g

Indian White Cabbage Stew

Prep time: 8 minutes | Cook time: 22 minutes | Serves 3

6 ounces (170 g) Goan chorizo sausage, sliced
2 cloves garlic, finely chopped
1 teaspoon Indian spice blend
1 pound (454 g) white cabbage, outer leaves removed and finely shredded
¾ cup cream of celery soup

1. Heat a large-sized wok over a moderate flame. Now, sear the Goan chorizo sausage until no longer pink; reserve.
2. Cook the garlic and Indian spice blend in the pan drippings until they are aromatic. Now, stir in the cabbage and cream of celery soup.
3. Turn the temperature to medium-low, cover, and continue simmering an additional 22 minutes or until tender and heated through.
4. Add the reserved Goan chorizo sausage; ladle into individual bowls and serve. Enjoy!

Per Serving
calories: 236 | fat: 17.7g | protein: 9.8g
carbs: 6.1g | net carbs: 3.7g | fiber: 2.4g

Pumpkin and Cauliflower Curry

Prep time: 15 minutes | Cook time: 7 to 8 hours | Serves 6

1 tablespoon extra-virgin olive oil
4 cups coconut milk
1 cup diced pumpkin
1 cup cauliflower florets
1 red bell pepper, diced
1 zucchini, diced
1 sweet onion, chopped
2 teaspoons grated fresh ginger
2 teaspoons minced garlic
1 tablespoon curry powder
2 cups shredded spinach
1 avocado, diced, for garnish

1. Lightly grease the insert of the slow cooker with the olive oil.
2. Add the coconut milk, pumpkin, cauliflower, bell pepper, zucchini, onion, ginger, garlic, and curry powder.
3. Cover and cook on low for 7 to 8 hours.
4. Stir in the spinach.
5. Garnish each bowl with a spoonful of avocado and serve.

Per Serving
calories: 501 | fat: 44.0g | protein: 7.0g
carbs: 19.0g | net carbs: 9.0g | fiber: 10.0g

Creamy Spinach

Prep time: 5 minutes | Cook time: 5 minutes | Serves 4

1 tablespoon butter, room temperature
1 clove garlic, minced
10 ounces (283 g) spinach
½ teaspoon garlic salt
¼ teaspoon ground black pepper, or more to taste
½ teaspoon cayenne pepper
3 ounces (85 g) cream cheese
½ cup double cream

1. Melt the butter in a saucepan that is preheated over medium heat. Once hot. Cook garlic for 30 seconds.
2. Now, add the spinach; cover the pan for 2 minutes to let the spinach wilt. Season with salt, black pepper, and cayenne pepper
3. Stir in cheese and cream; stir until the cheese melts. Serve immediately.

Per Serving
calories: 167 | fat: 15.1g | protein: 4.4g
carbs: 5.0g | net carbs: 3.3g | fiber: 1.7g

Cauliflower Egg Bake

Prep time: 10 minutes | Cook time: 25 minutes | Serves 6

1½ pounds (680 g) cauliflower, broken into small florets
½ cup Greek yogurt
4 eggs, beaten
6 ounces (170 g) ham, diced
1 cup Swiss cheese, preferably freshly grated

1. Place the cauliflower into a deep saucepan; cover with water and bring to a boil over high heat; immediately reduce the heat to medium-low.
2. Let it simmer, covered, approximately 6 minutes. Drain and mash with a potato masher.
3. Add in the yogurt, eggs and ham; stir until everything is well combined and incorporated.
4. Scrape the mixture into a lightly greased casserole dish. Top with the grated Swiss cheese and transfer to a preheated at 390ºF (199ºC) oven.
5. Bake for 15 to 20 minutes or until cheese bubbles and browns. Bon appétit!

Per Serving
calories: 237 | fat: 13.6g | protein: 20.2g
carbs: 7.1g | net carbs: 4.8g | fiber: 2.3g

Bell Pepper and Tomato Sataraš

Prep time: 5 minutes | Cook time: 15 minutes | Serves 3

3 teaspoons olive oil
1 onion, chopped
2 garlic cloves, minced
3 bell peppers, deveined and sliced
1 tomato, puréed

1. Heat the olive oil in a saucepan over moderate flame. Then, sweat the onion until translucent.
2. Stir in the garlic and bell peppers and sauté for 2 minutes more or until aromatic. Stir in the puréed tomato.
3. Cover, reduce the temperature to medium-low and continue to cook for 12 minutes or until the peppers have softened and the cooking liquid has evaporated.
4. Salt to taste and serve in individual bowls. Bon appétit!

Per Serving
calories: 84 | fat: 4.6g | protein: 1.6g
carbs: 6.5g | net carbs: 4.7g | fiber: 1.8g

Balsamic Glazed Brussels Sprouts

Prep time: 5 minutes | Cook time: 30 minutes | Serves 4

3 tablespoons balsamic vinegar
1 tablespoon erythritol
½ tablespoon olive oil
Salt and black pepper, to taste
1 pound (454 g) Brussels sprouts, halved
5 slices prosciutto, chopped

1. Preheat oven to 400ºF and line a baking sheet with parchment paper. Mix balsamic vinegar, erythritol, olive oil, salt, and black pepper and combine with the Brussels sprouts in a bowl.
2. Spread the mixture on the baking sheet and roast for 30 minutes until tender on the inside and crispy on the outside. Toss with prosciutto, share among 4 plates, and serve with chicken breasts.

Per Serving
calories: 143 | fat: 5g | protein: 10g
carbs: 16g | net carbs: 11g | fiber: 5g

Cheddar Buffalo Chicken Bake

Prep time: 5 minutes | Cook time: 28 minutes | Serves 6

2 tablespoons olive oil
8 ounces (227 g) cream cheese
1 pound (454 g) ground chicken
1 cup buffalo sauce
1 cup ranch dressing
3 cups grated yellow Cheddar cheese

1. Preheat oven to 350ºF. Lightly grease a baking sheet with a cooking spray. Warm the oil in a skillet over medium heat and brown the chicken for 5 minutes, take off the heat, and set aside.
2. Spread cream cheese at the bottom of the baking sheet, top with chicken, pour buffalo sauce over, add ranch dressing, and sprinkle with Cheddar cheese. Bake for 23 minutes until cheese has melted and golden brown on top. Remove and serve with veggie sticks.

Per Serving
calories: 618 | fat: 49g | protein: 33g
carbs: 14g | net carbs: 12g | fiber: 2g

Mushroom Stroganoff

Prep time: 5 minutes | Cook time: 10 minutes | Serves 3

2 tablespoons olive oil
½ shallot, diced
3 cloves garlic, chopped
12 ounces (340 g) brown mushrooms, thinly sliced
2 cups tomato sauce

1. Heat the olive oil in a stockpot over medium-high heat. Then, sauté the shallot for about 3 minutes until tender and fragrant.
2. Now, stir in the garlic and mushrooms and cook them for 1 minute more until aromatic.
3. Fold in the tomato sauce and bring to a boil; turn the heat to medium-low, cover, and continue to simmer for 5 to 6 minutes.
4. Salt to taste and serve over cauliflower rice if desired. Enjoy!

Per Serving
calories: 137 | fat: 9.3g | protein: 3.4g
carbs: 7.1g | net carbs: 5.3g | fiber: 1.8g

Classic Devilled Eggs with Sriracha Mayo

Prep time: 5 minutes | Cook time: 10 minutes | Serves 4

8 large eggs
3 cups water
3 tablespoons sriracha sauce
4 tablespoons mayonnaise
Salt, to taste
¼ teaspoon smoked paprika

1. Bring eggs to boil in salted water in a pot over high heat, and then reduce the heat to simmer for 10 minutes. Transfer eggs to an ice water bath, let cool completely and peel the shells.
2. Slice the eggs in half height wise and empty the yolks into a bowl. Smash with a fork and mix in sriracha sauce, mayonnaise, and half of the paprika until smooth. Spoon filling into a piping bag with a round nozzle and fill the egg whites to be slightly above the brim.
3. Garnish with remaining paprika and serve.

Per Serving
calories: 180 | fat: 12g | protein: 13g
carbs: 4g | net carbs: 4g | fiber: 0g

Broccoli and Cauliflower Mash

Prep time: 2 minutes | Cook time: 13 minutes | Serves 3

½ pound (227 g) broccoli florets
½ pound (227 g) cauliflower florets
Kosher salt and ground black pepper, to season
½ teaspoon garlic powder
1 teaspoon shallot powder
4 tablespoons whipped cream cheese
1½ tablespoons butter

1. Microwave the broccoli and cauliflower for about 13 minutes until they have softened completely. Transfer to a food processor and add in the remaining ingredients.
2. Process the ingredients until everything is well combined.
3. Taste and adjust the seasoning. Bon appétit!

Per Serving
calories: 163 | fat: 12.8g | protein: 4.7g carbs: 7.2g | net carbs: 3.7g | fiber: 3.5g

Zucchini Fritters

Prep time: 10 minutes | Cook time: 5 minutes | Serves 6

1 pound (454 g) zucchini, grated and drained
1 egg
1 teaspoon fresh Italian parsley
½ cup almond meal
½ cup goat cheese, crumbled
Sea salt and ground black pepper, to taste
½ teaspoon red pepper flakes, crushed
2 tablespoons olive oil

1. Mix all ingredients, except for the olive oil, in a large bowl. Let it sit in your refrigerator for 30 minutes.
2. Heat the oil in a non-stick frying pan over medium heat; scoop the heaped tablespoons of the zucchini mixture into the hot oil.
3. Cook for 3 to 4 minutes; then, gently flip the fritters over and cook on the other side. Cook in a couple of batches.
4. Transfer to a paper towel to soak up any excess grease. Serve and enjoy!

Per Serving
calories: 110 | fat: 8.8g | protein: 5.8g carbs: 3.2g | net carbs: 2.2g | fiber: 1.0g

Spinach Cheese Balls

Prep time: 10 minutes | Cook time: 10 to 12 minutes | Serves 8

⅓ cup crumbled ricotta cheese
¼ teaspoon nutmeg
¼ teaspoon pepper
3 tablespoons heavy cream
1 teaspoon garlic powder
1 tablespoon onion powder
2 tablespoons butter, melted
⅓ cup Parmesan cheese, shredded
2 eggs
1 cup spinach
1 cup almond flour

1. Place all ingredients in a food processor. Process until smooth. Place in the freezer for about 10 minutes.
2. Make balls out of the mixture and arrange them on a lined baking sheet. Bake in the oven at 350ºF for about 10-12 minutes.

Per Serving
calories: 149 | fat: 9g | protein: 6g carbs: 3g | net carbs: 1g | fiber: 2g

Braised Cream Kale

Prep time: 4 minutes | Cook time: 11 minutes | Serves 5

2 tablespoons olive oil
1 shallot, chopped
6 cups kale, torn into pieces
½ teaspoon fresh garlic, minced
2 tablespoons dry white wine
¼ teaspoon red pepper flakes, crushed
Sea salt and ground black pepper, to taste
½ cup double cream

1. Heat the olive oil in a large, heavy-bottomed sauté pan over moderate heat. Now, sauté the shallot until it is tender or about 4 minutes.
2. Stir in the kale and continue to cook for 2 minutes more. Remove any excess liquid and stir in the garlic; continue to cook for a minute or so.
3. Add a splash of wine to deglaze the pan. Then, add the red pepper, salt, black pepper, and double cream to the pan.
4. Turn the heat to simmer. Continue to simmer, covered, for a further 4 minutes. Serve warm and enjoy!

Per Serving
calories: 130 | fat: 10.5g | protein: 3.7g carbs: 6.1g | net carbs: 3.1g | fiber: 3.0g

Colby Bacon-Wrapped Jalapeño Peppers

Prep time: 5 minutes | Cook time: 25 minutes | Serves 6

12 jalapeño peppers
¼ cup shredded Colby cheese
6 ounces (170 g) cream cheese, softened
6 slices bacon, halved

1. Cut the jalapeño peppers in half, and then remove the membrane and seeds. Combine cheeses and stuff into the pepper halves. Wrap each pepper with a bacon strip and secure with toothpicks.
2. Place the filled peppers on a baking sheet lined with a piece of foil. Bake at 350ºF for 25 minutes until bacon has browned, and crispy and cheese is golden brown on the top. Remove to a paper towel lined plate to absorb grease, arrange on a serving plate, and serve warm.

Per Serving
calories: 219 | fat: 20g | protein: 7g
carbs: 3g | net carbs: 2g | fiber: 1g

Roasted Cauliflower with Serrano Ham

Prep time: 5 minutes | Cook time: 20 minutes | Serves 6

1 head cauliflower, cut into 1-inch slices
2 tablespoons olive oil
Salt and chili pepper, to taste
1 teaspoon garlic powder
10 slices Serrano ham, chopped
¼ cup pine nuts, chopped
1 teaspoon capers
1 teaspoon parsley

1. Preheat oven to 450ºF and line a baking sheet with foil. Brush the cauli steaks with olive oil and season with chili pepper, garlic, and salt. Spread the cauli slices on the baking sheet.
2. Roast in the oven for 10 minutes until tender and lightly browned. Remove the sheet and sprinkle the ham and pine nuts all over the cauli. Bake for another 10 minutes until the ham is crispy and a nutty aroma is perceived. Take out, sprinkle with capers and parsley and serve.

Per Serving
calories: 180 | fat: 13g | protein: 11g
carbs: 8g | net carbs: 5g | fiber: 3g

Crispy Chorizo with Parsley

Prep time: 5 minutes | Cook time: 15 minutes | Serves 6

7 ounces (198 g) Spanish chorizo, sliced
4 ounces (113 g) cream cheese
¼ cup chopped parsley

1. Preheat oven to 325ºF (163ºC). Line a baking dish with waxed paper. Bake chorizo for 15 minutes until crispy. Remove and let cool. Arrange on a serving platter. Top with cream cheese. Serve sprinkled with parsley.

Per Serving
calories: 207 | fat: 18g | protein: 9g
carbs: 1g | net carbs: 1g | fiber: 0g

Mashed Cauliflower with Bacon and Chives

Prep time: 5 minutes | Cook time: 16 minutes | Serves 6

6 slices bacon
3 heads cauliflower, leaves removed
2 cups water
2 tablespoons melted butter
½ cup coconut milk
Salt and black pepper, to taste
¼ cup grated yellow Cheddar cheese
2 tablespoons chopped chives

1. Preheat oven to 350ºF. Fry bacon in a heated skillet over medium heat for 5 minutes until crispy. Remove to a paper towel-lined plate, allow to cool, and crumble. Set aside and keep bacon fat. Boil cauli heads in water in a pot over high heat for 7 minutes, until tender. Drain and put in a bowl.
2. Include butter, coconut milk, salt, black pepper, and purée using a hand blender until smooth and creamy. Lightly grease a casserole dish with the bacon fat and spread the mash on it.
3. Sprinkle with Cheddar cheese and place under the broiler for 4 minutes on high until the cheese melts. Remove and top with bacon and chopped chives. Serve with pan-seared scallops.

Per Serving
calories: 206 | fat: 17g | protein: 8g
carbs: 8g | net carbs: 5g | fiber: 3g

Chicken-Stuffed Cucumber Bites

Prep time: 5 minutes | Cook time: 0 minutes | Serves 6

2 cucumbers, sliced with a 3-inch thickness
2 cups small dices leftover chicken
¼ jalapeño pepper, seeded and minced
1 tablespoon Dijon mustard
⅓ cup mayonnaise
Salt and black pepper, to taste

1. Cut mid-level holes in cucumber slices with a knife and set aside. Combine chicken, jalapeño pepper, mustard, mayonnaise, salt, and black pepper to be evenly mixed. Fill cucumber holes with chicken mixture and serve.

Per Serving
calories: 115 | fat: 14g | protein: 14g
carbs: 5g | net carbs: 4g | fiber: 1g

Herbed Eggplant

Prep time: 15 minutes | Cook time: 20 minutes | Serves 2

1 teaspoon basil
½ teaspoon oregano
½ teaspoon rosemary
½ teaspoon coarse sea salt
1 large-sized eggplant, curt into slices lengthwise
2 tablespoons coconut aminos
1 teaspoon balsamic vinegar
1 tablespoon olive oil
½ teaspoon Sriracha sauce
¼ cup fresh chives, chopped

1. Toss your eggplant with the basil, oregano, rosemary, and salt.
2. Place the eggplant on a parchment-lined roasting pan. Roast in the preheated oven at 420ºF (216ºC) approximately 15 minutes.
3. Meanwhile, mix the coconut aminos, vinegar, oil, and Sriracha sauce. Drizzle the Sriracha mixture over the eggplant slices.
4. Place under the preheated broil for 3 to 5 minutes. Garnish with fresh chives and serve warm.

Per Serving
calories: 102 | fat: 7.0g | protein: 1.6g
carbs: 8.0g | net carbs: 3.3g | fiber: 4.7g

Tuna-Mayo Topped Dill Pickles

Prep time: 5 minutes | Cook time: 0 minutes | Serves 12

18 ounces (510 g) canned and drained tuna
6 large dill pickles
¼ teaspoon garlic powder
⅓ cup sugar-free mayonnaise
1 tablespoon onion flakes

1. Combine the mayonnaise, tuna, onion flakes, and garlic powder in a bowl. Cut the pickles in half lengthwise. Top each half with tuna mixture. Place in the fridge for 30 minutes before serving.

Per Serving
calories: 59 | fat: 2g | protein: 9g
carbs: 3g | net carbs: 2g | fiber: 1g

Cheese Stuffed Spaghetti Squash

Prep time: 15 minutes | Cook time: 50 to 60 minutes | Serves 4

½ pound (227 g) spaghetti squash, halved, scoop out seeds
1 teaspoon olive oil
½ cup Mozzarella cheese, shredded
½ cup cream cheese
½ cup full-fat Greek yogurt
2 eggs
1 garlic clove, minced
½ teaspoon cumin
½ teaspoon basil
½ teaspoon mint
Sea salt and ground black pepper, to taste

1. Place the squash halves in a baking pan; drizzle the insides of each squash half with olive oil.
2. Bake in the preheated oven at 370ºF (188ºC) for 45 to 50 minutes or until the interiors are easily pierced through with a fork
3. Now, scrape out the spaghetti squash "noodles" from the skin in a mixing bowl. Add the remaining ingredients and mix to combine well.
4. Carefully fill each of the squash half with the cheese mixture. Bake at 350ºF (180ºC) for 5 to 10 minutes, until the cheese is bubbling and golden brown. Bon appétit!

Per Serving
calories: 220 | fat: 17.6g | protein: 9.0g
carbs: 6.8g | net carbs: 5.9g | fiber: 0.9g

Spiced Cauliflower Cheese Bake

Prep time: 20 minutes | Cook time: 20 minutes | Serves 4

½ teaspoon butter, melted
1 (½-pound / 227-g) head cauliflower, broken into florets
½ cup Swiss cheese, shredded
½ cup Mexican blend cheese, room temperature
½ cup Greek yogurt
1 cup cooked ham, chopped
1 roasted chili pepper, chopped
½ teaspoon porcini powder
1 teaspoon garlic powder
1 teaspoon shallot powder
½ teaspoon cayenne pepper
¼ teaspoon dried sage
½ teaspoon dried oregano
Sea salt and ground black pepper, to taste

1. Start by preheating your oven to 340ºF (171ºC). Then, coat the bottom and sides of a casserole dish with ½ teaspoon of melted butter.
2. Empty the cauliflower into a pot and cover it with water. Let it cook for 6 minutes until it is nice and tender (mashable). Mash the prepared cauliflower with a potato ricer press or potato masher.
3. Now, stir in the cheese; stir until the cheese has melted. Add Greek yogurt, chopped ham, roasted pepper, and spices.
4. Place the mixture in the prepared casserole dish; bake in the preheated oven for 20 minutes. Let it sit for about 10 minutes before cutting. Serve and enjoy!

Per Serving
calories: 189 | fat: 11.3g | protein: 14.9g
carbs: 5.7g | net carbs: 4.6g | fiber: 1.1g

Zucchini Casserole

Prep time: 15 minutes | Cook time: 45 minutes | Serves 4

Nonstick cooking spray
2 cups zucchini, thinly sliced
2 tablespoons leeks, sliced
½ teaspoon salt
Freshly ground black pepper, to taste
½ teaspoon dried basil
½ teaspoon dried oregano
½ cup Cheddar cheese, grated
¼ cup heavy cream
4 tablespoons Parmesan cheese, freshly grated
1 tablespoon butter, room temperature
1 teaspoon fresh garlic, minced

1. Start by preheating your oven to 370ºF (188ºC). Lightly grease a casserole dish with a nonstick cooking spray.
2. Place 1 cup of the zucchini slices in the dish; add 1 tablespoon of leeks; sprinkle with salt, pepper, basil, and oregano. Top with ¼ cup of Cheddar cheese. Repeat the layers one more time.
3. In a mixing dish, thoroughly whisk the heavy cream with Parmesan, butter, and garlic. Spread this mixture over the zucchini layer and cheese layers.
4. Place in the preheated oven and bake for about 40 to 45 minutes until the edges are nicely browned. Sprinkle with chopped chives, if desired. Bon appétit!

Per Serving
calories: 156 | fat: 12.8g | protein: 7.5g
carbs: 3.6g | net carbs: 2.8g | fiber: 0.8g

Cumin Green Cabbage Stir-Fry

Prep time: 10 minutes | Cook time: 20 minutes | Serves 2

2 tablespoons olive oil
1 (1-inch) piece fresh ginger, grated
½ teaspoon cumin seeds
1 shallot, chopped
½ cup chicken stock
¾ pound (340 g) green cabbage, sliced
¼ teaspoon turmeric powder
½ teaspoon coriander powder
Kosher salt and cayenne pepper, to taste

1. Heat the olive oil in a saucepan over medium heat; then, sauté the ginger and cumin seeds until fragrant.
2. Add in the shallot and continue sautéing an additional 2 to 3 minutes or until just tender and aromatic. Pour in the chicken stock to deglaze the pan.
3. Add the cabbage wedges, turmeric, coriander, salt, and cayenne pepper. Cover and cook for 15 to 18 minutes or until your cabbage has softened. Make sure to stir occasionally.
4. Serve in individual bowls and enjoy!

Per Serving
calories: 169 | fat: 13.0g | protein: 2.6g
carbs: 7.0g | net carbs: 2.9g | fiber: 4.1g

Riced Cauliflower Stuffed Bell Peppers

Prep time: 15 minutes | Cook time: 45 minutes | Serves 6

2 tablespoons vegetable oil	¼ teaspoon red pepper flakes, crushed
2 tablespoons yellow onion, chopped	½ teaspoon ground black pepper
1 teaspoon fresh garlic, crushed	1 teaspoon dried parsley flakes
½ pound (227 g) ground pork	6 medium-sized bell peppers, deveined and cleaned
½ pound (227 g) ground turkey	½ cup tomato sauce
1 cup cauliflower rice	½ cup Cheddar cheese, shredded
½ teaspoon sea salt	

1. Heat the oil in a pan over medium flame. Once hot, sauté the onion and garlic for 2 to 3 minutes.
2. Add the ground meat and cook for 6 minutes longer or until it is nicely browned. Add cauliflower rice and seasoning. Continue to cook for a further 3 minutes.
3. Divide the filling between the prepared bell peppers. Cover with a piece of foil. Place the peppers in a baking pan; add tomato sauce.
4. Bake in the preheated oven at 380ºF (193ºC) for 20 minutes. Uncover, top with cheese, and bake for 10 minutes more. Bon appétit!

Per Serving
calories: 245 | fat: 12.8g | protein: 16.6g
carbs: 3.3g | net carbs: 2.3g | fiber: 1.0g

Herbed Eggplant and Kale Bake

Prep time: 20 minutes | Cook time: 40 minutes | Serves 6

1 (¾-pound / 340-g) eggplant, cut into ½-inch slices	sugar
1 tablespoon olive oil	⅓ cup cream cheese
1 tablespoon butter, melted	1 cup Asiago cheese, shredded
8 ounces (227 g) kale leaves, torn into pieces	½ cup Gorgonzola cheese, grated
14 ounces (397 g) garlic-and-tomato pasta sauce, without	2 tablespoons ketchup, without sugar
	1 teaspoon hot pepper
	1 teaspoon basil
	1 teaspoon oregano
	½ teaspoon rosemary

1. Place the eggplant slices in a colander and sprinkle them with salt. Allow it to sit for 2 hours. Wipe the eggplant slices with paper towels.
2. Brush the eggplant slices with olive oil; cook in a cast-iron grill pan until nicely browned on both sides, about 5 minutes.
3. Melt the butter in a pan over medium flame. Now, cook the kale leaves until wilted. In a mixing bowl, combine the three types of cheese.
4. Transfer the grilled eggplant slices to a lightly greased baking dish. Top with the kale. Then, add a layer of ½ of cheese blend.
5. Pour the tomato sauce over the cheese layer. Top with the remaining cheese mixture. Sprinkle with seasoning.
6. Bake in the preheated oven at 350ºF (180ºC) until cheese is bubbling and golden brown, about 35 minutes. Bon appétit!

Per Serving
calories: 231 | fat: 18.6g | protein: 10.5g
carbs: 6.7g | net carbs: 4.3g | fiber: 2.4g

Vegetable Mix

Prep time: 10 minutes | Cook time: 15 to 20 minutes | Serves 4

1 butternut squash, cut into chunks	1 sprig thyme, chopped
¼ pound (113 g) shallots, peeled	4 cloves garlic, peeled only
¼ pound (113 g) Brussels sprouts	3 tablespoons olive oil
1 sprig rosemary, chopped	Salt and black pepper, to taste

1. Preheat the oven to 450ºF (235ºC).
2. Pour the butternut squash, shallots, garlic cloves, and Brussels sprouts in a bowl. Season with salt, black pepper, olive oil, and toss. Pour the mixture on a baking sheet and sprinkle with the chopped thyme and rosemary. Roast the vegetables for 15–20 minutes.
3. Once ready, remove and spoon into a serving bowl. Serve with oven roasted chicken thighs.

Per Serving
calories: 159 | fat: 10g | protein: 3g
carbs: 14g | net carbs: 10g | fiber: 4g

Zucchini Sticks with Garlic Aioli

Prep time: 5 minutes | Cook time: 15 minutes | Serves 4

¼ cup pork rind crumbs
1 teaspoon sweet paprika
¼ cup shredded Parmesan cheese
Aioli:
½ cup mayonnaise
1 garlic clove, minced
Salt and chili pepper, to taste
3 fresh eggs
2 zucchinis, cut into strips
Juice and zest from ½ lemon

1. Preheat oven to 425ºF and line a baking sheet with foil. Grease with cooking spray and set aside.
2. Mix the pork rinds, paprika, Parmesan cheese, salt, and chili pepper in a bowl. Beat the eggs in another bowl.
3. Coat zucchini strips in eggs, then in Parmesan mixture, and arrange on the baking sheet. Grease lightly with cooking spray and bake for 15 minutes to be crispy.
4. To make the aioli, combine in a bowl mayonnaise, lemon juice, and garlic, and gently stir until everything is well incorporated. Add the lemon zest, adjust the seasoning and stir again. Cover and place in the refrigerator until ready to serve.
5. Serve the zucchini strips with garlic aioli for dipping.

Per Serving
calories: 186 | fat: 11g | protein: 8g
carbs: 7g | net carbs: 5g | fiber: 2g

Italian Tomato and Cheese Stuffed Peppers

Prep time: 15 minutes | Cook time: 10 minutes | Serves 2

1 tablespoon canola oil
1 garlic clove, pressed
½ cup celery, finely chopped
½ Spanish onion, finely chopped
4 ounces (113 g) pork, ground
Sea salt, to taste
1 teaspoon Italian seasoning mix
2 sweet Italian peppers, deveined and halved
1 large-sized Roma tomato, puréed
½ cup Cheddar cheese, grated

1. Heat the canola oil in a sauté pan over medium-high heat. Now, sauté the garlic, celery, and onion until they have softened.
2. Stir in the ground pork and cook for a further 3 minutes or until no longer pink. Sprinkle with salt and Italian seasoning mix. Divide the filling mixture between the pepper halves.
3. Add the puréed tomato to a lightly greased baking dish; place the stuffed peppers in the baking dish.
4. Bake in the preheated oven at 390ºF (199ºC) for 20 minutes. Top with the Cheddar cheese and bake an additional 4 to 6 minutes or until the cheese is bubbling. Serve warm and enjoy!

Per Serving
calories: 312 | fat: 21.4g | protein: 20.2g
carbs: 5.7g | net carbs: 3.8g | fiber: 1.9g

Broccoli Cheese

Prep time: 10 minutes | Cook time: 15 minutes | Serves 5

3 tablespoons olive oil
1 teaspoon garlic, minced
1½ pounds (680 g) broccoli florets
½ teaspoon flaky salt
½ teaspoon ground black pepper
½ teaspoon paprika
½ cup cream of mushrooms soup
6 ounces (170 g) Swiss cheese, shredded

1. Heat 1 tablespoon of the olive oil in a nonstick frying pan over a moderate flame. Then, sauté the garlic until just tender and fragrant.
2. Preheat your oven to 390ºF (199ºC). Now, brush the sides and bottom of a casserole dish with 1 tablespoon of olive oil.
3. Parboil the broccoli in salted water until it is crisp-tender; discard any excess water and transfer the boiled broccoli florets to the prepared casserole dish. Scatter the sautéed garlic around the broccoli florets.
4. Drizzle the remaining tablespoon of olive oil; sprinkle the salt, black pepper, and paprika over your broccoli. Pour in the cream of mushroom soup.
5. Top with the Swiss cheese and bake approximately 18 minutes until the cheese bubbled all over. Bon appétit!

Per Serving
calories: 180 | fat: 10.3g | protein: 13.5g
carbs: 7.6g | net carbs: 4.0g | fiber: 3.6g

Duo-Cheese Broccoli Croquettes

Prep time: 10 minutes | Cook time: 10 minutes | Serves 5

1 pound (454 g) broccoli florets
1 tablespoon fresh parsley, minced
½ teaspoon paprika
Sea salt and ground black pepper, to taste
3 eggs
1 cup Romano cheese, preferably freshly grated
5 ounces (142 g) Swiss cheese, sliced
2 tablespoons olive oil

1. Pulse the broccoli florets in your food processor until small rice-sized pieces are formed.
2. Mix the chopped broccoli florets with the parsley, paprika, salt, pepper, eggs, and Romano cheese. Shape the mixture into bite-sized balls; flatten the balls with your hands or fork.
3. Heat the olive oil in a frying pan over a moderate flame.
4. Cook for 4 to 5 minutes; turn over, top with the Swiss cheese and continue to cook on the other side for a further 4 minutes or until thoroughly cooked. Bon appétit!

Per Serving
calories: 324 | fat: 24.1g | protein: 19.9g carbs: 5.8g | net carbs: 3.5g | fiber: 2.3g

Mascarpone Turkey Pastrami Pinwheels

Prep time: 5 minutes | Cook time: 0 minutes | Serves 4

Cooking spray
8 ounces (227 g) mascarpone cheese
10 ounces (284 g) turkey pastrami, sliced
10 canned pepperoncini peppers, sliced and drained

1. Lay a 12 x 12 plastic wrap on a flat surface and arrange the pastrami all over slightly overlapping each other. Spread the cheese on top of the salami layers and arrange the pepperoncini on top.
2. Hold two opposite ends of the plastic wrap and roll the pastrami. Twist both ends to tighten and refrigerate for 2 hours. Unwrap the salami roll and slice into 2-inch pinwheels. Serve.

Per Serving
calories: 549 | fat: 49g | protein: 29g carbs: 10g | net carbs: 7g | fiber: 3g

Duo-Cheese Lettuce Rolls

Prep time: 5 minutes | Cook time: 5 minutes | Serves 6

½ pound (227 g) gouda cheese, grated
½ pound (227 g) feta cheese, crumbled
1 teaspoon taco seasoning mix
2 tablespoons olive oil
1½ cups guacamole
1 cup coconut milk
A head lettuce

1. Mix both types of cheese with taco seasoning mix. Set a pan over medium heat and warm the olive oil. Spread the shredded cheese mixture all over the pan. Fry for 5 minutes, turning once. Arrange some of the cheese mixture on each lettuce leaf, top with coconut milk and guacamole, then roll up folding in the ends to secure and serve.

Per Serving
calories: 401 | fat: 30g | protein: 18g carbs: 10g | net carbs: 5g | fiber: 5g

Pecorino Cauli Bake with Mayo

Prep time: 5 minutes | Cook time: 25 minutes | Serves 6

2 heads cauliflower, cut into florets
¼ cup melted butter
Salt and black pepper to taste
1 pinch red pepper flakes
½ cup mayonnaise
¼ teaspoon Dijon mustard
3 tablespoons grated pecorino cheese

1. Preheat oven to 400ºF (205ºC) and grease a baking dish with cooking spray.
2. Combine the cauli florets, butter, salt, black pepper, and red pepper flakes in a bowl until well mixed. Mix the mayonnaise and Dijon mustard in a bowl, and set aside until ready to serve.
3. Arrange cauliflower florets on the prepared baking dish. Sprinkle with grated pecorino cheese and bake for 25 minutes until the cheese has melted and golden brown on the top.
4. Remove, let sit for 3 minutes to cool, and serve with the mayo sauce.

Per Serving
calories: 171 | fat: 13g | protein: 5g carbs: 13g | net carbs: 9g | fiber: 4g

Roasted Asparagus

Prep time: 10 minutes | Cook time: 15 minutes | Serves 5

4 tablespoons butter, melted
4 tablespoons Pecorino Romano cheese, grated
1½ pounds (680 g) asparagus, trimmed
½ teaspoon cayenne pepper
Sea salt and cracked black pepper, to taste
1 tablespoon Sriracha sauce
1 tablespoon fresh cilantro, roughly chopped

1. Toss your asparagus with the melted butter, cheese, cayenne pepper, salt, black pepper, and Sriracha sauce; toss until well coated.
2. Place the asparagus on a roasting pan. Roast in the preheated oven at 420ºF (216ºC) for 10 minutes.
3. Rotate the pan and continue to cook an additional 4 to 5 minutes. Serve immediately garnished with fresh cilantro. Bon appétit!

Per Serving
calories: 141 | fat: 11.5g | protein: 5.6g
carbs: 5.5g | net carbs: 2.6g | fiber: 2.9g

Chicken Breast Fritters with Dill Dip

Prep time: 10 minutes | Cook time: 8 minutes | Serves 4

1 pound (454 g) chicken breasts, thinly sliced
1¼ cup mayonnaise
¼ cup coconut flour
2 eggs
Salt and black pepper, to taste
1 cup Mozzarella cheese, grated
4 tablespoons dill, chopped
3 tablespoons olive oil
1 cup sour cream
1 teaspoon garlic powder
1 tablespoon parsley, chopped
1 onion, finely chopped

1. In a bowl, mix 1 cup of the mayonnaise, 3 tablespoons of dill, sour cream, garlic powder, onion, and salt. Cover the bowl with plastic wrap and refrigerate for 30 minutes.
2. Mix the chicken, remaining mayonnaise, coconut flour, eggs, salt, black pepper, Mozzarella, and remaining dill, in a bowl. Cover the bowl with plastic wrap and refrigerate it for 2 hours. After the marinating time is over, remove from the fridge.
3. Place a skillet over medium fire and heat the olive oil. Fetch 2 tablespoons of chicken mixture into the skillet, use the back of a spatula to flatten the top. Cook for 4 minutes, flip, and fry for 4 more.
4. Remove onto a wire rack and repeat the cooking process until the batter is finished, adding more oil as needed. Garnish the fritters with parsley and serve with dill dip.

Per Serving
calories: 671 | fat: 42g | protein: 45g
carbs: 15g | net carbs: 13g | fiber: 2g

Mozzarella Prosciutto Wraps with Basil

Prep time: 5 minutes | Cook time: 0 minutes | Serves 6

6 thin prosciutto slices
18 basil leaves
18 ciliegine Mozzarella balls
2 tablespoons extra-virgin olive oil

1. Cut the prosciutto slices into three strips each. Place basil leaves at the end of each strip. Top with a ciliegine Mozzarella ball. Wrap the Mozzarella in prosciutto. Secure with toothpicks. Arrange on a platter, drizzle with olive oil, and serve.

Per Serving
calories: 211 | fat: 16g | protein: 14g
carbs: 2g | net carbs: 1g | fiber: 1g

Buttered Broccoli

Prep time:5 minutes | Cook time: 3 minutes | Serves 6

1 broccoli head, florets only
Kosher salt and black pepper, to taste
¼ cup butter

1. Place the broccoli in a pot filled with salted water and bring to a boil. Cook for about 3 minutes until crisp-tender. Drain the broccoli and transfer to a plate.
2. Melt the butter in a microwave. Drizzle the butter over and season with some salt and black pepper.

Per Serving
calories: 102 | fat: 8g | protein: 3g
carbs: 7g | net carbs: 4g | fiber: 3g

Feta Zucchini and Pepper Gratin

Prep time: 5 minutes | Cook time: 30 to 40 minutes | Serves 6

2 pounds (907 g) zucchinis, sliced
2 red bell peppers, seeded and sliced
Salt and black pepper, to taste
1½ cups crumbled feta cheese
2 tablespoons butter, melted
½ cup heavy whipping cream

1. Preheat oven to 370ºF. Place the sliced zucchinis in a colander over the sink, sprinkle with salt and let sit for 20 minutes. Transfer to paper towels to drain the excess liquid.
2. Grease a baking dish with cooking spray and make a layer of zucchini and bell peppers overlapping one another. Season with pepper, and sprinkle with feta cheese. Repeat the layering process a second time.
3. Combine the butter and whipping cream in a bowl, stir to mix completely, and pour over the vegetables. Bake for 30-40 minutes or until golden brown on top.

Per Serving

calories: 211 | fat: 16g | protein: 10g | carbs: 9g | net carbs: 6g | fiber: 3g

Pecorino Mushroom Burgers

Prep time: 15 minutes | Cook time: 13 minutes | Serves 4

2 tablespoons butter, softened
2 tablespoons olive oil
2 garlic cloves, minced
2 cups portobello mushrooms, chopped
4 tablespoons blanched almond flour
4 tablespoons ground flax seeds
4 tablespoons hemp seeds
4 tablespoons sunflower seeds
1 tablespoon Cajun seasoning
1 teaspoon mustard
2 eggs, whisked
½ cup Pecorino cheese, shredded

1. Set a pan over medium heat and warm the olive oil. Add in mushrooms and garlic and sauté until there is no more water in mushrooms. Remove to a plate and let cool for a few minutes.
2. In a bowl, place Pecorino cheese, almond flour, hemp seeds, mustard, eggs, sunflower seeds, flax seeds, mushrooms, and Cajun seasoning. Create 4 burgers from the mixture.
3. To the same pan, add and warm the butter; fry the burgers for 7 minutes. Flip them over with a wide spatula and cook for 6 more minutes. Serve with guacamole.

Per Serving

calories: 368 | fat: 30g | protein: 14g | carbs: 15g | net carbs: 11g | fiber: 4g

Parmesan Cauliflower Fritters

Prep time: 5 minutes | Cook time: 6 minutes | Serves 4

1 pound (454 g) grated cauliflower
½ cup Parmesan cheese, grated
3 ounces (85 g) chopped onion
½ teaspoon baking powder
½ cup almond flour
2 eggs
½ teaspoon lemon juice
2 tablespoons olive oil
⅓ teaspoon salt

1. Sprinkle the salt over the cauliflower in a bowl, and let it stand for 10 minutes. Add in the other ingredients. Mix with your hands to combine. Place a skillet over medium heat, and heat olive oil.
2. Shape fritters out of the cauliflower mixture. Fry in batches, for about 3 minutes per side.

Per Serving

calories: 231 | fat: 13g | protein: 11g | carbs: 10g | net carbs: 6g | fiber: 4g

Prosciutto-Wrapped Piquillo Peppers

Prep time: 15 minutes | Cook time: 0 minutes | Serves 8

8 canned roasted piquillo peppers
1 tablespoon olive oil
Filling:
8 ounces (227 g) goat cheese
3 tablespoons heavy cream
3 tablespoons chopped parsley

3 slices prosciutto, cut into thin slices
1 tablespoon balsamic vinegar

½ teaspoon minced garlic
1 tablespoon olive oil
1 tablespoon chopped mint

1. Mix all filling ingredients in a bowl. Place in a freezer bag, press down and squeeze, and cut off the bottom. Drain and deseed the peppers. Squeeze about 2 tablespoons of the filling into each pepper.
2. Wrap a prosciutto slice onto each pepper. Secure with toothpicks. Arrange them on a serving platter. Sprinkle the olive oil and vinegar over.

Per Serving

calories: 216 | fat: 17g | protein: 11g | carbs: 6g | net carbs: 5g | fiber: 1g

Avocado Crostini Nori with Walnuts

Prep time: 5 minutes | Cook time: 2 minutes | Serves 4

8 slices low carb bread (baguette)
4 nori sheets
1 cup mashed avocado
⅓ teaspoon salt

1 teaspoon lemon juice
1½ tablespoons coconut oil
⅓ cup chopped raw walnuts
1 tablespoon chia seeds

1. In a bowl, flake the nori sheets into the smallest possible pieces.
2. In another bowl, mix the avocado, salt, and lemon juice, and stir in half of the nori flakes. Set aside.
3. Place the bread slices on a baking sheet and toast in a broiler on medium heat for 2 minutes, making sure not to burn. Remove the crostini after and brush with coconut oil on both sides. Top each crostini with the avocado mixture and garnish with the chia seeds, chopped walnuts, Serve.

Per Serving

calories: 317 | fat: 18g | protein: 9g | carbs: 10g | net carbs: 3g | fiber: 7g

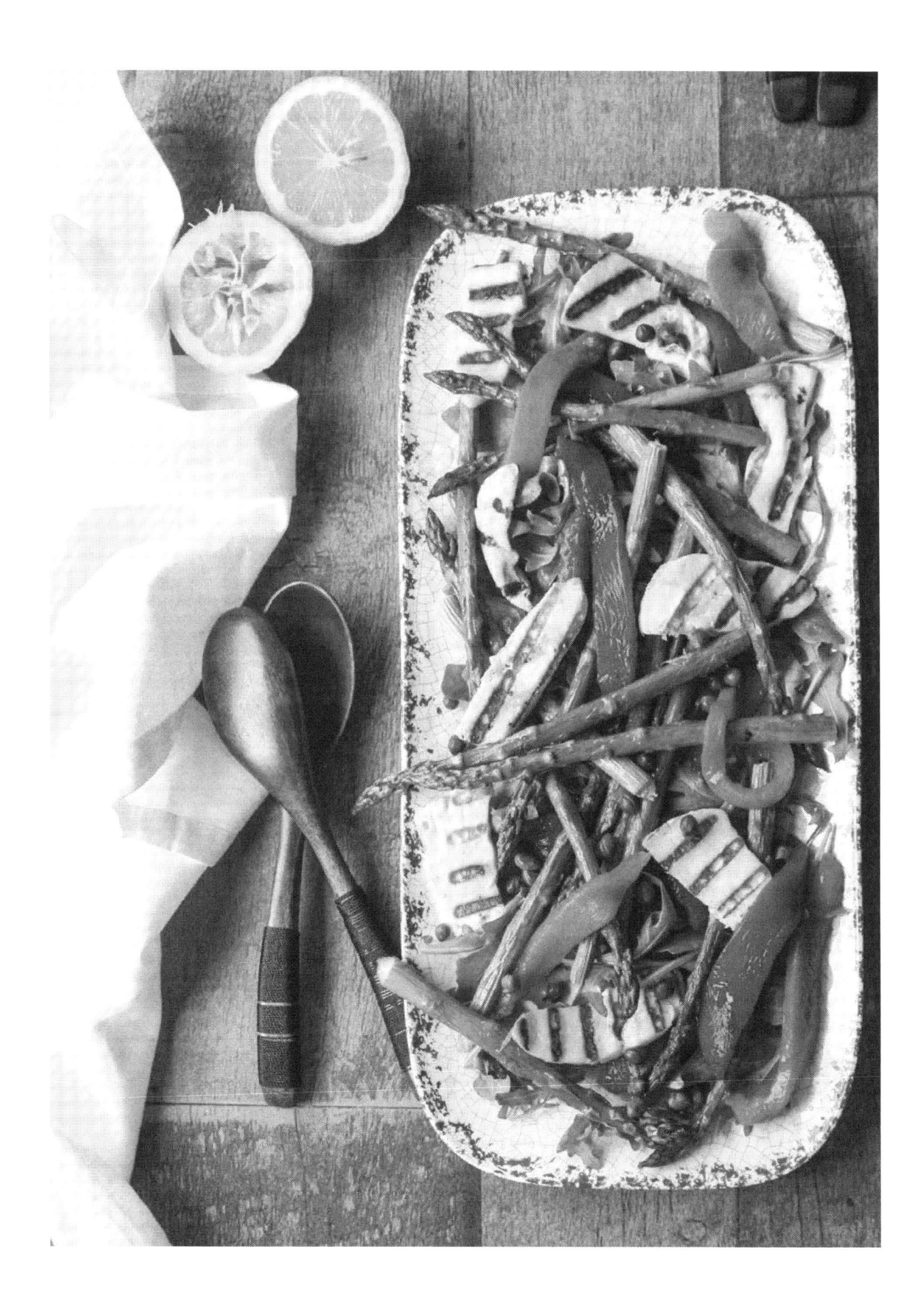

Chapter 6 Vegan and Vegetarian

Cauliflower and Celery Soup

Prep time: 5 minutes | Cook time: 15 minutes | Serves 4

2 green onions, chopped
½ teaspoon ginger-garlic paste
1 celery stalk, chopped
1 pound (454 g) cauliflower florets
3 cups vegetable broth

1. Heat up a lightly oiled soup pot over a medium-high flame. Now, sauté the green onions for 2 minutes, until they have softened.
2. Stir in the ginger-garlic paste, celery, cauliflower, and vegetable broth; bring to a rapid boil. Turn the heat to medium-low.
3. Continue to simmer for 13 minutes more or until heated through; heat off.
4. purée the soup in your blender until creamy and uniform. Enjoy!

Per Serving
calories: 69 | fat: 2g | protein: 6g
carbs: 7g | net carbs: 4g | fiber: 3g

Mushroom and Zucchini Stew

Prep time: 5 minutes | Cook time: 15 minutes | Serves 4

½ cup leeks, chopped
1 pound (454 g) brown mushrooms, chopped
1 teaspoon garlic, minced
1 medium-sized zucchini, diced
2 ripe tomatoes, puréed

1. Heat up a lightly greased soup pot over medium-high heat. Now, sauté the leeks until just tender about 3 minutes.
2. Stir in the mushrooms, garlic, and zucchini. Continue to sauté an additional 2 minutes or until tender and aromatic.
3. Add in the tomatoes and 2 cups of water. Season with Sazón spice, if desired. Reduce the temperature to simmer and continue to cook, covered, for 10 to 12 minutes more. Bon appétit!

Per Serving
calories: 108 | fat: 8g | protein: 3g
carbs: 7g | net carbs: 4g | fiber: 3g

Lemony Cucumber-Avocado Salad

Prep time: 5 minutes | Cook time: 0 minutes | Serves 6

1 avocado, peeled, pitted and sliced
½ white onion, chopped
1 Lebanese cucumber, sliced
3 teaspoons fresh lemon juice
2 tablespoons extra-virgin olive oil

1. Toss all ingredients in a nice salad bowl.
2. Transfer to your refrigerator until ready to serve.
3. Serve well chilled and enjoy!

Per Serving
calories: 149 | fat: 14g | protein: 2g
carbs: 6g | net carbs: 2g | fiber: 4g

Swiss Cheese Broccoli

Prep time: 5 minutes | Cook time: 27 minutes | Serves 6

6 eggs
6 ounces (170 g) sour cream
1 cup vegetable broth
¾ pound (340 g) broccoli florets
6 ounces (170 g) Swiss cheese, shredded

1. Start by preheating your oven to 360ºF (182ºC). Then, spritz a baking pan with nonstick cooking spray.
2. Thoroughly combine the eggs, sour cream, and vegetable broth.
3. Bring a pot with lightly salted water to a boil. Add the broccoli florets to the boiling water and cook for 2 minutes.
4. Arrange the broccoli florets on the bottom of the prepared pan. Pour the egg/cream mixture over the broccoli. Top with the shredded cheese.
5. Bake for 25 to 28 minutes, turning your pan once or twice. Bon appétit!

Per Serving
calories: 241 | fat: 16g | protein: 16g
carbs: 6g | net carbs: 4g | fiber: 2g

Creamy Cabbage and Cauliflower

Prep time: 5 minutes | Cook time: 13 minutes | Serves 4

2 tablespoons olive oil
1 white onion, chopped
½ pound (227 g) savoy cabbage, shredded
½ pound (227 g) cauliflower florets
1 bell pepper
1 cup cream of mushroom soup
1 cup heavy whipping cream
Sea salt and red pepper flakes, to taste

1. Heat the olive oil in a saucepan over a moderate flame. Now, sauté the onion for 3 minutes, until just tender and fragrant.
2. Stir in the cabbage, cauliflower, bell pepper, and cream of mushroom soup. Reduce the heat to medium-low; let it cook for 8 minutes more until the vegetables have softened.
3. Fold in the heavy whipping cream and continue to simmer for 2 to 3 minutes more. Sprinkle with salt and red pepper to taste. Serve warm.

Per Serving
calories: 256 | fat: 24g | protein: 3g
carbs: 7g | net carbs: 4g | fiber: 3g

Mushroom and Bell Pepper Omelet

Prep time: 5 minutes | Cook time: 10 minutes | Serves 4

2 tablespoons olive oil
1 cup Chanterelle mushrooms, chopped
2 bell peppers, chopped
1 white onion, chopped
6 eggs

1. Heat the olive oil in a nonstick skillet over moderate heat. Now, cook the mushrooms, peppers, and onion for 5 minutes, until they have softened.
2. In a mixing bowl, whisk the eggs until frothy. Add the eggs to the skillet, reduce the heat to medium-low, and cook for approximately 5 minutes until the center starts to look dry. Do not overcook.
3. Taste and season with salt to taste. Bon appétit!

Per Serving
calories: 239 | fat: 18g | protein: 12g
carbs: 6g | net carbs: 4g | fiber: 2g

Egg-Stuffed Avocados

Prep time: 5 minutes | Cook time: 15 minutes | Serves 4

2 avocados, pitted and halved
4 eggs
Sea salt and freshly ground black pepper, to taste
1 cup Asiago cheese, grated
½ teaspoon red pepper flakes
½ teaspoon dried rosemary
1 tablespoon fresh chives, chopped

1. Crack the eggs into the avocado halves, keeping the yolks intact. Sprinkle with salt and black pepper.
2. Top with cheese, red pepper flakes, and rosemary. Arrange the stuffed avocado halves in a baking pan.
3. Bake in the preheated oven at 420°F (216°C) for about 15 minutes. Serve garnished with fresh chives. Enjoy!

Per Serving
calories: 300 | fat: 25g | protein: 15g
carbs: 6g | net carbs: 1g | fiber: 5g

Summer Stew with Chives

Prep time: 10 minutes | Cook time: 28 minutes | Serves 4

2 teaspoons sesame oil
2 bell peppers, seeded and chopped
1 small-sized shallot, chopped
1 summer zucchini, chopped
4 cups vegetable broth
2 vine-ripe tomatoes
4 tablespoons sour cream, well-chilled
2 tablespoons fresh chives, minced

1. Heat the sesame oil in a heavy pot over moderate flame. Sauté the bell peppers and shallot for 3 minutes, until just tender and aromatic.
2. Stir in the zucchini, broth, tomatoes, and stir to combine. Bring to a rolling boil. Immediately reduce the heat to medium-low and let it simmer for 25 minutes until everything is thoroughly cooked.
3. Ladle into individual bowls and garnish with sour cream and fresh chives. Enjoy!

Per Serving
calories: 67 | fat: 4g | protein: 2g
carbs: 6g | net carbs: 4g | fiber: 2g

Citrus Asparagus and Cherry Tomato Salad

Prep time: 10 minutes | Cook time: 16 minutes | Serves 3

1 pound (454 g) asparagus, trimmed
¼ teaspoon ground black pepper
Flaky salt, to season
3 tablespoons sesame seeds
1 tablespoon Dijon mustard
½ lime, freshly squeezed
3 tablespoons extra-virgin olive oil
2 garlic cloves, minced
1 tablespoon fresh tarragon, snipped
1 cup cherry tomatoes, sliced

1. Start by preheating your oven to 395ºF (202ºC). Spritz a roasting pan with nonstick cooking spray.
2. Roast the asparagus for about 13 minutes, turning the spears over once or twice. Sprinkle with salt, pepper, and sesame seeds; roast an additional 3 to 4 minutes.
3. To make the dressing, whisk the Dijon mustard, lime juice, olive oil, and minced garlic.
4. Chop the asparagus spears into bite-sized pieces and place them in a nice salad bowl. Add the tarragon and tomatoes to the bowl; gently toss to combine.
5. Dress your salad and serve at room temperature. Enjoy!

Per Serving

calories: 159 | fat: 12g | protein: 6g
carbs: 6g | net carbs: 2g | fiber: 4g

Shirataki Mushroom Ramen

Prep time: 10 minutes | Cook time: 13 to 18 minutes | Serves 4

1½ tablespoons butter, melted
1 pound (454 g) brown mushrooms, chopped
1 teaspoon ginger-garlic paste
½ teaspoon ground cumin
½ teaspoon ground coriander
¼ teaspoon ground black pepper, or more to taste
Sea salt, to taste
2 tablespoons green onions, chopped
4 cups roasted vegetable broth
8 ounces (227 g) shirataki noodles

1. Melt the butter in a soup pot over moderate heat. Then, sauté the mushrooms for about 3 minutes or until they are just tender.
2. Stir in the ginger-garlic paste, cumin, coriander, black pepper, salt, and green onions. Pour in the roasted vegetable broth and bring to a boil.
3. Immediately reduce the heat to medium-low. Let it simmer for 8 to 11 minutes. Fold in the shirataki noodles and cook for 2 to 4 minutes more.
4. Serve hot and enjoy!

Per Serving

calories: 76 | fat: 5g | protein: 4g
carbs: 5g | net carbs: 4g | fiber: 1g

Cauliflower Chowder with Fresh Dill

Prep time: 10 minutes | Cook time: 31 minutes | Serves 4

1 tablespoon butter, softened at room temperature
½ stalk celery, chopped
1 white onion, chopped
1 teaspoon ginger-garlic paste
1 pound (454 g) cauliflower florets
Sea salt and white pepper, to taste
1 teaspoon ground sumac
4 cups roasted vegetable broth
1 cup heavy whipping cream
2 tablespoons fresh dill, chopped

1. Melt the butter in a heavy pot over medium-high heat. Then, sauté the celery and onions for 5 minutes, until just tender and fragrant.
2. Stir in the ginger-garlic paste, cauliflower, salt, white pepper, and sumac; continue to sauté for 1 minute more.
3. Pour in the vegetable broth, bringing to a rapid boil. Immediately turn the heat to medium-low. Cover part-way and continue to simmer for about 25 minutes.
4. Purée the chowder using an immersion blender or food processor until you achieve your desired smoothness. Return the chowder to the pot and fold in the heavy whipping cream.
5. Cook briefly until your chowder is all warmed through. Test and adjust seasonings as needed.
6. Garnish with fresh dill and serve warm.

Per Serving

calories: 172 | fat: 15g | protein: 3g
carbs: 7g | net carbs: 4g | fiber: 3g

Parmesan Veggie Fritters

Prep time: 10 minutes | Cook time: 5 to 6 minutes | Serves 5

1 pound (454 g) cauliflower florets
1 celery stalk, chopped
1 small-sized zucchini, cut into rounds
1 shallot, chopped
Sea salt and freshly ground black pepper, to taste
½ teaspoon cayenne pepper
2 garlic cloves, minced
1 cup Parmesan cheese, shredded
1 egg, beaten
½ cup almond meal
2 tablespoons sesame oil

1. Pulse the cauliflower florets and celery in a food processor until they've broken down into "rice". Then, pulse the zucchini and shallot in your food processor for 30 to 40 seconds.
2. Mix the grated vegetables with the salt, black pepper, cayenne pepper, garlic, parmesan cheese, egg, and almond meal. Shape the mixture into small patties.
3. Heat the sesame oil in a frying pan and fry the patties for 5 to 6 minutes until golden brown and thoroughly cooked. Bon appétit!

Per Serving
calories: 173 | fat: 11g | protein: 11g
carbs: 7g | net carbs: 4g | fiber: 3g

Italian Broccoli and Spinach Soup

Prep time: 15 minutes | Cook time: 30 minutes | Serves 3

4 ounces (113 g) broccoli
2 tablespoons sesame oil
1 small-sized onion, chopped
2 garlic cloves, minced
1 teaspoon cayenne pepper
Sea salt and ground black pepper, to taste
1 cup spinach leaves, torn into pieces
1 celery stalk, peeled and chopped
2 cups vegetable broth
1 cup water
1 tomato, puréed
1 jalapeño pepper, minced
1 tablespoon Italian seasonings

1. Pulse the broccoli in your food processor until rice-sized pieces are formed; work in batches; reserve.
2. Then, heat the oil in a saucepan over medium heat. Then, sauté the onion and garlic for 3 minutes, until tender and aromatic.
3. Add the broccoli and cook for 2 minutes more. Add the remaining ingredients, except the spinach.
4. Bring to a rapid boil and then, immediately reduce the heat to medium-low. Now, simmer the soup approximately 25 minutes.
5. Add spinach, turn off the heat, and cover with the lid; let it wilt. Bon appétit!

Per Serving
calories: 137 | fat: 11g | protein: 6g
carbs: 6g | net carbs: 5g | fiber: 1g

Mexican-Flavored Stuffed Peppers

Prep time: 5 minutes | Cook time: 40 minutes | Serves 3

3 bell peppers, halved, seeded
3 eggs, whisked
1 cup Mexican cheese blend
1 teaspoon chili powder
1 garlic clove, minced
1 teaspoon onion powder
1 ripe tomato, puréed
1 teaspoon mustard powder

1. Start by preheating your oven to 370ºF (188ºC). Spritz the bottom and sides of a baking pan with a cooking oil.
2. In a mixing bowl, thoroughly combine the eggs, cheese, chili powder, garlic, and onion powder. Divide the filling between the bell peppers.
3. Mix the tomatoes with mustard powder and transfer the mixture to the baking pan. Cover with foil and bake for 40 minutes, until the peppers are tender and the filling is thoroughly heated. Bon appétit!

Per Serving
calories: 194 | fat: 14g | protein: 13g
carbs: 4g | net carbs: 3g | fiber: 1g

Peppery Omelet with Cheddar Cheese

Prep time: 10 minutes | Cook time: 8 minutes | Serves 2

2 tablespoons olive oil
1 onion, sliced
2 bell peppers, chopped
1 jalapeño pepper, chopped
4 eggs, whisked
4 tablespoons full-fat yogurt
½ teaspoon red pepper flakes
Sea salt and ground black pepper, to season
3 ounces (85 g) Cheddar cheese, shredded

1. Heat the olive oil in a frying pan over a moderate flame. Sauté the onion and peppers for 3 minutes, until tender and fragrant.
2. Then, mix the eggs with the full-fat yogurt. Now, pour the egg mixture into the frying pan. Season with red pepper, salt, and black pepper.
3. Move the pan around to spread it out evenly.
4. Continue to cook for about 5 minutes until the eggs are fully set and the surface is smooth. Top with cheese and serve immediately. Bon appétit!

Per Serving
calories: 439 | fat: 37g | protein: 23g
carbs: 4g | net carbs: 4g | fiber: 0g

Greek Aubergine-Egg Casserole

Prep time: 5 minutes | Cook time: 57 minutes | Serves 5

1 pound (454 g) aubergine, cut into rounds
2 vine-ripe tomatoes, sliced
5 eggs, beaten
1 cup Greek-style yogurt
1½ cups feta cheese, grated

1. Place the aubergine on a large pan lined with paper towel; toss with 1 teaspoon of sea salt and let it stand for 25 minutes in a colander.
2. Pat your aubergine dry and transfer to a lightly oiled baking sheet. Brush them with olive oil. Bake in the preheated oven at 390ºF (199ºC) for about 40 minutes, or until they are golden brown.
3. Layer the rounds of roasted aubergine on the bottom of a lightly oiled casserole dish. Top with sliced tomatoes.
4. In a mixing dish, whisk the eggs with the yogurt. Pour the mixture over the prepared vegetables. Top with feta cheese and bake in the preheated oven at 360ºF (182ºC) for 17 minutes. Enjoy!

Per Serving
calories: 226 | fat: 14g | protein: 16g
carbs: 7g | net carbs: 4 g | fiber: 3g

Halloumi Asparagus Frittata

Prep time: 10 minutes | Cook time: 20 minutes | Serves 4

1 tablespoon olive oil
½ red onion, sliced
4 ounces (113 g) asparagus, cut into small chunks
1 tomato, chopped
5 whole eggs, beaten
10 ounces (284 g) Halloumi cheese, crumbled
2 tablespoons green olives, pitted and sliced
1 tablespoon fresh parsley, chopped

1. Heat the oil in a skillet over medium-high heat; then, cook the onion and asparagus about 3 minutes, stirring continuously.
2. Next, add the tomato and cook for 2 minutes longer. Transfer the sautéed vegetables to a baking pan that is lightly greased with cooking oil.
3. Mix the eggs with cheese until well combined. Pour the mixture over the vegetables. Scatter sliced olives over the top. Bake in the preheated oven at 350ºF (180ºC) for 15 minutes.
4. Garnish with fresh parsley and serve immediately. Enjoy!

Per Serving
calories: 376 | fat: 29g | protein: 25g
carbs: 4g | net carbs: 3g | fiber: 1g

Swiss Zucchini Gratin

Prep time: 10 minutes | Cook time: 10 minutes | Serves 5

10 large eggs
3 tablespoons yogurt
2 zucchinis, sliced
½ medium-sized leek, sliced
Sea salt and ground black pepper, to taste
1 teaspoon cayenne pepper
1 cup cream cheese
2 garlic cloves, minced
1 cup Swiss cheese, shredded

1. Start by preheating your oven to 360°F (182°C). Then, spritz the bottom and sides of an oven proof pan with a nonstick cooking spray. Then, mix the eggs with yogurt until well combined.
2. Overlap ½ of the zucchini and leek slices in the pan. Season with salt, black pepper, and cayenne pepper. Add cream cheese and minced garlic.
3. Add the remaining zucchini slices and leek. Add the egg mixture. Top with Swiss cheese. Bake for 40 minutes, until the top is golden brown. Bon appétit!

Per Serving
calories: 371 | fat: 32g | protein: 16g
carbs: 5g | net carbs: 4g | fiber: 1g

Colby Broccoli Bake

Prep time: 10 minutes | Cook time: 26 minutes | Serves 5

1 pound (454 g) broccoli florets
1 cup yellow onion, sliced
2 cloves garlic, smashed
½ cup heavy cream
1 cup vegetable broth
1 cup Colby cheese, shredded
1 teaspoon cayenne pepper
½ teaspoon dried oregano
½ teaspoon basil
½ teaspoon ground bay laurel
Sea salt and ground black pepper, to taste

1. Bring a saucepan with salted water to a boil. Parboil your broccoli for 2 to 3 minutes until crisp-tender. Throw the broccoli into a lightly oiled baking dish.
2. Add in the onion and garlic. In a mixing dish, whisk the heavy cream with the vegetable broth. Season with cayenne pepper, oregano, basil, ground bay laurel, salt, and black pepper.
3. Pour the cream mixture over the vegetables in the baking dish. Bake in the preheated oven at 390°F (199°C) for 18 minutes.
4. Top with the cheese and continue to bake an additional 6 minutes or until bubbling. Bon appétit!

Per Serving
calories: 194 | fat: 14g | protein: 9g
carbs: 7g | net carbs: 4g | fiber: 3g

Double Cheese Kale Bake

Prep time: 10 minutes | Cook time: 30 to 35 minutes | Serves 4

Nonstick cooking spray
6 ounces (170 g) kale, torn into pieces
4 eggs, whisked
1 cup Cheddar cheese, grated
1 cup Romano cheese
2 tablespoons sour cream
1 garlic clove, minced
Sea salt, to taste
½ teaspoon ground black pepper, or more to taste
½ teaspoon cayenne pepper

1. Start by preheating your oven to 365°F (185°C). Spritz the sides and bottom of a baking pan with a nonstick cooking spray.
2. Mix all ingredients and pour the mixture into the baking pan.
3. Bake for 30 to 35 minutes or until it is thoroughly heated. Bon appétit!

Per Serving
calories: 384 | fat: 29g | protein: 25g
carbs: 6g | net carbs: 4g | fiber: 2g

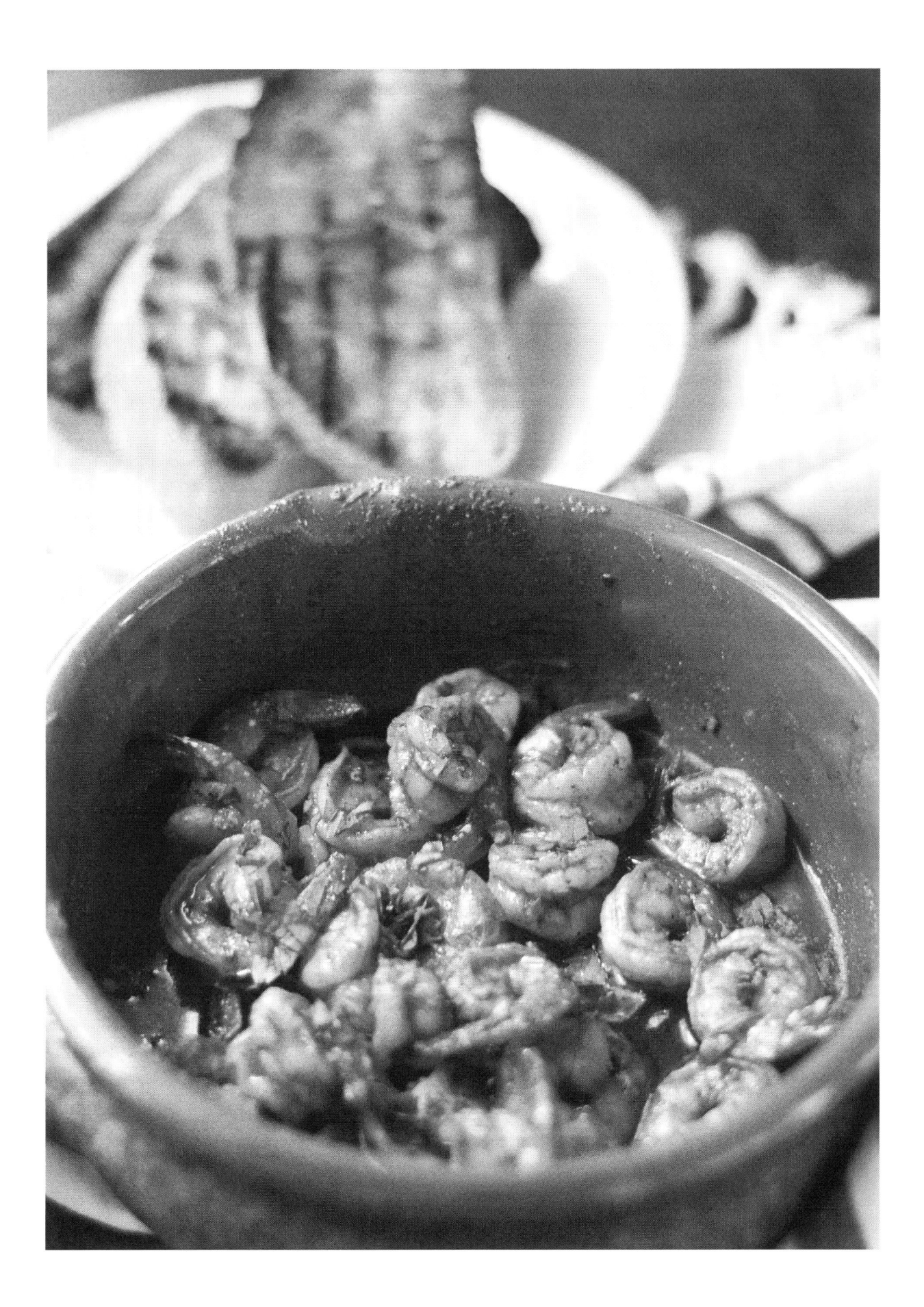

Chapter 7 Fish and Seafood

Pistachio Nut Salmon with Shallot Sauce

Prep time: 15 minutes | Cook time: 30 minutes | Serves 4

4 salmon fillets
½ teaspoon pepper
1 teaspoon salt
Sauce:
1 shallot, chopped
2 teaspoons lemon zest
¼ cup mayonnaise
½ cup pistachios, chopped
1 tablespoon olive oil
A pinch of pepper
1 cup heavy cream

1. Preheat the oven to 375ºF (190ºC). Brush the salmon with mayonnaise and season with salt and pepper. Coat with pistachios. Place in a lined baking dish, and bake, for 15 minutes.
2. Heat the olive oil in a saucepan, and sauté the shallots, for a few minutes. Stir in the rest of the sauce ingredients. Bring to a boil, and cook until thickened. Serve the salmon topped with the sauce.

Per Serving
calories: 564 | fat: 47.0g | protein: 34.0g
carbs: 8.1g | net carbs: 6.0g | fiber: 2.1g

Greek Tilapia with Tomatoes and Olives

Prep time: 10 minutes | Cook time: 15 minutes | Serves 4

4 tilapia fillets
2 garlic cloves, minced
2 teaspoons oregano
14 ounces (397 g) tomatoes, diced
1 tablespoon olive oil
½ red onion, chopped
2 tablespoons parsley
¼ cup kalamata olives

1. Heat olive oil in a skillet over medium heat, and cook onion, garlic, and oregano for 3 minutes. Stir in tomatoes and bring the mixture to a boil. Reduce the heat and simmer, for 5 minutes. Add olives and tilapia. Cook, for about 8 minutes. Serve the tilapia with the tomato sauce.

Per Serving
calories: 183 | fat: 15.0g | protein: 22.9g
carbs: 7.9g | net carbs: 6.2g | fiber: 1.7g

Tuna Fillet Salade Niçoise

Prep time: 5 minutes | Cook time: 7 minutes | Serves 2

¾ pound (340 g) tuna fillet, skinless
1 white onion, sliced
1 teaspoon Dijon mustard
8 Niçoise olives, pitted and sliced
½ teaspoon anchovy paste

1. Brush the tuna with nonstick cooking oil; season with salt and freshly cracked black pepper. Then, grill your tuna on a lightly oiled rack approximately 7 minutes, turning over once or twice.
2. Let the fish stand for 3 to 4 minutes and break into bite-sized pieces. Transfer to a nice salad bowl.
3. Toss the tuna pieces with the white onion, Dijon mustard, Niçoise olives, and anchovy paste. Serve well chilled and enjoy!

Per Serving
calories: 194 | fat: 3g | protein: 37g
carbs: 1g | net carbs: 1g | fiber: 0g

Anchovies with Caesar Dressing

Prep time: 5 minutes | Cook time: 3 minutes | Serves 3

6 anchovies, cleaned and deboned
1 fresh garlic clove, peeled
1 teaspoon Dijon
mustard
2 egg yolks
⅓ cup extra-virgin olive oil

1. Place the anchovies onto a lightly oiled grill pan; place under the grill for 2 minutes. Turn them over and cook for a further minute or so; remove from the grill.
2. Process the garlic, Dijon mustard, egg yolks, and extra-virgin olive oil in your blender. Blend until creamy and uniform.
3. Serve the warm grilled anchovies with the Caesar dressing on the side. Bon appétit!

Per Serving
calories: 449 | fat: 34g | protein: 33g
carbs: 1g | net carbs: 1g | fiber: 0g

Coconut Shrimp Stew

Prep time: 15 minutes | Cook time: 15 minutes | Serves 6

1 cup coconut milk
2 tablespoons lime juice
¼ cup diced roasted peppers
1½ pounds (680 g) shrimp, peeled and deveined
¼ cup olive oil
1 garlic clove, minced
14 ounces (397 g) diced tomatoes
2 tablespoons sriracha sauce
¼ cup onions, chopped
¼ cup cilantro, chopped
Fresh dill, chopped to garnish
Salt and black pepper to taste

1. Heat the olive oil in a pot over medium heat. Add onions and, cook for 3 minutes, or until translucent. Add the garlic and cook, for another minute, until soft. Add tomatoes, shrimp, and cilantro. Cook until the shrimp becomes opaque, about 3-4 minutes. Stir in sriracha and coconut milk, and cook, for 2 more minutes. Do NOT bring to a boil. Stir in the lime juice, and season with salt and pepper to taste. Spoon the stew in bowls, garnish with fresh dill, and serve warm.

Per Serving
calories: 325 | fat: 20.9g | protein: 22.8g
carbs: 6.2g | net carbs: 5.1g | fiber: 1.1g

Dijon Crab Cakes

Prep time: 10 minutes | Cook time: 5 minutes | Serves 4

1 tablespoon coconut oil
1 pound (454 g) lump crab meat
1 teaspoon Dijon mustard
1 egg
¼ cup mayonnaise
1 tablespoon coconut flour
1 tablespoon cilantro, chopped

1. In a bowl, add crab meat, mustard, mayonnaise, coconut flour, egg, cilantro, salt, and pepper; mix to combine. Make patties out of the mixture. Melt coconut oil in a skillet over medium heat. Add crab patties and cook for 2-3 minutes per side. Remove to kitchen paper.
2. Serve.

Per Serving
calories: 316 | fat: 24.3g | protein: 15.2g
carbs: 1.8g | net carbs: 1.5g | fiber: 0.3g

Smoked Salmon and Avocado Omelet

Prep time: 10 minutes | Cook time: 5 minutes | Serves 1

½ avocado, sliced
2 tablespoons chives, chopped
2 ounces (57 g) smoked salmon, cut into strips
1 spring onion, sliced
3 eggs
2 tablespoons cream cheese
1 tablespoon butter
Salt and black pepper to taste

1. In a small bowl, combine the chives and cream cheese. Set aside. Beat the eggs in a large bowl and season with salt and pepper. Melt the butter in a pan over medium heat. Add the eggs to the pan and cook, for about 3 minutes. Carefully flip the omelet over and continue cooking for 2 minutes until golden. Remove the omelet to a plate and spread the chive mixture over. Arrange the salmon, avocado, and onion slices. Wrap the omelet. Serve immediately.

Per Serving
calories: 512 | fat: 47.9g | protein: 36.8g
carbs: 12.9g | net carbs: 5.6g | fiber: 7.3g

Haddock with Mediterranean Sauce

Prep time: 10 minutes | Cook time: 20 minutes | Serves 4

1 pound haddock fillets
1 tablespoon olive oil
Sea salt and freshly cracked black pepper, to taste Mediterranean Sauce:
2 scallions, chopped
½ teaspoon dill weed
½ teaspoon oregano
1 teaspoon basil
¼ cup mayonnaise
¼ cup cream cheese, at room temperature

1. Start by preheating your oven to 360ºF (182ºC). Toss the haddock fillets with the olive oil, salt, and black pepper.
2. Cover with foil and bake for 20 to 25 minutes.
3. In the meantime, make the sauce by whisking all ingredients until well combined. Serve with the warm haddock fillets and enjoy!

Per Serving
calories: 260 | fat: 19g | protein: 20g
carbs: 1g | net carbs: 1g | fiber: 0g

Tilapia Tacos with Cabbage Slaw

Prep time: 10 minutes | Cook time: 5 minutes | Serves 4

1 tablespoon olive oil	2 tilapia fillets
1 teaspoon chili powder	1 teaspoon paprika
	4 keto tortillas

Slaw:

½ cup red cabbage, shredded	1 teaspoon apple cider vinegar
1 tablespoon lemon juice	1 tablespoon olive oil

1. Season tilapia with chili powder and paprika. Heat the olive oil in a skillet over medium heat. Add tilapia, and cook until blackened, about 3 minutes per side. Cut into strips. Divide the tilapia between the tortillas. Combine all of the slaw ingredients in a bowl. Divide the slaw between the tortillas.

Per Serving
calories: 261 | fat: 20.1g | protein: 13.9g
carbs: 5.5g | net carbs: 3.6g | fiber: 1.9g

Tilapia and Riced Cauliflower Cabbage Tortillas

Prep time: 10 minutes | Cook time: 15 minutes | Serves 4

1 teaspoon avocado oil	paprika to taste
1 cup cauli rice	2 whole cabbage leaves
4 tilapia fillets, cut into cubes	2 tablespoons guacamole
¼ teaspoon taco seasoning	1 tablespoon cilantro, chopped
Sea salt and hot	

1. Microwave the cauli rice in microwave safe bowl for 4 minutes. Fluff with a fork and set aside.
2. Warm avocado oil in a skillet over medium heat, rub the tilapia with the taco seasoning, salt, and hot paprika, and fry until brown on all sides, for about 8 minutes in total. Divide the fish among the cabbage leaves, top with cauli rice, guacamole and cilantro.

Per Serving
calories: 171 | fat: 6.5g | protein: 24.4g
carbs: 2.8g | net carbs: 1.5g | fiber: 1.3g

Catalan Shrimp

Prep time: 5 minutes | Cook time: 20 minutes | Serves 4

¼ cup olive oil, divided	pepper
1 pound (454 g) shrimp, deveined	3 garlic cloves, sliced
Salt to taste	2 tablespoons chopped parsley
¼ teaspoon cayenne	

1. Warm olive oil in a large skillet over medium heat. Reduce the heat and add the garlic; cook for 6-8 minutes, but make sure it doesn't brown or burn. Add the shrimp, season with salt and cayenne pepper, stir for one minute and turn off the heat. Let the shrimp finish cooking with the heat of the hot oil for about 8-10 minutes. Serve garnished with parsley.

Per Serving
calories: 442 | fat: 28.9g | protein: 43.2g
carbs: 1.2g | net carbs: 1.1g | fiber: 0.1g

Halibut Tacos with Cabbage Slaw

Prep time: 15 minutes | Cook time: 6 minutes | Serves 4

1 tablespoon olive oil	4 halibut fillets, skinless, sliced
1 teaspoon chili powder	2 low carb tortillas

Slaw:

2 tablespoons red cabbage, shredded	½ tablespoon extra-virgin olive oil
1 tablespoon lemon juice	½ carrot, shredded
Salt to taste	1 tablespoon cilantro, chopped

1. Combine red cabbage with salt in a bowl; massage cabbage to tenderize. Add in the remaining slaw ingredient, toss to coat and set aside.
2. Rub the halibut with olive oil, chili powder and paprika. Heat a grill pan over medium heat.
3. Add halibut and cook until lightly charred and cooked through, about 3 minutes per side.
4. Divide between the tortillas. Combine all slaw ingredients in a bowl. Split the slaw among the tortillas.

Per Serving
calories: 386 | fat: 25.9g | protein: 23.7g
carbs: 12.6g | net carbs: 6.4g | fiber: 6.2g

Tuna Shirataki Pad Thai

Prep time: 15 minutes | Cook time: 5 minutes | Serves 4

1 (7-ounce / 198-g) pack shirataki noodles
4 cups water
1 red bell pepper, sliced
2 tablespoons soy sauce, sugar-free
1 tablespoon ginger-garlic paste
1 teaspoon chili powder
1 tablespoon water
4 tuna steaks
Salt and black pepper to taste
1 tablespoon olive oil
1 tablespoon parsley, chopped

1. In a colander, rinse the shirataki noodles with running cold water. Bring a pot of salted water to a boil; blanch the noodles for 2 minutes. Drain and set aside.
2. Preheat a grill on medium-high. Season the tuna with salt and black pepper, brush with olive oil, and grill covered. Cook for 3 minutes on each side.
3. In a bowl, whisk soy sauce, ginger-garlic paste, olive oil, chili powder, and water. Add bell pepper, and noodles and toss to coat. Assemble noodles and tuna in serving plate and garnish with parsley.

Per Serving
calories: 288 | fat: 16.1g | protein: 23.2g
carbs: 7.7g | net carbs: 6.7g | fiber: 1.0g

Sardines with Zoodles

Prep time: 10 minutes | Cook time: 15 minutes | Serves 4

2 tablespoons olive oil
4 cups zoodles (spiralized zucchini)
1 pound (454 g) whole fresh sardines, gutted
and cleaned
½ cup sundried tomatoes, chopped
1 tablespoon dill
1 garlic clove, minced

1. Preheat the oven to 350ºF (180ºC) and line a baking sheet with parchment paper. Arrange the sardines on the dish, drizzle with olive oil, sprinkle with salt and pepper. Bake for 10 minutes until the skin is crispy.
2. Warm oil in a skillet and stir-fry zucchini, garlic and tomatoes for 5 minutes. Transfer the sardines to a plate and serve with the veggie pasta.

Per Serving
calories: 432 | fat: 28.2g | protein: 32.3g
carbs: 7.1g | net carbs: 5.4g | fiber: 1.7g

White Chowder

Prep time: 5 minutes | Cook time: 15 minutes | Serves 4

2 teaspoons butter, at room temperature
½ white onion, chopped
1 tablespoon Old Bay
seasoning
¾ pound (340 g) sea bass, broken into chunks
1 cup heavy cream

1. Melt the butter in a soup pot over a moderate flame. Now, sweat the white onion until tender and translucent.
2. Then, add in the Old Bay seasoning and 3 cups of water; bring to a rapid boil. Reduce the heat to medium-low and let it simmer, covered, for 9 to 12 minutes.
3. Fold in the sea bass and heavy cream; continue to cook until everything is thoroughly heated or about 5 minutes. Serve warm and enjoy!

Per Serving
calories: 257 | fat: 18g | protein: 21g
carbs: 4g | net carbs: 4g | fiber: 0g

Cajun Tilapia Fish Burgers

Prep time: 5 minutes | Cook time: 46 minutes | Serves 5

1½ pounds tilapia fish, broken into chunks
2 eggs, whisked
½ cup shallots,
chopped
½ cup almond flour
1 tablespoon Cajun seasoning mix

1. Mix all of the above ingredients in a bowl. Shape the mixture into 10 patties and place in your refrigerator for about 40 minutes.
2. Cook in the preheated frying pan that is previously greased with nonstick cooking spray.
3. Cook for 3 minutes until golden brown on the bottom. Carefully flip over and cook the other side for a further 3 minutes. Remove to a paper towel-lined plate until ready to serve.
4. Serve with fresh lettuce, if desired. Bon appétit!

Per Serving
calories: 238 | fat: 11g | protein: 33g
carbs: 3g | net carbs: 2g | fiber: 1g

Salmon Fillets with Broccoli

Prep time: 10 minutes | Cook time: 30 minutes | Serves 4

4 salmon fillets
Salt and black pepper to taste
2 tablespoons mayonnaise
2 tablespoons fennel seeds, crushed
½ head broccoli, cut in florets
1 red bell pepper, sliced
1 tablespoon olive oil
2 lemon wedges

1. Brush the salmon with mayonnaise and season with salt and black pepper. Coat with fennel seeds, place in a lined baking dish and bake for 15 minutes at 370ºF (188ºC). Steam the broccoli and carrot for 3-4 minutes, or until tender, in a pot over medium heat.
2. Heat the olive oil in a saucepan and sauté the red bell pepper for 5 minutes. Stir in the broccoli and turn off the heat. Let the pan sit on the warm burner for 2-3 minutes. Serve with baked salmon garnished with lemon wedges.

Per Serving
calories: 564 | fat: 36.8g | protein: 53.9g
carbs: 8.3g | net carbs: 5.9g | fiber: 2.4g

Italian Haddock Fillet

Prep time: 5 minutes | Cook time: 10 minutes | Serves 6

2 pounds (907 g) haddock fillets
1 tablespoon Italian seasoning blend
Sea salt and freshly ground black pepper, to taste
2 tablespoons olive oil
½ cup marinara sauce

1. Season the haddock fillets and brush them on all sides with olive oil and marinara sauce.
2. Grill over medium heat for 9 to 11 minutes until golden with brown edges.
3. Use a metal spatula to gently lift the haddock fillets, place them on serving plates and serve with the remaining marinara sauce. Bon appétit!

Per Serving
calories: 226 | fat: 6g | protein: 38g
carbs: 2g | net carbs: 1g | fiber: 1g

Dijon-Tarragon Salmon

Prep time: 10 minutes | Cook time: 10 minutes | Serves 4

4 salmon fillets
¾ teaspoon fresh thyme
1 tablespoon butter
Sauce:
¼ cup Dijon mustard
2 tablespoons white wine
¾ teaspoon tarragon
Salt and black pepper to taste
½ teaspoon tarragon
¼ cup heavy cream

1. Season the salmon with thyme, tarragon, salt, and black pepper. Melt the butter in a pan over medium heat. Add salmon and cook for about 4-5 minutes on both sides until the salmon is cooked through. Remove to a warm dish and cover.
2. To the same pan, add the sauce ingredients over low heat and simmer until the sauce is slightly thickened, stirring continually. Cook for 60 seconds to infuse the flavors and adjust the seasoning. Serve the salmon, topped with the sauce.

Per Serving
calories: 538 | fat: 26.5g | protein: 66.9g
carbs: 2.1g | net carbs: 1.4g | fiber: 0.7g

Chive-Sauced Chili Cod

Prep time: 10 minutes | Cook time: 20 minutes | Serves 4

1 teaspoon chili powder
4 cod fillets
Salt and black pepper to taste
1 tablespoon olive oil
1 garlic clove, minced
⅓ cup lemon juice
2 tablespoons vegetable stock
2 tablespoons chives, chopped

1. Preheat oven to 400ºF (205ºC) and grease a baking dish with cooking spray. Rub the cod fillets with chili powder, salt, and pepper and lay in the dish. Bake for 10-15 minutes.
2. In a skillet over low heat, warm olive oil and sauté garlic for 1 minute. Add lemon juice, vegetable stock, and chives. Season with salt, pepper, and cook for 3 minutes until the stock slightly reduces. Divide fish into 2 plates, top with sauce, and serve.

Per Serving
calories: 450 | fat: 35.2g | protein: 20.1g
carbs: 7.0g | net carbs: 6.4g | fiber: 0.6g

Lobster and Cauliflower Salad Rolls

Prep time: 15 minutes | Cook time: 0 minutes | Serves 4

5 cups cauliflower florets
1/3 cup celery, diced
2 cups large shrimp, cooked
1 tablespoon dill, chopped
½ cup mayonnaise
1 teaspoon apple cider vinegar
¼ teaspoon celery seeds
2 tablespoons lemon juice
2 teaspoons Swerve
Salt and black pepper to taste

1. Combine cauliflower, celery, shrimp, and dill in a large bowl. Whisk mayonnaise, vinegar, celery seeds, sweetener, and lemon juice in another bowl. Season with salt. Pour the dressing over the salad, and gently toss to combine. Serve cold.

Per Serving
calories: 181 | fat: 15.1g | protein: 11.9g
carbs: 5.4g | net carbs: 1.9g | fiber: 3.5g

Salmon with Radish and Arugula Salad

Prep time: 15 minutes | Cook time: 10 minutes | Serves 4

1 pound (454 g) salmon, cut into 4 steaks each
1 cup radishes, sliced
Salt and black pepper to taste
8 green olives, pitted and chopped
1 cup arugula
2 large tomatoes, diced
3 tablespoons red wine vinegar
2 green onions, sliced
3 tablespoons olive oil
2 slices zero carb bread, cubed
¼ cup parsley, chopped

1. In a bowl, mix the radishes, olives, black pepper, arugula, tomatoes, wine vinegar, green onion, olive oil, bread, and parsley. Let sit for the flavors to incorporate. Season the salmon steaks with salt and pepper; grill on both sides for 8 minutes in total. Serve the salmon on a bed of the radish salad.

Per Serving
calories: 339 | fat: 21.6g | protein: 28.4g
carbs: 5.3g | net carbs: 3.0g | fiber: 2.3g

Tuna Omelet Wraps

Prep time: 10 minutes | Cook time: 10 minutes | Serves 4

1 avocado, sliced
1 tablespoon chopped chives
1 cup canned tuna, drained
2 spring onions, sliced
8 eggs, beaten
4 tablespoons mascarpone cheese
1 tablespoon butter
Salt and black pepper, to taste

1. In a small bowl, combine the chives and mascarpone cheese; set aside. Melt the butter in a pan over medium heat. Add the eggs to the pan and cook for about 3 minutes. Flip the omelet over and continue cooking for another 2 minutes until golden. Season with salt and black pepper.
2. Remove the omelet to a plate and spread the chive mixture over. Arrange the tuna, avocado, and onion slices. Wrap the omelet and serve immediately.

Per Serving
calories: 480 | fat: 37.8g | protein: 26.8g
carbs: 9.9g | net carbs: 6.3g | fiber: 3.6g

Gambas al Ajillo

Prep time: 5 minutes | Cook time: 3 minutes | Serves 5

2 tablespoons butter
2 cloves garlic, minced
2 small cayenne pepper pods
2 pounds (907 g) shrimp, peeled and deveined
¼ cup Manzanilla
Sea salt and ground black pepper, to taste

1. Melt the butter in a sauté pan over moderate heat. Add the garlic and cayenne peppers and cook for 40 seconds.
2. Add the shrimp and cook for about a minute. Pour in the Manzanilla; season with salt and black pepper.
3. Continue to cook for a minute or so, until the shrimp are cooked through. Add lemon slices to each serving if desired. Enjoy!

Per Serving
calories: 203 | fat: 6g | protein: 37g
carbs: 2g | net carbs: 2g | fiber: 0g

Swedish Herring and Spinach Salad

Prep time: 10 minutes | Cook time: 0 minutes | Serves 3

6 ounces (170 g) pickled herring pieces, drained and flaked
½ cup baby spinach
2 tablespoons fresh basil leaves
2 tablespoons fresh chives, chopped
1 teaspoon garlic, minced
1 bell pepper, chopped
1 red onion, chopped
2 tablespoons key lime juice, freshly squeezed
Sea salt and ground black pepper, to taste

1. In a salad bowl, combine the herring pieces with spinach, basil leaves, chives, garlic, bell pepper, and red onion.
2. Then, drizzle key lime juice over the salad; add salt and pepper to taste and toss to combine. Smaklig maltid! Bon appétit!

Per Serving
calories: 134 | fat: 8g | protein: 10g
carbs: 5g | net carbs: 4g | fiber: 1g

Baked Tilapia with Black Olives

Prep time: 15 minutes | Cook time: 25 minutes | Serves 4

4 tilapia fillets
2 garlic cloves, minced
1 teaspoon basil, chopped
1 cup canned tomatoes
¼ tablespoon chili powder
2 tablespoons white wine
1 tablespoon olive oil
½ red onion, chopped
2 tablespoons parsley
10 black olives, pitted and halved

1. Preheat oven to 350°F (180°C).
2. Heat the olive oil in a skillet over medium heat and cook the onion and garlic for about 3 minutes. Stir in tomatoes, olives, chili powder, and white wine and bring the mixture to a boil. Reduce the heat and simmer for 5 minutes. Put the tilapia in a baking dish, pour over the sauce and bake in the oven for 10-15 minutes. Serve garnished with basil.

Per Serving
calories: 281 | fat: 15.0g | protein: 23.0g
carbs: 7.2g | net carbs: 6.0g | fiber: 1.2g

Garlicky Mackerel Fillet

Prep time: 5 minutes | Cook time: 5 minutes | Serves 2

1 tablespoon olive oil
2 mackerel fillets
2 garlic cloves, minced
Sea salt and ground
black pepper, to taste
½ teaspoon thyme
1 teaspoon rosemary
½ teaspoon basil

1. Heat the olive oil in a frying pan over a moderate flame and swirl to coat the bottom of the pan. Pat dry the mackerel fillets.
2. Now, brown the fish fillets for 5 minutes per side until golden and crisp, shaking the pan lightly.
3. During the last minutes, add the garlic, salt, black pepper, and herbs. Bon appétit!

Per Serving
calories: 481 | fat: 15g | protein: 80g
carbs: 1g | net carbs: 1g | fiber: 0g

Seared Scallops with Sausage

Prep time: 10 minutes | Cook time: 10 minutes | Serves 4

2 tablespoons butter
12 fresh scallops, rinsed
8 ounces (227 g) sausage, chopped
1 red bell pepper, sliced
1 red onion, finely chopped
1 cup Grana Padano, grated
Salt and black pepper to taste

1. Melt half of the butter in a skillet over medium heat, and cook the onion and bell pepper for 5 minutes until tender. Add the sausage and stir-fry for another 5 minutes. Remove and set aside.
2. Pat dry scallops with paper towels, and season with salt and pepper. Add the remaining butter to the skillet and sear scallops for 2 minutes on each side to have a golden brown color. Add the sausage mixture back, and warm through. Transfer to serving platter and top with Grana Padano cheese.

Per Serving
calories: 835 | fat: 61.9g | protein: 55.9g
carbs: 10.5g | net carbs: 9.4g | fiber: 1.1g

Tuna, Ham and Avocado Wraps

Prep time: 10 minutes | Cook time: 3 minutes | Serves 3

½ cup dry white wine
½ cup water
½ teaspoon mixed peppercorns
½ teaspoon dry mustard powder
½ pound Ahi tuna steak
6 slices of ham
½ Hass avocado, peeled, pitted and sliced
1 tablespoon fresh lemon juice
6 lettuce leaves

1. Add wine, water, peppercorns, and mustard powder to a skillet and bring to a boil. Add the tuna and simmer gently for 3 minutes to 5 minutes per side.
2. Discard the cooking liquid and slice tuna into bite-sized pieces. Divide the tuna pieces between slices of ham.
3. Add avocado and drizzle with fresh lemon. Roll the wraps up and place each wrap on a lettuce leaf. Serve well chilled. Bon appétit!

Per Serving
calories: 308 | fat: 20g | protein: 28g
carbs: 4g | net carbs: 1g | fiber: 3g

Anchovies and Veggies Wraps

Prep time: 10 minutes | Cook time: 0 minutes | Serves 4

2 (2-ounce / 57-g) can anchovies in olive oil, drained
1 cucumber, sliced
2 cups red cabbage, shredded
1 red onion, chopped
1 teaspoon Dijon mustard
4 tablespoons mayonnaise
¼ teaspoon ground black pepper
1 large-sized tomato, diced
12 lettuce leaves

1. In a mixing bowl, combine the anchovies with the cucumber, cabbage, onion, mustard, mayonnaise, black pepper, and tomatoes.
2. Arrange the lettuce leaves on a tray. Spoon the anchovy/vegetable mixture into the center of a lettuce leaf, taco-style.
3. Repeat until you run out of ingredients. Bon appétit!

Per Serving
calories: 191 | fat: 13g | protein: 3g
carbs: 10g | net carbs: 7g | fiber: 3g

Grilled Salmon Steak

Prep time: 5 minutes | Cook time: 10 minutes | Serves 4

4 (5-ounce / 142-g) salmon steaks
2 cloves garlic, pressed
4 tablespoons olive oil
1 tablespoon Taco seasoning mix
2 tablespoons fresh lemon juice

1. Place all of the above ingredients in a ceramic dish; cover and let it marinate for 40 minutes in your refrigerator.
2. Place the salmon steaks onto a lightly oiled grill pan; place under the grill for 6 minutes.
3. Turn them over and cook for a further 5 to 6 minutes, basting with the reserved marinade; remove from the grill.
4. Serve immediately and enjoy!

Per Serving
calories: 331 | fat: 21g | protein: 30g
carbs: 2g | net carbs: 2g | fiber: 0g

Tiger Shrimp with Chimichurri

Prep time: 15 minutes | Cook time: 35 minutes | Serves 4

1 pound (454 g) tiger shrimp, peeled and deveined
2 tablespoons olive oil
Chimichurri:
Salt and black pepper to taste
¼ cup extra-virgin olive oil
2 garlic cloves, minced
1 lime, juiced
1 garlic clove, minced
Juice of 1 lime
Salt and black pepper to taste
¼ cup red wine vinegar
2 cups parsley, minced
¼ teaspoon red pepper flakes

1. Combine the shrimp, olive oil, garlic, and lime juice, in a bowl, and let marinate in the fridge for 30 minutes. To make the chimichurri dressing, blitz the chimichurri ingredients in a blender until smooth; set aside. Preheat your grill to medium. Add shrimp and cook about 2 minutes per side. Serve shrimp drizzled with the chimichurri dressing.

Per Serving
calories: 524 | fat: 30.2g | protein: 48.8g
carbs: 8.3g | net carbs: 7.1g | fiber: 1.2g

Mediterranean Halibut Fillet

Prep time: 5 minutes | Cook time: 30 minutes | Serves 4

1½ pounds (680 g) halibut fillets
2 tablespoons olive oil
2 tablespoons fresh lemon juice
1 tablespoon Greek seasoning blend
½ cup Kalamata olives, pitted and sliced

1. Start by preheating your oven to 380ºF (193ºC).
2. Toss the halibut fillets with the olive oil, fresh lemon juice, and Greek seasoning blend. Arrange the halibut fillets in a baking pan and cover with foil.
3. Bake approximately 30 minutes, flipping once or twice.
4. Garnish with Kalamata olives and serve warm. Bon appétit!

Per Serving
calories: 397 | fat: 32g | protein: 25g
carbs: 2g | net carbs: 1g | fiber: 1g

Goan Sole Fillet Stew

Prep time: 5 minutes | Cook time: 20 minutes | Serves 3

1 tablespoon butter, at room temperature
1 shallot, chopped
1 teaspoon curry paste
1 cup tomatoes, pureed
¾ pound (340 g) sole fillets, cut into 1-inch pieces

1. Melt the butter in a stockpot over a medium-high flame. Sauté the shallot until softened.
2. Add the curry paste and pureed tomatoes along with 2 cups of water to the pot; bring to a rolling boil.
3. Immediately reduce the heat to medium-low and continue to simmer, covered, for 12 minutes longer; make sure to stir periodically.
4. Fold in the chopped sole fillets; continue to cook for a further 8 minutes or until the fish flakes easily with a fork. Enjoy!

Per Serving
calories: 191 | fat: 9g | protein: 24g
carbs: 3g | net carbs: 2g | fiber: 1g

Parsley-Lemon Salmon

Prep time: 10 minutes | Cook time: 20 minutes | Serves 4

4 salmon fillets
½ cup heavy cream
1 tablespoon mayonnaise
½ tablespoon parsley, chopped
½ lemon, zested and juiced
Salt and black pepper to season
1 tablespoon Parmesan cheese, grated

1. In a bowl, mix the heavy cream, parsley, mayonnaise, lemon zest, lemon juice, salt and pepper, and set aside. Season the fish with salt and black pepper, drizzle lemon juice on both sides of the fish and arrange them in a parchment paper–lined baking sheet. Spread the parsley mixture and sprinkle with Parmesan cheese. Bake in the oven for 15 minutes at 400ºF (205ºC). Great served with steamed broccoli.

Per Serving
calories: 555 | fat: 30.3g | protein: 56.1g
carbs: 2.2g | net carbs: 2.1g | fiber: 0.1g

Spanish Cod à La Nage

Prep time: 5 minutes | Cook time: 15 minutes | Serves 5

2 tablespoons olive oil
1 Spanish onion, chopped
1 medium-sized zucchini, diced
1 vine-ripe tomatoes, pureed
1½ pounds (680 g) cod fish fillets

1. Heat the olive oil in a stockpot over medium-high flame. Now, cook the Spanish onion until tender and translucent.
2. Pour in the pureed tomatoes along with 2 cups of water. Bring to a boil and reduce the heat to medium-low. Let it simmer an additional 10 to 13 minutes.
3. Now, fold in the cod fish fillets. Cook, covered, an additional 5 to 6 minutes or until the codfish is just cooked through and an instant-read thermometer registers 140 ºF (60ºC).
4. Place the fish in individual bowls; ladle the fish broth over each serving, and serve hot. Enjoy!

Per Serving
calories: 177 | fat: 6g | protein: 25g
carbs: 4g | net carbs: 3g | fiber: 1g

Asian Scallop and Vegetable

Prep time: 10 minutes | Cook time: 5 minutes | Serves 4

4 teaspoons sesame oil
½ cup yellow onion, sliced
1 cup asparagus spears, sliced
½ cup celery, chopped
½ cup enoki mushrooms
1 pound (454 g) bay scallops
1 tablespoon fresh parsley, chopped
Kosher salt and ground black pepper, to taste
½ teaspoon red pepper flakes, crushed
1 tablespoon coconut aminos
2 tablespoons rice wine
½ cup dry roasted peanuts, roughly chopped

1. Heat 1 teaspoon of the sesame oil in a wok over a medium-high flame. Now, fry the onion until crisp-tender and translucent; reserve.
2. Heat another teaspoon of the sesame oil and fry the asparagus and celery for about 3 minutes until crisp-tender; reserve.
3. Then, heat another teaspoon of the sesame oil and cook the mushrooms for 2 minutes more or until they start to soften; reserve.
4. Lastly, heat the remaining teaspoon of sesame oil and cook the bay scallops just until they are opaque.
5. Return all reserved vegetables to the wok. Add in the remaining ingredients and toss to combine. Serve warm and enjoy!

Per Serving
calories: 236 | fat: 13g | protein: 27g
carbs: 6g | net carbs: 4g | fiber: 2g

Shrimp and Vegetable Bowl

Prep time: 10 minutes | Cook time: 4 minutes | Serves 4

2 pounds (907 g) large shrimp, peeled and deveined
1 teaspoon cayenne pepper
Sea salt and freshly ground black pepper, to taste
1 red onion, sliced
2 garlic cloves, sliced
2 Italian peppers, sliced
1 tablespoon fresh lemon juice
2 tablespoons olive oil
1 cup arugula

1. Gently pat the shrimp dry with a paper towel. Add the cayenne pepper, salt, black pepper, and toss to evenly coat.
2. Grill the shrimp over medium-high heat for 2 minutes; flip them and cook for a further 2 minutes.
3. Transfer to a bowl; add in the remaining ingredients and toss to combine. Serve immediately.

Per Serving
calories: 268 | fat: 8g | protein: 46g
carbs: 4g | net carbs: 3g | fiber: 1g

Shrimp and Pork Rind Stuffed Zucchini

Prep time: 15 minutes | Cook time: 25 minutes | Serves 4

4 medium zucchinis
1 pound (454 g) small shrimp, peeled, deveined
1 tablespoon minced onion
2 teaspoons butter
¼ cup chopped tomatoes
Salt and black pepper to taste
1 cup pork rinds, crushed
1 tablespoon chopped basil leaves
2 tablespoons melted butter

1. Preheat the oven to 350ºF (180ºC) and trim off the top and bottom ends of the zucchinis. Lay them flat on a chopping board, and cut a ¼-inch off the top to create a boat for the stuffing. Scoop out the seeds with a spoon and set the zucchinis aside.
2. Melt the firm butter in a small skillet and sauté the onion and tomato for 6 minutes. Transfer the mixture to a bowl and add the shrimp, half of the pork rinds, basil leaves, salt, and black pepper.
3. Combine the ingredients and stuff the zucchini boats with the mixture. Sprinkle the top of the boats with the remaining pork rinds and drizzle the melted butter over them.
4. Place on a baking sheet and bake for 15 to 20 minutes. The shrimp should no longer be pink by this time. Remove the zucchinis after and serve with a tomato and Mozzarella salad.

Per Serving
calories: 136 | fat: 14.2g | protein: 24.4g
carbs: 3.4g | net carbs: 3.1g | fiber: 0.3g

Red Snapper Fillet and Salad

Prep time: 10 minutes | Cook time: 18 minutes | Serves 4

1 pound (454 g) red snapper fillets
5 eggs
1 bell pepper, deseeded and sliced
1 tomato, sliced
1 cucumber, sliced
2 scallions, sliced
½ cup radishes, sliced
4 cups lettuce salad
4 tablespoons olive oil
4 tablespoons apple cider vinegar
½ cup Kalamata olives, pitted and halved

1. Steam the red snapper fillets until done and cooked through, approximately 10 minutes. Slice the fish fillets into bite-sized strips.
2. Cook the eggs in a saucepan for about 8 minutes; peel the eggs under running water and carefully slice them.
3. Place your veggies in a salad bowl; add the olive oil and vinegar and toss to combine. Top with the fish and boiled eggs. Salt to taste.
4. Garnish with Kalamata olives and serve well-chilled or at room temperature. Bon appétit!

Per Serving
calories: 300 | fat: 19g | protein: 27g
carbs: 4g | net carbs: 3g | fiber: 1g

Hazelnut Haddock Bake

Prep time: 15 minutes | Cook time: 25 minutes | Serves 4

1 tablespoon butter
1 shallot, sliced
1 pound (454 g) haddock fillet
2 eggs, hard-boiled, chopped
½ cup water
3 tablespoons hazelnut flour
2 cups sour cream
1 tablespoon parsley, chopped
½ cup pork rinds, crushed
1 cup Mozzarella cheese, grated
Salt and black pepper to taste

1. Melt butter in a saucepan over medium heat and sauté the shallots for about 3 minutes.
2. Reduce the heat to low and stir the hazelnut flour into it to form a roux. Cook the roux to be golden brown and stir in the sour cream until the mixture is smooth. Season with salt and pepper, and stir in the parsley.
3. Spread the haddock fillet in a greased baking dish, sprinkle the eggs on top, and spoon the sauce over. In a bowl, mix the pork rinds with the Mozzarella cheese, and sprinkle it over the sauce.
4. Bake in the oven for 20 minutes at 370°F (188°C) until the top is golden and the sauce and cheese are bubbly.

Per Serving
calories: 786 | fat: 56.9g | protein: 64.9g
carbs: 9.5g | net carbs: 8.4g | fiber: 1.1g

Provençal Lemony Fish Stew

Prep time: 15 minutes | Cook time: 6 minutes | Serves 2

1 tablespoon olive oil
1 shallot, sliced
3 garlic cloves, minced
1 cup tomato purée
5 cups white fish stock
1 teaspoon basil
½ teaspoon rosemary
½ California bay leaf
⅓ teaspoon saffron threads, crumbled
Sea salt and freshly
cracked black pepper, to taste
1 pound (454 g) grouper fish
⅓ pound (151 g) cockles, scrubbed
⅓ pound (151 g) prawns
1 tablespoon fresh lemon juice

1. Heat the olive oil in a stockpot over a moderate flame. Now, sauté the shallot for 3 minutes or until tender; add in the garlic and cook an additional 30 seconds or until aromatic.
2. Pour in the tomato purée and white fish stock; bring everything to a boil. Stir in the basil, rosemary, California bay leaf, saffron threads, salt, and black pepper.
3. Turn the heat to medium-low. Fold in the grouper and cockles; gently stir to combine and allow it to simmer for 2 to 3 minutes. Next, add in the prawns; continue to simmer for 3 minutes more or until everything is thoroughly warmed.
4. Drizzle each serving with fresh lemon juice and enjoy!

Per Serving
calories: 176 | fat: 5g | protein: 24g
carbs: 5g | net carbs: 4g | fiber: 1g

Shirataki Noodles with Grilled Tuna

Prep time: 10 minutes | Cook time: 25 minutes | Serves 4

1 (7-ounce / 198-g) pack shirataki noodles
3 cups water
1 red bell pepper, seeded and halved
4 tuna steaks
Salt and black pepper to taste
Olive oil for brushing
2 tablespoons pickled ginger
2 tablespoons chopped cilantro

1. In a colander, rinse the shirataki noodles with running cold water. Bring a pot of salted water to a boil; blanch the noodles for 2 minutes. Drain and transfer to a dry skillet over medium heat. Dry roast for a minute until opaque.
2. Grease a grill's grate with cooking spray and preheat on medium heat. Season the red bell pepper and tuna with salt and black pepper, brush with olive oil, and grill covered. Cook both for 3 minutes on each side. Transfer to a plate to cool. Dice bell pepper with a knife.
3. Assemble the noodles, tuna, and bell pepper in serving plate. Top with pickled ginger and garnish with cilantro. Serve with roasted sesame sauce.

Per Serving
calories: 312 | fat: 18.3g | protein: 22.1g
carbs: 2.5g | net carbs: 1.8g | fiber: 0.7g

Almond Breaded Hoki

Prep time: 15 minutes | Cook time: 25 minutes | Serves 4

1 cup flaked smoked hoki, bones removed
1 cup cubed hoki fillets, cubed
4 eggs
1 cup water
3 tablespoons almond flour
1 onion, sliced
2 cups sour cream
1 tablespoon chopped parsley
1 cup pork rinds, crushed
1 cup grated Cheddar cheese
Salt and black pepper to taste
2 tablespoons butter

1. Preheat the oven to 360ºF (182ºC) and lightly grease a baking dish with cooking spray.
2. Then, boil the eggs in water in a pot over medium heat to be well done for 10 minutes, run the eggs under cold water and peel the shells. After, place on a cutting board and chop them.
3. Melt the butter in a saucepan over medium heat and sauté the onion for 4 minutes. Turn the heat off and stir in the almond flour to form a roux. Turn the heat back on and cook the roux to be golden brown and stir in the cream until the mixture is smooth. Season with salt and black pepper, and stir in the parsley.
4. Spread the smoked and cubed fish in the baking dish, sprinkle the eggs on top, and spoon the sauce over. In a bowl, mix the pork rinds with the Cheddar cheese, and sprinkle it over the sauce.
5. Bake the casserole in the oven for 20 minutes until the top is golden and the sauce and cheese are bubbly. Remove the bake after and serve with a steamed green vegetable mix.

Per Serving
calories: 384 | fat: 27.1g | protein: 28.4g
carbs: 3.9g | net carbs: 3.6g | fiber: 0.3g

Asparagus and Trout Foil Packets

Prep time: 15 minutes | Cook time: 15 minutes | Serves 4

1 pound (454 g) asparagus spears
1 tablespoon garlic purée
1 pound (454 g) deboned trout, butterflied
Salt and black pepper to taste
3 tablespoons olive oil
2 sprigs rosemary
2 sprigs thyme
2 tablespoons butter
½ medium red onion, sliced
2 lemon slices

1. Preheat the oven to 400ºF (205ºC). Rub the trout with garlic purée, salt and black pepper.
2. Prepare two aluminum foil squares. Place the fish on each square. Divide the asparagus and onion between the squares, top with a pinch of salt and pepper, a sprig of rosemary and thyme, and 1 tablespoon of butter. Also, lay the lemon slices on the fish. Wrap and close the fish packets securely, and place them on a baking sheet. Bake in the oven for 15 minutes, and remove once ready.

Per Serving
calories: 495 | fat: 39.2g | protein: 26.9g
carbs: 7.5g | net carbs: 4.9g | fiber: 2.6g

Coconut and Pecorino Fried Shrimp

Prep time: 15 minutes | Cook time: 10 minutes | Serves 4

2 teaspoons coconut flour
2 tablespoons grated Pecorino cheese
1 egg, beaten in a bowl
¼ teaspoon curry powder
1 pound (454 g) shrimp, shelled
3 tablespoons coconut oil
Salt to taste

Sauce:
2 tablespoons butter
2 tablespoons cilantro leaves, chopped
½ onion, diced
½ cup coconut cream
½ ounce (14 g) Paneer cheese, grated

1. Combine coconut flour, Pecorino cheese, curry powder, and salt in a bowl.
2. Melt the coconut oil in a skillet over medium heat. Dip the shrimp in the egg first, and then coat with the dry mixture. Fry until golden and crispy, about 5 minutes.
3. In another skillet, melt the butter. Add onion and cook for 3 minutes. Add curry and cilantro and cook for 30 seconds. Stir in coconut cream and Paneer cheese and cook until thickened. Add the shrimp and coat well. Serve warm.

Per Serving
calories: 740 | fat: 63.8g | protein: 34.2g
carbs: 5.2g | net carbs:4.2 g | fiber: 1.0g

Seafood Chowder

Prep time: 10 minutes | Cook time: 20 minutes | Serves 4

2 tablespoons coconut oil
2 garlic cloves, pressed
1 shallot, chopped
1 cup broccoli, broken into small florets
1 bell peppers, chopped
4 cups fish broth
4 tablespoons dry sherry
6 ounces (170 g) scallops
6 ounces (170 g) shrimp, peeled and deveined
1 cup heavy cream
1 tablespoon fresh chives, chopped

1. Melt the coconut oil in a soup pot over a moderate flame. Now, cook the garlic and shallot for 3 to 4 minutes or until they have softened.
2. Stir in the broccoli florets, bell peppers, and fish broth; bring to a boil. Turn the heat to medium-low, partially cover, and let it cook for 12 minutes more.
3. Add in the dry sherry, scallops, shrimp, and heavy cream. Continue to cook an additional 7 minutes or until heated through.
4. Taste and adjust the seasonings. Serve garnished with fresh chives. Bon appétit!

Per Serving
calories: 272 | fat: 20g | protein: 17g
carbs: 7g | net carbs: 6g | fiber: 1g

Curry White Fish Fillet

Prep time: 10 minutes | Cook time: 15 minutes | Serves 6

2 tablespoons sesame oil
1 shallot, chopped
2 bell peppers, deveined and sliced
1 teaspoon coriander, ground
1 teaspoon cumin, ground
4 tablespoons red curry paste
1 teaspoon ginger-garlic paste
1 ½ pounds (680 g) white fish fillets, skinless, boneless
½ cup tomato purée
½ cup haddi ka shorba (Indian bone broth)
1 cup coconut milk
½ teaspoon red chili powder
Kosher salt and ground black pepper, to taste

1. Heat the sesame oil in a saucepan over moderate heat; then, sauté the shallot and peppers until they have softened or about 4 minutes.
2. Now, stir in the coriander, cumin, red curry paste, and ginger-garlic paste; continue to sauté an additional 4 minutes, stirring frequently.
3. After that, fold in the fish and tomato purée; pour in the haddi ka shorba and coconut milk. Season with red chili powder, salt, and black pepper.
4. Turn the heat to simmer and let it cook for 5 minutes longer or until everything is cooked through. Enjoy!

Per Serving
calories: 349 | fat: 25g | protein: 23g
carbs: 6g | net carbs: 3g | fiber: 4g

Sardine Burgers

Prep time: 10 minutes | Cook time: 6 minutes | Serves 3

2 (5.5-ounce / 156-g) canned sardines, drained
2 ounces (57 g) Romano cheese, preferably freshly grated
1 egg, beaten
3 tablespoons flaxseed meal
1 tablespoon dry Italian seasoning blend
1 teaspoon fresh garlic, peeled and minced
½ onion, chopped
½ teaspoon celery salt
Freshly ground black pepper, to taste
½ teaspoon smoked paprika
2 tablespoons butter

1. In a mixing dish, thoroughly combine the sardines with the cheese, egg, flaxseed meal, dry Italian seasoning blend, garlic, and onion.
2. Season with the celery salt, black pepper, and smoked paprika. Form the mixture into six equal patties.
3. Melt the butter in a frying pan over a moderate flame. Once hot, fry the fish burgers for 4 to
4. 6 minutes on each side. Serve garnished with fresh lemon slices. Bon appétit!

Per Serving
calories: 267 | fat: 21g | protein: 14g
carbs: 6g | net carbs: 2g | fiber: 3g

Coconut Mussel Curry

Prep time: 15 minutes | Cook time: 20 minutes | Serves 4

2 tablespoons cup coconut oil
2 green onions, chopped
1 pound (454 g) mussels, cleaned, de-bearded
1 shallot, chopped
1 garlic clove, minced
½ cup coconut milk
½ cup white wine
1 teaspoon red curry powder
2 tablespoons parsley, chopped

1. Cook the shallots and garlic in the wine over low heat. Stir in the coconut milk and red curry powder and cook for 3 minutes.
2. Add the mussels and steam for 7 minutes or until their shells are opened. Then, use a slotted spoon to remove to a bowl leaving the sauce in the pan. Discard any closed mussels at this point.
3. Stir the coconut oil into the sauce, turn the heat off, and stir in the parsley and green onions. Serve the sauce immediately with a butternut squash mash.

Per Serving
calories: 354 | fat: 20.4g | protein: 21.0g
carbs: 2.2g | net carbs: 0.2g | fiber: 2.0g

Old Bay Sea Bass Fillet

Prep time: 10 minutes | Cook time: 15 minutes | Serves 6

2 tablespoons butter, at room temperature
1 leek, chopped
1 bell pepper, chopped
1 serrano pepper, chopped
2 garlic cloves, minced
2 tablespoons fresh coriander, chopped
2 vine-ripe tomatoes, pureed
4 cups fish stock
2 pounds (907 g) sea bass fillets, chopped into small chunks
1 tablespoon Old Bay seasoning
½ teaspoon sea salt, to taste
1 bay laurels

1. Melt the butter in a heavy-bottomed pot over moderate heat. Stir in the leek and peppers and sauté them for about 5 minutes or until tender.
2. Stir in the garlic and continue to sauté for 30 to 40 seconds more.
3. Add in the remaining ingredients; gently stir to combine. Turn the heat to medium-low and partially cover the pot.
4. Now, let it cook until thoroughly heated, approximately 10 minutes longer. Lastly, discard the bay laurels and serve warm. Bon appétit!

Per Serving
calories: 227 | fat: 8g | protein: 32g
carbs: 5g | net carbs: 4g | fiber: 1g

Cheesy Shrimp Stuffed Mushrooms

Prep time: 10 minutes | Cook time: 17 minutes | Serves 6

1 tablespoon butter
1 yellow onion, finely minced
1 cloves garlic, minced
Flaky salt and ground black pepper, to taste
16 ounces (454 g) fresh Bay shrimp, chopped
8 ounces (227 g) ricotta cheese, softened
6 tablespoons mayonnaise
1 ½ pounds (680 g) large-sized button mushroom cups
1 cup cheddar cheese, shredded

1. Melt the butter in a frying pan over moderate heat. Then, sauté the onion and garlic for 2 to 3 minutes or until just tender and fragrant.
2. Stir in the salt, black pepper, fresh Bay shrimp, ricotta cheese, and mayo; gently stir to combine well.
3. Bake the mushroom cups in the preheated oven at 390ºF (199ºC) until they have softened slightly.
4. Spoon the shrimp mixture into each mushroom cup. Return to the oven and bake for 8 to 11 minutes more. Top each mushroom cup with cheddar cheese.
5. Bake for a further 7 minutes or until bubbly. Bon appétit!

Per Serving
calories: 354 | fat: 24g | protein: 28g
carbs: 5g | net carbs: 3g | fiber: 2g

Fennel and Trout Parcels

Prep time: 10 minutes | Cook time: 15 minutes | Serves 4

½ pound (227 g) deboned trout, butterflied
Salt and black pepper to season
3 tablespoons olive oil plus extra for tossing
4 sprigs rosemary
4 sprigs thyme
4 butter cubes
1 cup thinly sliced fennel
1 medium red onion, sliced
8 lemon slices
3 teaspoons capers to garnish

1. Preheat the oven to 400ºF (205ºC). Cut out parchment paper wide enough for each trout. In a bowl, toss the fennel and onion with a little bit of olive oil and share into the middle parts of the papers.
2. Place the fish on each veggie mound, top with a drizzle of olive oil each, a pinch of salt and black pepper, a sprig of rosemary and thyme, and 1 cube of butter. Also, lay the lemon slices on the fish. Wrap and close the fish packets securely, and place them on a baking sheet. Bake in the oven for 15 minutes, and remove once ready. Plate them and garnish the fish with capers and serve with a squash mash.

Per Serving
calories: 235 | fat: 9.1g | protein: 17.1g
carbs: 3.7g | net carbs: 2.7g | fiber: 1.0g

Salmon and Cucumber Panzanella

Prep time: 15 minutes | Cook time: 10 minutes | Serves 4

1 pound (454 g) skinned salmon, cut into 4 steaks each
1 cucumber, peeled, seeded, cubed
Salt and black pepper to taste
8 black olives, pitted and chopped
1 tablespoon capers, rinsed
2 large tomatoes, diced
3 tablespoons red wine vinegar
¼ cup thinly sliced red onion
3 tablespoons olive oil
2 slices zero carb bread, cubed
¼ cup thinly sliced basil leaves

1. Preheat a grill to 350ºF (180ºC) and prepare the salad. In a bowl, mix the cucumbers, olives, pepper, capers, tomatoes, wine vinegar, onion, olive oil, bread, and basil leaves. Let sit for the flavors to incorporate.
2. Season the salmon steaks with salt and pepper; grill them on both sides for 8 minutes in total. Serve the salmon steaks warm on a bed of the veggies' salad.

Per Serving
calories: 339 | fat: 21.6g | protein: 28.6g
carbs: 5.3g | net carbs: 3.2g | fiber: 2.1g

Shrimp Jambalaya

Prep time: 5 minutes | Cook time: 20 minutes | Serves 4

1 shallot, chopped
1 cup ham, cut into 1/2-inch cubes
1½ cups tomatoes, crushed
1½ cups vegetable broth
¾ pound (340 g) shrimp

1. Heat up a lightly greased soup pot over a moderate flame. Now, sauté the shallots until they have softened or about 4 minutes.
2. Add in the ham, tomatoes, and vegetable broth and bring to a boil. Turn the heat to simmer, cover and continue to cook for 13 minutes longer.
3. Fold in the shrimp and continue to simmer until they are thoroughly cooked and the cooking liquid has thickened slightly, about 3 to 4 minutes.
4. Serve in individual bowls and enjoy!

Per Serving
calories: 170 | fat: 5g | protein: 26g carbs: 6g | net carbs: 5g | fiber: 1g

Thai Tuna Fillet

Prep time: 15 minutes | Cook time: 20 minutes | Serves 4

1 tablespoon peanut oil
4 tuna fillets
1 teaspoon freshly grated ginger
Kosher salt and freshly ground black pepper,
Sauce:
1 scallions, chopped
2 garlic cloves, minced
1 tablespoon fresh cilantro, chopped
1 teaspoon Sriracha sauce
to taste
1 teaspoon cayenne pepper
½ teaspoon cumin seeds
¼ teaspoon ground cinnamon
4 tablespoons mayonnaise
½ cup sour cream
1 teaspoon stone-ground mustard

1. Preheat your oven to 375ºF (190ºC). Line a baking sheet with foil.
2. Place the tuna fillets onto the prepared baking sheet; now, fold up all 4 sides of the foil.
3. Add peanut oil, grated ginger, salt, black pepper, cayenne pepper, cumin, and cinnamon.
4. Fold the sides of the foil over the fish fillets, sealing the packet. Bake until cooked through, approximately 20 minutes.
5. To make the sauce, whisk together all of the sauce ingredients. Serve immediately and enjoy!

Per Serving
calories: 389 | fat: 18g | protein: 50g carbs: 4g | net carbs: 4g | fiber: 0g

Alaskan Cod Fillet

Prep time: 10 minutes | Cook time: 2 minutes | Serves 4

1 tablespoon coconut oil
4 Alaskan cod fillets
Salt and freshly ground black pepper,
Sauce:
1 teaspoon yellow mustard
1 teaspoon paprika
¼ teaspoon ground bay leaf
3 tablespoons cream cheese
½ cup Greek-style
to taste
6 leaves basil, chiffonade Mustard Cream
yogurt
1 garlic clove, minced
1 teaspoon lemon zest
1 tablespoon fresh parsley, minced
Sea salt and ground black pepper, to taste

1. Heat coconut oil in a pan over medium heat. Sear the fish for 2 to 3 minutes per side. Season with salt and ground black pepper.
2. Mix all ingredients for the sauce until everything is well combined. Top the fish fillets with the sauce and serve garnished with fresh basil leaves. Bon appétit!

Per Serving
calories: 166 | fat: 8g | protein: 20g carbs: 3g | net carbs: 3g | fiber: 0g

Catfish Flakes and Cauliflower Casserole

Prep time: 10 minutes | Cook time: 25 minutes | Serves 4

1 tablespoon sesame oil	1 sprigs dried thyme, crushed
11 ounces (312 g) cauliflower	1 sprig rosemary, crushed
4 scallions	24 ounces (680 g) catfish, cut into pieces
1 garlic clove, minced	½ cup cream cheese
1 teaspoon fresh ginger root, grated	½ cup heavy cream
Salt and ground black pepper, to taste	1 egg
Cayenne pepper, to taste	1 ounce (28 g) butter, cold

1. Start by preheating your oven to 390°F (199°C). Now, lightly grease a casserole dish with a nonstick cooking spray.
2. Then, heat the oil in a pan over medium-high heat; once hot, cook the cauliflower and scallions until tender or 5 to 6 minutes. Add the garlic and ginger; continue to sauté 1 minute more.
3. Transfer the vegetables to the prepared casserole dish. Sprinkle with seasonings. Add catfish to the top.
4. In a mixing bowl, thoroughly combine the cream cheese, heavy cream, and egg. Spread this creamy mixture over the top of your casserole.
5. Top with slices of butter. Bake in the preheated oven for 18 to 22 minutes or until the fish flakes easily with a fork. Bon appétit!

Per Serving
calories: 510 | fat: 40g | protein: 31g carbs: 6g | net carbs: 4g | fiber: 2g

Smoked Haddock Burgers

Prep time: 10 minutes | Cook time: 6 minutes | Serves 4

2 tablespoons extra virgin olive oil	1 teaspoon dried parsley flakes
8 ounces (227 g) smoked haddock	¼ cup scallions, chopped
1 egg	1 teaspoon fresh garlic, minced
¼ cup Parmesan cheese, grated	Salt and ground black pepper, to taste
1 teaspoon chili powder	4 lemon wedges

1. Heat 1 tablespoon of oil in a pan over medium-high heat. Cook the haddock for 6 minutes or until just cooked through; discard the skin and bones and flake into small pieces.
2. Mix the smoked haddock, egg, cheese, chili powder, parsley, scallions, garlic, salt, and black pepper in a large bowl.
3. Heat the remaining tablespoon of oil and cook fish burgers until they are well cooked in the middle or about 6 minutes. Garnish each serving with a lemon wedge.

Per Serving
calories: 174 | fat: 11g | protein: 15g carbs: 2g | net carbs: 2g | fiber: 0g

Cod Patties with Creamed Horseradish

Prep time: 10 minutes | Cook time: 13 minutes | Serves 4

1 pound (454 g) cod fillets	4 tablespoons parmesan cheese, grated
2 eggs, beaten	2 tablespoons olive oil
1 tablespoon flax seeds meal	
Sauce:	
4 tablespoons mayonnaise	horseradish
4 tablespoons Ricotta cheese	2 green onions, chopped
1 teaspoon creamed	1 tablespoon fresh basil, chopped

1. Steam the cod fillets until done and cooked through, approximately 10 minutes. Flake the fish with a fork; add in the beaten eggs, flax seeds meal, and parmesan.
2. Shape the mixture into 4 equal patties. Heat the olive oil in a nonstick skillet. Fry the fish patties over moderate heat for 3 minutes per side.
3. In the meantime, whisk the sauce ingredients until everything is well incorporated. Bon appétit!

Per Serving
calories: 346 | fat: 23g | protein: 26g carbs: 7g | net carbs: 6g | fiber: 1g

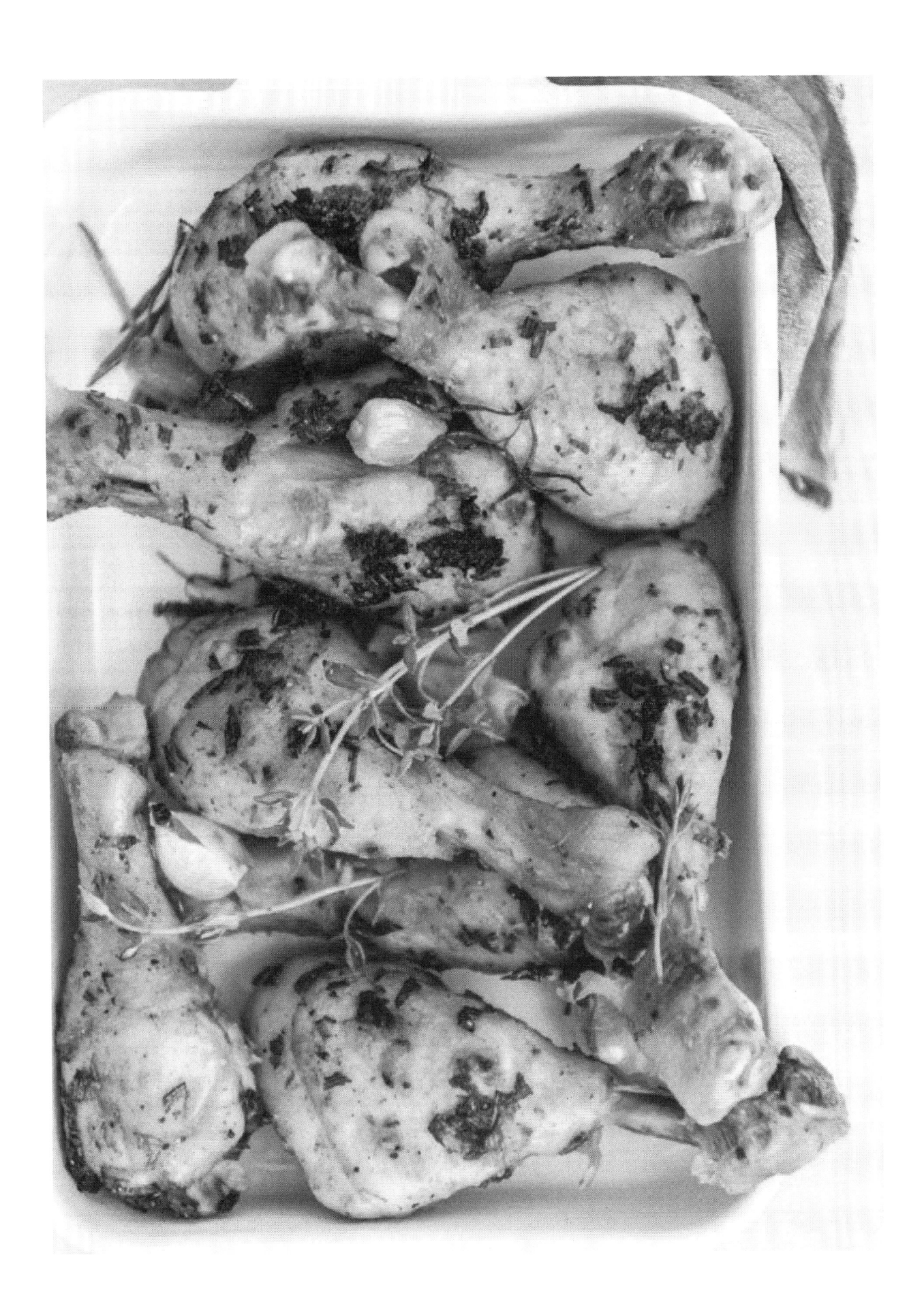

Chapter 8 Poultry

Tikka Masala

Prep time: 10 minutes | Cook time: 25 minutes | Serves 5

1½ pounds (680 g) chicken breasts, cut into bite-sized pieces
1 onion, chopped
10 ounces (283 g) tomato purée
1 teaspoon garam masala
½ cup heavy cream

1. Heat a wok that is greased with a nonstick cooking spray over medium-high heat. Now, sear the chicken breasts until golden brown on all sides.
2. Add the onions and sauté them for 2 to 3 minutes more or until tender and fragrant. Stir in the tomato purée and garam masala. Cook for 10 minutes until the sauce turns into a dark red color.
3. Fold in the heavy cream and stir to combine. Cook for 10 to 13 minutes more or until heated through.
4. Serve with cauliflower rice if desired and enjoy!

Per Serving
calories: 293 | fat: 17.1g | protein: 29.1g
carbs: 4.8g | net carbs: 3.6g | fiber: 1.2g

Italian Turkey Meatballs with Leeks

Prep time: 10 minutes | Cook time: 20 minutes | Serves 4

1 pound (454 g) ground turkey
1 tablespoon Italian seasoning blend
2 cloves garlic, minced
½ cup leeks, minced
1 egg

1. Throw all ingredients into a mixing bowl; mix to combine well.
2. Form the mixture into bite-sized balls and arrange them on a parchment-lined baking pan. Spritz the meatballs with cooking spray.
3. Bake in the preheated oven at 400ºF (205ºC) for 18 to 22 minutes. Serve with cocktail sticks and enjoy!

Per Serving
calories: 217 | fat: 11.1g | protein: 24.1g
carbs: 3.4g | net carbs: 2.8g | fiber: 0.6g

Grilled Lemony Chicken Wings

Prep time: 10 minutes | Cook time: 12 minutes | Serves 4

2 pounds (907 g) chicken wings
Juice from 1 lemon
½ cup fresh parsley, chopped
2 garlic cloves, peeled and minced
1 Serrano pepper, chopped
1 tablespoon olive oil
Salt and black pepper, to taste
Lemon wedges, for serving
Ranch dip, for serving
½ teaspoon cilantro

In a bowl, stir together lemon juice, garlic, salt, serrano pepper, cilantro, olive oil, and black pepper. Place in the chicken wings and toss well to coat. Refrigerate for 2 hours. Set a grill over high heat and add on the chicken wings; cook each side for 6 minutes. Remove to a plate and serve alongside lemon wedges and ranch dip.

Per Serving
calories: 326 | fat: 12g | protein: 50g
carbs: 3g | net carbs: 2g | fiber: 1g

Simple White Wine Drumettes

Prep time: 10 minutes | Cook time: 35 minutes | Serves 4

1 pound (454 g) chicken drumettes
1 tablespoon olive oil
2 tablespoons butter, melted
1 garlic cloves, sliced
Fresh juice of ½ lemon
2 tablespoons white wine
Salt and ground black pepper, to taste
1 tablespoon fresh scallions, chopped

1. Start by preheating your oven to 450ºF (235ºC). Place the chicken in a parchment-lined baking pan. Drizzle with olive oil and melted butter.
2. Add the garlic, lemon, wine, salt, and black pepper.
3. Bake in the preheated oven for about 35 minutes. Serve garnished with fresh scallions. Enjoy!

Per Serving
calories: 210 | fat: 12.3g | protein: 23.3g
carbs: 0.5g | net carbs: 0.4g | fiber: 0.1g

Asian Turkey and Bird's Eye Soup

Prep time: 10 minutes | Cook time: 15 minutes | Serves 5

2 tablespoons canola oil
2 Oriental sweets peppers, deseeded and chopped
1 Bird's eye chili, deseeded and chopped
2 green onions, chopped
5 cups vegetable broth
1 pound (454 g) turkey thighs, deboned and cut into halves
½ teaspoon five-spice powder
1 teaspoon oyster sauce
Kosher salt, to taste

1. Heat the olive oil in a stockpot over a moderate flame. Then, sauté the peppers and onions until they have softened or about 4 minutes
2. Add in the other ingredients and bring to a boil. Turn the heat to simmer, cover, and continue to cook an additional 12 minutes.
3. Ladle into individual bowls and serve warm. Enjoy!

Per Serving
calories: 180 | fat: 7.5g | protein: 21.4g
carbs: 6.7g | net carbs: 5.5g | fiber: 1.2g

Turkey and Canadian Bacon Pizza

Prep time: 10 minutes | Cook time: 32 minutes | Serves 4

½ pound (227 g) ground turkey
½ cup Parmesan cheese, freshly grated
½ cup Mozzarella cheese, grated
Salt and ground black pepper, to taste
1 bell pepper, sliced
2 slices Canadian bacon, chopped
1 tomato, chopped
1 teaspoon oregano
½ teaspoon basil

1. In mixing bowl, thoroughly combine the ground turkey, cheese, salt, and black pepper.
2. Then, press the cheese-chicken mixture into a parchment-lined baking pan. Bake in the preheated oven, at 390ºF (199ºC) for 22 minutes.
3. Add bell pepper, bacon, tomato, oregano, and basil. Bake an additional 10 minutes and serve warm. Bon appétit!

Per Serving
calories: 361 | fat: 22.6g | protein: 32.5g
carbs: 5.8g | net carbs: 5.2g | fiber: 0.6g

Grilled Rosemary Wings with Leeks

Prep time: 10 minutes | Cook time: 20 minutes | Serves 4

8 chicken wings
2 tablespoons butter, melted The Marinade:
2 garlic cloves, minced
¼ cup leeks, chopped
2 tablespoons lemon juice
Salt and ground black pepper, to taste
½ teaspoon paprika
1 teaspoon dried rosemary

1. Thoroughly combine all ingredients for the marinade in a ceramic bowl. Add the chicken wings to the bowl.
2. Cover and allow it to marinate for 1 hour.
3. Then, preheat your grill to medium-high heat. Drizzle melted butter over the chicken wings. Grill the chicken wings for 20 minutes, turning them periodically.
4. Taste, adjust the seasonings, and serve warm. Enjoy!

Per Serving
calories: 132 | fat: 7.9g | protein: 13.3g
carbs: 1.9g | net carbs: 1.6g | fiber: 0.3g

Thyme Roasted Drumsticks

Prep time: 10 minutes | Cook time: 40 minutes | Serves 6

1 stick unsalted butter, softened
4 cloves garlic, minced
Sea salt and ground black pepper, to taste
1 tablespoon fresh thyme leaves
2 pounds (907 g) chicken drumsticks

1. In a mixing bowl, thoroughly combine the butter, garlic, salt, black pepper, and thyme. Rub this mixture all over the chicken drumsticks.
2. Lay the chicken drumsticks on a parchment-lined baking tray. Bake in the preheated oven at 390ºF (199ºC) until an instant-read thermometer reads 165ºF (74ºC) about 40 minutes.
3. Place under the preheated broiler for 1 to 2 minutes if you'd like the golden, crisp skin. Bon appétit!

Per Serving
calories: 342 | fat: 24.3g | protein: 28.1g
carbs: 1.7g | net carbs: 1.4g | fiber: 0.3g

Herbed Turkey with Cucumber Salsa

Prep time: 15 minutes | Cook time: 6 minutes | Serves 4

2 spring onions, thinly sliced
1 pound (454 g) ground turkey
1 egg
2 garlic cloves, minced
1 tablespoon chopped herbs
1 small chili pepper, deseeded and diced
1 tablespoon butter

Cucumber Salsa:
1 tablespoon apple cider vinegar
1 tablespoon chopped dill
1 garlic clove, minced
2 cucumbers, grated
1 cup sour cream
1 jalapeño pepper, minced
1 tablespoon olive oil

1. Place all turkey ingredients, except the butter, in a bowl. Mix to combine. Make patties out of the mixture.
2. Melt the butter in a skillet over medium heat. Cook the patties for 3 minutes per side. Place all salsa ingredients in a bowl and mix to combine. Serve the patties topped with salsa.

Per Serving
calories: 350 | fat: 23g | protein: 27g
carbs: 7g | net carbs: 5g | fiber: 2g

Lemony Rosemary Chicken Thighs

Prep time: 10 minutes | Cook time: 14 minutes | Serves 4

8 chicken thighs
1 teaspoon salt
1 tablespoon lemon juice
1 teaspoon lemon zest
1 tablespoon olive oil
1 tablespoon chopped rosemary
¼ teaspoon black pepper
1 garlic clove, minced

1. Combine all ingredients in a bowl. Place in the fridge for one hour. Heat a skillet over medium heat. Add the chicken along with the juices and cook until crispy, about 7 minutes per side.
2. Serve immediately.

Per Serving
calories: 477 | fat: 31g | protein: 31g
carbs: 3g | net carbs: 3g | fiber: 0g

Asiago Drumsticks with Spinach

Prep time: 10 minutes | Cook time: 12 minutes | Serves 2

1 tablespoon peanut oil
2 chicken drumsticks
½ cup vegetable broth
½ cup cream cheese
2 cups baby spinach
Sea salt and ground black pepper, to taste
½ teaspoon parsley flakes
½ teaspoon shallot powder
½ teaspoon garlic powder
½ cup Asiago cheese, grated

1. Heat the oil in a pan over medium-high heat. Then cook the chicken for 7 minutes, turning occasionally; reserve.
2. Pour in broth; add cream cheese and spinach; cook until spinach has wilted. Add the chicken back to the pan.
3. Add seasonings and Asiago cheese; cook until everything is thoroughly heated, an additional 4 minutes. Serve immediately and enjoy!

Per Serving
calories: 588 | fat: 46.0g | protein: 37.6g
carbs: 5.7g | net carbs: 4.7g | fiber: 1.0g

Greek Drumettes with Olives

Prep time: 10 minutes | Cook time: 20 minutes | Serves 2

1 pound (454 g) chicken drumettes
1 teaspoon Greek seasoning blend
1 tablespoon olive oil
6 ounces (170 g) tomato sauce
6 Kalamata olives, pitted and sliced

1. Place the chicken drumettes and Greek seasoning blend in a Ziploc bag. Shake the bag, ensuring even coating.
2. Heat the olive oil in a saucepan over medium-high heat. Sear the chicken drumettes until golden brown, flipping them occasionally to ensure even cooking.
3. After that, stir in the tomato sauce and Kalamata olives. Continue to cook until the chicken is tender and everything is thoroughly heated or about 20 minutes. Bon appétit!

Per Serving
calories: 342 | fat: 14.2g | protein: 47.0g
carbs: 3.5g | net carbs: 2.4g | fiber: 1.1g

Chipotle Tomato and Pumpkin Chicken Chili

Prep time: 20 minutes | Cook time: 7 to 8 hours | Serves 6

3 tablespoons extra-virgin olive oil, divided
1 pound (454 g) ground chicken
½ sweet onion, chopped
2 teaspoons minced garlic
1 (28-ounce / 794-g) can diced tomatoes
1 cup chicken broth
1 cup diced pumpkin
1 green bell pepper, diced
3 tablespoons chili powder
1 teaspoon chipotle chili powder
1 cup sour cream, for garnish
1 cup shredded Cheddar cheese, for garnish

1. Lightly grease the insert of the slow cooker with 1 tablespoon of the olive oil.
2. In a large skillet over medium-high heat, heat the remaining 2 tablespoons of the olive oil. Add the chicken and sauté until it is cooked through, about 6 minutes.
3. Add the onion and garlic and sauté for an additional 3 minutes.
4. Transfer the chicken mixture to the insert and stir in the tomatoes, broth, pumpkin, bell pepper, chili powder, and chipotle chili powder.
5. Cover and cook on low for 7 to 8 hours.
6. Serve topped with the sour cream and cheese.

Per Serving
calories: 390 | fat: 30.0g | protein: 22.0g carbs: 14.0g | net carbs: 9.0g | fiber: 5.0g

Chicken Thigh and Kale Stew

Prep time: 20 minutes | Cook time: 6 hours | Serves 6

3 tablespoons extra-virgin olive oil, divided
1 pound (454 g) boneless chicken thighs, diced into 1½-inch pieces
½ sweet onion, chopped
2 teaspoons minced garlic
2 cups chicken broth
2 celery stalks, diced
1 carrot, diced
1 teaspoon dried thyme
1 cup shredded kale
1 cup coconut cream
Salt, for seasoning
Freshly ground black pepper, for seasoning

1. Lightly grease the insert of the slow cooker with 1 tablespoon of the olive oil.
2. In a large skillet over medium-high heat, heat the remaining 2 tablespoons of the olive oil. Add the chicken and sauté until it is just cooked through, about 7 minutes.
3. Add the onion and garlic and sauté for an additional 3 minutes.
4. Transfer the chicken mixture to the insert, and stir in the broth, celery, carrot, and thyme.
5. Cover and cook on low for 6 hours.
6. Stir in the kale and coconut cream.
7. Season with salt and pepper, and serve warm.

Per Serving
calories: 277 | fat: 22.0g | protein: 17.0g carbs: 6.0g | net carbs: 4.0g | fiber: 2.0g

Bell Pepper Turkey Casserole

Prep time: 10 minutes | Cook time: 25 minutes | Serves 5

3 teaspoons olive oil
1 cup bell peppers, sliced
1 yellow onion, thinly sliced
1½ pounds (680 g) turkey breast
Se salt and ground black pepper, to taste
1 cup chicken bone broth
1 cup double cream
½ cup Swiss cheese, shredded

1. Heat 2 teaspoons of the olive oil in a sauté pan over a moderate flame. Sauté the peppers and onion until they have softened; reserve.
2. In the same sauté pan, heat the remaining teaspoon of olive oil and sear the turkey breasts until no longer pink.
3. Layer the peppers and onions in a lightly greased baking pan. Add the turkey breast; sprinkle with salt and pepper.
4. Mix the chicken bone broth with the double cream; pour the mixture over the turkey breasts. Bake in the preheated oven at 350ºF (180ºC) for 20 minutes; top with the Swiss cheese.
5. Bake an additional 5 minutes or until golden brown on top. Bon appétit!

Per Serving
calories: 465 | fat: 28.5g | protein: 45.4g carbs: 4.5g | net carbs: 4.2g | fiber: 0.3g

Chicken and Bell Pepper Kabobs

Prep time: 10 minutes | Cook time: 10 minutes | Serves 6

2 tablespoons olive oil
4 tablespoons dry sherry
1 tablespoon stone-ground mustard
1½ pounds (680 g) chicken, skinless, boneless and cubed
2 red onions, cut into wedges
1 green bell pepper, cut into 1-inch pieces
1 red bell pepper, cut into 1-inch pieces
1 yellow bell pepper, cut into 1-inch pieces
½ teaspoon sea salt
¼ teaspoon ground black pepper, or more to taste

1. In a mixing bowl, combine the olive oil, dry sherry, mustard and chicken until well coated.
2. Alternate skewering the chicken and vegetables until you run out of ingredients. Season with salt and black pepper.
3. Preheat your grill to medium-high heat.
4. Place the kabobs on the grill, flipping every 2 minutes and cook to desired doneness. Serve warm.

Per Serving
calories: 201 | fat: 8.2g | protein: 24.3g
carbs: 7.0 g | net carbs: 5.7g | fiber: 1.3g

Chicken Mélange

Prep time: 15 minutes | Cook time: 35 minutes | Serves 3

2 ounces (57 g) bacon, diced
¾ pound (340 g) whole chicken, boneless and chopped
½ medium-sized leek, chopped
1 teaspoon ginger garlic paste
1 teaspoon poultry seasoning mix
Sea salt, to taste
1 bay leaf
1 thyme sprig
1 rosemary sprig
1 cup chicken broth
½ cup cauliflower, chopped into small florets
2 vine-ripe tomatoes, puréed

1. Heat a medium-sized pan over medium-high heat; once hot, fry the bacon until it is crisp or about 3 minutes. Add in the chicken and cook until it is no longer pink; reserve.
2. Then, sauté the leek until tender and fragrant. Stir in the ginger garlic paste, poultry seasoning mix, salt, bay leaf, thyme, and rosemary.
3. Pour in the chicken broth and reduce the heat to medium; let it cook for 15 minutes, stirring periodically.
4. Add in the cauliflower and tomatoes along with the reserved bacon and chicken. Decrease the temperature to simmer and let it cook for a further 15 minutes or until warmed through. Bon appétit!

Per Serving
calories: 353 | fat: 14.4g | protein: 44.1g
carbs: 5.9g | net carbs: 3.5g | fiber: 2.4g

Rind and Cheese Crusted Chicken

Prep time: 10 minutes | Cook time: 10 minutes | Serves 3

2 tablespoons double cream
1 egg
2 ounces (57 g) pork rinds, crushed
2 ounces (57 g) Romano cheese, grated
Sea salt and ground black pepper, to taste
1 teaspoon cayenne pepper
1 teaspoon dried parsley
1 garlic clove, halved
½ pound (227 g) chicken fillets
2 tablespoons olive oil
1 large-sized Roma tomato, puréed

1. In a mixing bowl, whisk the cream and egg.
2. In another bowl, mix the crushed pork rinds, Romano cheese, salt, black pepper, cayenne pepper, and dried parsley.
3. Rub the garlic halves all over the chicken. Dip the chicken fillets into the egg mixture; then, coat the chicken with breading on all sides.
4. Heat the olive oil in a pan over medium-high heat; add butter. Once hot, cook chicken fillets until no longer pink, 2 to 4 minutes on each side.
5. Transfer the prepared chicken fillets to a baking pan that is lightly greased with a nonstick cooking spray. Cover with the puréed tomato. Bake for 2 to 3 minutes until everything is thoroughly warmed. Bon appétit!

Per Serving
calories: 360 | fat: 23.5g | protein: 30.5g
carbs: 5.7g | net carbs: 3.4g | fiber: 1.3g

Leek and Pumpkin Turkey Stew

Prep time: 20 minutes | Cook time: 7 to 8 hours | Serves 6

3 tablespoons extra-virgin olive oil, divided
1 pound (454 g) boneless turkey breast, cut into 1-inch pieces
1 leek, thoroughly cleaned and sliced
2 teaspoons minced garlic
2 cups chicken broth
1 cup coconut milk
2 celery stalks, chopped
2 cups diced pumpkin
1 carrot, diced
2 teaspoons chopped thyme
Salt, for seasoning
Freshly ground black pepper, for seasoning
1 scallion, white and green parts, chopped, for garnish

1. Lightly grease the insert of the slow cooker with 1 tablespoon of the olive oil.
2. In a large skillet over medium-high heat, heat the remaining 2 tablespoons of the olive oil. Add the turkey and sauté until browned, about 5 minutes.
3. Add the leek and garlic and sauté for an additional 3 minutes.
4. Transfer the turkey mixture to the insert and stir in the broth, coconut milk, celery, pumpkin, carrot, and thyme.
5. Cover and cook on low for 7 to 8 hours.
6. Season with salt and pepper.
7. Serve topped with the scallion.

Per Serving
calories: 357 | fat: 27.0g | protein: 21.0g
carbs: 11.0g | net carbs: 7.0g | fiber: 4.0g

Teriyaki Turkey with Peppers

Prep time: 15 minutes | Cook time: 10 minutes | Serves 3

¾ pound (340 g) lean ground turkey
1 brown onion, chopped
1 red bell pepper, deveined and chopped
1 serrano pepper, deveined and chopped
1 tablespoon rice vinegar
1 garlic clove, pressed
1 tablespoon sesame oil
½ teaspoon ground cumin
½ teaspoon hot sauce
2 tablespoons peanut butter
Sea salt and cayenne pepper, to season
½ teaspoon celery seeds
½ teaspoon mustard seeds
1 rosemary sprig, leaves chopped
2 tablespoons fresh Thai basil, snipped

1. Heat a medium-sized pan over medium-high heat; once hot, brown the ground turkey for 4 to 6 minutes; reserve.
2. Then cook the onion and peppers in the pan drippings for a further 2 to 3 minutes.
3. Add ¼ cup of cold water to another saucepan and heat over medium heat. Now, stir in vinegar, garlic, sesame oil, cumin, hot sauce, peanut butter, salt, cayenne pepper, celery seeds, and mustard seeds.
4. Let it simmer, stirring occasionally, until the mixture begins to bubble slightly. Bring the mixture to a boil; then, immediately remove from the heat and add the cooked ground turkey and sautéed onion/pepper mixture.
5. Ladle into serving bowls and garnish with the rosemary and Thai basil. Enjoy!

Per Serving
calories: 411 | fat: 27.2g | protein: 36.6g
carbs: 6.5g | net carbs: 5.5g | fiber: 1.0g

Chicken Drumsticks in Capocollo

Prep time: 10 minutes | Cook time: 35 minutes | Serves 5

2 pounds (907 g) chicken drumsticks, skinless and boneless
1 garlic clove, peeled and halved
½ teaspoon smoked paprika
Coarse sea salt and ground black pepper, to taste
10 thin slices of capocollo

1. Using a sharp kitchen knife, butterfly cut the chicken drumsticks in half.
2. Lay each chicken drumstick flat on a cutting board and rub garlic halves over the surface of chicken drumsticks. Season with paprika, salt, and black pepper.
3. Lay a slice of capocollo on each piece, pressing lightly. Roll them up and secure with toothpicks.
4. Bake in the preheated oven at 420ºF (216ºC) for about 15 minutes until the edges of the chicken begin to brown.
5. Turn over and bake for a further 15 to 20 minutes. Bon appétit!

Per Serving
calories: 486 | fat: 33.7g | protein: 39.1g
carbs: 3.6g | net carbs: 2.6g | fiber: 1.0g

Olla Tapada

Prep time: 15 minutes | Cook time: 25 minutes | Serves 3

2 teaspoons canola oil
1 red bell pepper, deveined and chopped
1 shallot, chopped
½ cup celery rib, chopped
½ cup chayote, peeled and cubed
1 pound (454 g) duck breasts, boneless, skinless, and chopped into small chunks
1½ cups vegetable broth
½ stick Mexican cinnamon
1 thyme sprig
1 rosemary sprig
Sea salt and freshly ground black pepper, to taste

1. Heat the canola oil in a soup pot (or clay pot) over a medium-high flame. Now, sauté the bell pepper, shallot and celery until they have softened about 5 minutes.
2. Add the remaining ingredients and stir to combine. Once it starts boiling, turn the heat to simmer and partially cover the pot.
3. Let it simmer for 17 to 20 minutes or until thoroughly cooked. Enjoy!

Per Serving
calories: 230 | fat: 9.6g | protein: 30.5g carbs: 3.3g | net carbs: 2.3g | fiber: 1.0g

Chicken and Tomato Packets

Prep time: 15 minutes | Cook time: 40 minutes | Serves 4

1 cup goat cheese
½ cup chopped oil-packed sun-dried tomatoes
1 teaspoon minced garlic
½ teaspoon dried basil
½ teaspoon dried oregano
4 (4-ounce / 113-g) boneless chicken breasts
Sea salt, for seasoning
Freshly ground black pepper, for seasoning
3 tablespoons olive oil

1. Preheat the oven. Set the oven temperature to 375ºF (190ºC).
2. Prepare the filling. In a medium bowl, stir together the goat cheese, sun-dried tomatoes, garlic, basil, and oregano until everything is well blended.
3. Stuff the chicken. Make a horizontal slice in the middle of each chicken breast to make a pocket, making sure not to cut through the sides or ends. Spoon one-quarter of the filling into each breast, folding the skin and chicken meat over the slit to form packets. Secure the packets with a toothpick. Lightly season the breasts with salt and pepper.
4. Brown the chicken. In a large oven-safe skillet over medium heat, warm the olive oil. Add the breasts and sear them, turning them once, until they are golden, about 8 minutes in total.
5. Bake the chicken. Place the skillet in the oven and bake the chicken for 30 minutes or until it's cooked through.
6. Serve. Remove the toothpicks. Divide the chicken between four plates and serve them immediately.

Per Serving
calories: 388 | fat: 29g | protein: 28g carbs: 4g | net carbs: 3g | fiber: 1g

Creamy-Lemony Chicken Thighs

Prep time: 10 minutes | Cook time: 7 to 8 hours | Serves 6

3 tablespoons extra-virgin olive oil
2 tablespoons butter
1½ pounds (680 g) boneless chicken thighs
½ sweet onion, diced
2 teaspoons minced garlic
2 teaspoons dried oregano
½ teaspoon salt
⅛ teaspoon pepper, depending on taste
1½ cups chicken broth
Juice and zest of 1 lemon
1 tablespoon dijon mustard
1 cup heavy (whipping) cream

1. Lightly grease the insert of the slow cooker with 1 tablespoon of the olive oil.
2. In a large skillet over medium-high heat, heat the remaining 2 tablespoons of the olive oil and the butter. Add the chicken and brown for 5 minutes, turning once.
3. Transfer the chicken to the insert and add the onion, garlic, oregano, salt, and pepper.
4. In a small bowl, whisk together the broth, lemon juice and zest, and mustard. Pour the mixture over the chicken.
5. Cover and cook on low for 7 to 8 hours.
6. Remove from the heat, stir in the heavy cream, and serve.

Per Serving
calories: 400 | fat: 34g | protein: 22g carbs: 2g | net carbs: 2g | fiber: 0g

Slow Cooked Chicken Cacciatore

Prep time: 15 minutes | Cook time: 3 to 4 hours or 6 to 8 hours | Serves 4

¼ cup good-quality olive oil
4 (4-ounce /113-g) boneless chicken breasts, each cut into three pieces
1 onion, chopped
2 celery stalks, chopped
1 cup sliced mushrooms
2 tablespoons minced garlic
1 (28-ounce / 794-g) can sodium-free diced tomatoes
½ cup red wine
½ cup tomato purée
1 tablespoon dried basil
1 teaspoon dried oregano
⅛ teaspoon red pepper flakes

1. Brown the chicken. In a skillet over medium-high heat, warm the olive oil. Add the chicken breasts and brown them, turning them once, about 10 minutes in total.
2. Cook in the slow cooker. Place the chicken in the slow cooker and stir in the onion, celery, mushrooms, garlic, tomatoes, red wine, tomato purée, basil, oregano, and red pepper flakes. Cook it on high for 3 to 4 hours or on low for 6 to 8 hours, until the chicken is fully cooked and tender.
3. Serve. Divide the chicken and sauce between four bowls and serve it immediately.

Per Serving
calories: 383 | fat: 26g | protein: 26g
carbs: 11g | net carbs: 7g | fiber: 4g

Coconut Turkey Breast

Prep time: 25 minutes | Cook time: 7 to 8 hours | Serves 6

3 tablespoons extra-virgin olive oil, divided
1½ pounds (680 g) boneless turkey breasts
Salt, for seasoning
Freshly ground black pepper, for seasoning
1 cup coconut milk
2 teaspoons minced garlic
2 teaspoons dried thyme
1 teaspoon dried oregano
1 avocado, peeled, pitted, and chopped
1 tomato, diced
½ jalapeño pepper, diced
1 tablespoon chopped cilantro

1. Lightly grease the insert of the slow cooker with 1 tablespoon of the olive oil.
2. In a large skillet over medium-high heat, heat the remaining 2 tablespoons of the olive oil.
3. Lightly season the turkey with salt and pepper. Add the turkey to the skillet and brown for about 7 minutes, turning once.
4. Transfer the turkey to the insert and add the coconut milk, garlic, thyme, and oregano.
5. Cover and cook on low for 7 to 8 hours.
6. In a small bowl, stir together the avocado, tomato, jalapeño pepper, and cilantro.
7. Serve the turkey topped with the avocado salsa.

Per Serving
calories: 347 | fat: 27g | protein: 25g
carbs: 5g | net carbs: 2g | fiber: 3g

Turkey and Pumpkin Ragout

Prep time: 15 minutes | Cook time: 8 hours | Serves 6

1 tablespoon extra-virgin olive oil
1 pound (454 g) boneless turkey thighs, cut into 1½-inch chunks
3 cups cubed pumpkin, cut into 1-inch chunks
1 red bell pepper, diced
½ sweet onion, cut in half and sliced
1 tablespoon minced garlic
1½ cups chicken broth
1½ cups coconut milk
2 teaspoons chopped fresh thyme
½ cup coconut cream
Salt, for seasoning
Freshly ground black pepper, for seasoning
12 slices cooked bacon, chopped, for garnish

1. Lightly grease the insert of the slow cooker with the olive oil.
2. Add the turkey, pumpkin, red bell pepper, onion, garlic, broth, coconut milk, and thyme.
3. Cover and cook on low for 8 hours.
4. Stir in the coconut cream and season with salt and pepper.
5. Serve topped with the bacon.

Per Serving
calories: 418 | fat: 34g | protein: 25g
carbs: 6g | net carbs: 5g | fiber: 1g

Spiced Duck Goulash

Prep time: 15 minutes | Cook time: 5 minutes | Serves 2

2 (1-ounce / 28-g) slices bacon, chopped
½ pound (227 g) duck legs, skinless and boneless
2 cups chicken broth, preferably homemade
½ cup celery ribs, chopped
2 green garlic stalks, chopped
2 green onion stalks, chopped
1 ripe tomato, puréed
Kosher salt, to season
¼ teaspoon red pepper flakes
½ teaspoon Hungarian paprika
½ teaspoon ground black pepper
½ teaspoon mustard seeds
½ teaspoon sage
1 bay laurel

1. Heat a stockpot over medium-high heat; once hot, fry the bacon until it is crisp or about 3 minutes. Add in the duck legs and cook until they are no longer pink.
2. Chop the meat, discarding any remaining skin and bones. Then, reserve the bacon and meat.
3. Pour in a splash of chicken broth to deglaze the pan.
4. Now, sauté the celery, green garlic and onions for 2 to 3 minutes, stirring periodically. Add the remaining ingredients to the pot, including the reserved bacon and meat.
5. Stir to combine and reduce the heat to medium-low. Let it cook, covered, until everything is thoroughly heated or about 1 hour. Serve in individual bowls and enjoy!

Per Serving
calories: 364 | fat: 22.4g | protein: 33.2g
carbs: 5.1g | net carbs: 3.7g | fiber: 1.4g

Italian Asiago and Pepper Stuffed Turkey

Prep time: 15 minutes | Cook time: 50 minutes | Serves 6

2 tablespoons extra-virgin olive oil
1 tablespoon Italian seasoning mix
Sea salt and freshly ground black pepper, to season
2 garlic cloves, sliced
6 ounces (170 g) Asiago cheese, sliced
2 bell peppers, thinly sliced
1½ pounds (680 g) turkey breasts
2 tablespoons Italian parsley, roughly chopped

1. Brush the sides and bottom of a casserole dish with 1 tablespoon of extra-virgin olive oil. Preheat an oven to 360ºF (182ºC).
2. Sprinkle the turkey breast with the Italian seasoning mix, salt, and black pepper on all sides.
3. Make slits in each turkey breast and stuff with garlic, cheese, and bell peppers. Drizzle the turkey breasts with the remaining tablespoon of olive oil.
4. Bake in the preheated oven for 50 minutes or until an instant-read thermometer registers 165ºF (74ºC).
5. Garnish with Italian parsley and serve warm. Bon appétit!

Per Serving
calories: 350 | fat: 22.3g | protein: 32.1g
carbs: 3.0g | net carbs: 2.4g | fiber: 0.6g

Chicken, Pepper, and Tomato Bake

Prep time: 10 minutes | Cook time: 25 minutes | Serves 3

1 tablespoon olive oil
¾ pound (340 g) chicken breast fillets, chopped into bite-sized chunks
2 garlic cloves, sliced
¼ teaspoon Korean chili pepper flakes
¼ teaspoon Himalayan salt
½ teaspoon poultry seasoning mix
1 bell pepper, deveined and chopped
2 ripe tomatoes, chopped
¼ cup heavy whipping cream
¼ cup sour cream

1. Brush a casserole dish with olive oil. Add the chicken, garlic, Korean chili pepper flakes, salt, and poultry seasoning mix to the casserole dish.
2. Next, layer the pepper and tomatoes. Whisk the heavy whipping cream and sour cream in a mixing bowl.
3. Top everything with the cream mixture. Bake in the preheated oven at 390ºF (199ºC) for about 25 minutes or until thoroughly heated. Bon appétit!

Per Serving
calories: 411 | fat: 20.6g | protein: 50.0g
carbs: 6.2g | net carbs: 4.7g | fiber: 1.5g

Mediterranean Roasted Chicken Drumettes

Prep time: 15 minutes | Cook time: 20 minutes | Serves 5

2 tablespoons olive oil
1½ pounds (680 g) chicken drumettes
2 cloves garlic, minced
1 thyme sprig
1 rosemary sprig
½ teaspoon dried oregano
Sea salt and freshly ground black pepper, to taste
2 tablespoons Greek cooking wine
½ cup chicken bone broth
1 red onion, cut into wedges
2 bell peppers, sliced

1. Start by preheating your oven to 420ºF (216ºC). Brush the sides and bottom a baking dish with 1 tablespoon of olive oil.
2. Heat the remaining tablespoon of olive oil in a saucepan over a moderate flame. Brown the chicken drumettes for 5 to 6 minutes per side.
3. Transfer the warm chicken drumettes to a baking dish. Add the garlic, spices, wine and broth. Scatter red onion and peppers around chicken drumettes.
4. Roast in the preheated oven for about 13 minutes. Serve immediately and enjoy!

Per Serving
calories: 219 | fat: 9.2g | protein: 28.5g
carbs: 4.2g | net carbs: 3.5g | fiber: 0.7g

Classic Jerk Chicken

Prep time: 15 minutes | Cook time: 7 to 8 hours | Serves 6

½ cup extra-virgin olive oil, divided
2 pounds (907 g) boneless chicken (breast and thighs)
1 sweet onion, quartered
4 garlic cloves
2 scallions, white and green parts, coarsely chopped
2 habanero chiles, stemmed and seeded
2 tablespoons granulated erythritol
1 tablespoon grated fresh ginger
2 teaspoons allspice
1 teaspoon dried thyme
½ teaspoon cardamom
½ teaspoon salt
2 tablespoons chopped cilantro, for garnish

1. Lightly grease the insert of the slow cooker with 1 tablespoon of the olive oil.
2. Arrange the chicken pieces in the bottom of the insert.
3. In a blender, pulse the remaining olive oil, onion, garlic, scallions, chiles, erythritol, ginger, allspice, thyme, cardamom, and salt until a thick, uniform sauce forms.
4. Pour the sauce over the chicken, turning the pieces to coat.
5. Cover and cook on low for 7 to 8 hours.
6. Serve topped with the cilantro.

Per Serving
calories: 485 | fat: 40g | protein: 27g
carbs: 5g | net carbs: 4g | fiber: 1g

Marinated Chicken with Peanut Sauce

Prep time: 20 minutes | Cook time: 14 minutes | Serves 6

1 tablespoon wheat-free coconut aminos
1 tablespoon sugar-free fish sauce
1 tablespoon lime juice
1 teaspoon cilantro
1 teaspoon minced garlic
1 teaspoon minced ginger
1 tablespoon olive oil
1 tablespoon rice wine vinegar
1 teaspoon cayenne pepper
1 teaspoon erythritol
6 chicken thighs

Peanut sauce:
½ cup peanut butter
1 teaspoon minced garlic
1 tablespoon lime juice
1 tablespoon water
1 teaspoon minced ginger
1 tablespoon chopped jalapeño
1 tablespoon rice wine vinegar
1 tablespoon erythritol
1 tablespoon fish sauce

1. Combine all chicken ingredients in a large Ziploc bag. Seal the bag and shake to combine. Refrigerate for 1 hour. Remove from fridge about 15 minutes before cooking.
2. Preheat the grill to medium heat and cook the chicken for 7 minutes per side. Whisk together all sauce ingredients in a mixing bowl. Serve the chicken drizzled with peanut sauce.

Per Serving
calories: 492 | fat: 36g | protein: 35g
carbs: 5g | net carbs: 3g | fiber: 2g

Cheddar Bacon Stuffed Chicken Fillets

Prep time: 10 minutes | Cook time: 25 minutes | Serves 2

2 chicken fillets, skinless and boneless
½ teaspoon oregano
½ teaspoon tarragon
½ teaspoon paprika
¼ teaspoon ground black pepper
Sea salt, to taste
2 (1-ounce / 28-g) slices bacon
2 (1-ounce / 28-g) slices Cheddar cheese
1 tomato, sliced

1. Sprinkle the chicken fillets with oregano, tarragon, paprika, black pepper, and salt.
2. Place the bacon slices and cheese on each chicken fillet. Roll up the fillets and secure with toothpicks. Place the stuffed chicken fillets on a lightly greased baking pan. Scatter the sliced tomato around the fillets.
3. Bake in the preheated oven at 390°F (199°C) for 15 minutes; turn on the other side and bake an additional 5 to 10 minutes or until the meat is no longer pink.
4. Discard the toothpicks and serve immediately. Bon appétit!

Per Serving
calories: 400 | fat: 23.8g | protein: 41.3g
carbs: 3.6g | net carbs: 2.4g | fiber: 1.2g

Tuscan Chicken Breast Sauté

Prep time: 10 minutes | Cook time: 35 minutes | Serves 4

1 pound (454 g) boneless chicken breasts, each cut into three pieces
Sea salt, for seasoning
Freshly ground black pepper, for seasoning
3 tablespoons olive oil
1 tablespoon minced garlic
¾ cup chicken stock
1 teaspoon dried oregano
½ teaspoon dried basil
½ cup heavy (whipping) cream
½ cup shredded Asiago cheese
1 cup fresh spinach
¼ cup sliced Kalamata olives

1. Prepare the chicken. Pat the chicken breasts dry and lightly season them with salt and pepper.
2. Sauté the chicken. In a large skillet over medium-high heat, warm the olive oil. Add the chicken and sauté until it is golden brown and just cooked through, about 15 minutes in total. Transfer the chicken to a plate and set it aside.
3. Make the sauce. Add the garlic to the skillet and sauté until it's softened, about 2 minutes. Stir in the chicken stock, oregano, and basil, scraping up any browned bits in the skillet. Bring to a boil, then reduce the heat to low and simmer until the sauce is reduced by about one-quarter, about 10 minutes.
4. Finish the dish. Stir in the cream and Asiago and simmer, stirring the sauce frequently, until it has thickened, about 5 minutes. Return the chicken to the skillet along with any accumulated juices. Stir in the spinach and olives and simmer until the spinach is wilted, about 2 minutes.
5. Serve. Divide the chicken and sauce between four plates and serve it immediately.

Per Serving
calories: 483 | fat: 38g | protein: 31g
carbs: 5g | net carbs: 3g | fiber: 2g

Herbed Balsamic Turkey

Prep time: 15 minutes | Cook time: 15 minutes | Serves 2

1 turkey drumstick, skinless and boneless
1 tablespoon balsamic vinegar
1 tablespoon whiskey
3 tablespoons olive oil
1 tablespoon stone ground mustard
½ teaspoon tarragon
1 teaspoon rosemary
1 teaspoon sage
1 garlic clove, pressed
Kosher salt and ground black pepper, to season
1 brown onion, peeled and chopped

1. Place the turkey drumsticks in a ceramic dish. Toss them with the balsamic vinegar, whiskey, olive oil, mustard, tarragon, rosemary, sage, and garlic.
2. Cover with plastic wrap and refrigerate for 3 hours. Heat your grill to the hottest setting.
3. Grill the turkey drumsticks for about 13 minutes per side. Season with salt and pepper to taste and serve with brown onion. Bon appétit!

Per Serving
calories: 389 | fat: 19.6g | protein: 42.0g
carbs: 6.0g | net carbs: 4.6g | fiber: 1.4g

Turkish Chicken Thigh Kebabs

Prep time: 15 minutes | Cook time: 9 to 12 minutes | Serves 2

1 pound (454 g) chicken thighs, boneless, skinless and halved
½ cup Greek yogurt
Sea salt, to taste
1 tablespoon Aleppo red pepper flakes
½ teaspoon ground black pepper
¼ teaspoon dried oregano
½ teaspoon mustard seeds
⅛ teaspoon ground cinnamon
½ teaspoon sumac
2 Roma tomatoes, chopped
2 tablespoons olive oil
1½ ounces (43 g) Swiss cheese, sliced

1. Place the chicken thighs, yogurt, salt, red pepper flakes, black pepper, oregano, mustard seeds, cinnamon, sumac, tomatoes, and olive oil in a ceramic dish. Cover and let it marinate in your refrigerator for 4 hours.
2. Preheat your grill for medium-high heat and lightly oil the grate. Thread the chicken thighs onto skewers, making a thick log shape.
3. Cook your kebabs for 3 or 4 minutes; turn over and continue cooking for 3 to 4 minutes more. An instant-read thermometer should read about 165ºF (74ºC).
4. Add the cheese and let it cook for a further 3 to 4 minutes or until completely melted. Bon appétit!

Per Serving
calories: 500 | fat: 23.3g | protein: 61.0g
carbs: 6.2g | net carbs: 4.5g | fiber: 1.7g

Turkey Wing Curry

Prep time: 15 minutes | Cook time: 55 minutes | Serves 4

3 teaspoons sesame oil
1 pound (454 g) turkey wings, boneless and chopped
2 cloves garlic, finely chopped
1 small-sized red chili pepper, minced
½ teaspoon turmeric powder
½ teaspoon ginger powder
1 teaspoon red curry paste
1 cup unsweetened coconut milk, preferably homemade
½ cup water
½ cup turkey consommé
Kosher salt and ground black pepper, to taste

1. Heat sesame oil in a sauté pan. Add the turkey and cook until it is light brown about 7 minutes.
2. Add garlic, chili pepper, turmeric powder, ginger powder, and curry paste and cook for 3 minutes longer.
3. Add the milk, water, and consommé. Season with salt and black pepper. Cook for 45 minutes over medium heat. Bon appétit!

Per Serving
calories: 296 | fat: 19.6g | protein: 25.6g
carbs: 3.0g | net carbs: 3.0g | fiber: 0g

Chicken Paella and Chorizo

Prep time: 15 minutes | Cook time: 42 minutes | Serves 6

18 chicken drumsticks
12 ounces (340 g) chorizo, chopped
1 white onion, chopped
4 ounces (113 g) jarred Piquillo peppers, finely diced
1 tablespoon olive oil
½ cup chopped parsley
1 teaspoon smoked paprika
1 tablespoon tomato puree
½ cup white wine
1 cup chicken broth
2 cups cauli rice
1 cup chopped green beans
1 lemon, cut in wedges
Salt and pepper, to taste

1. Preheat the oven to 350ºF (180ºC).
2. Heat the olive oil in a cast iron pan over medium heat, meanwhile season the chicken with salt and black pepper, and fry in the hot oil on both sides for 10 minutes to lightly brown. After, remove onto a plate with a perforated spoon.
3. Then, add the chorizo and onion to the hot oil, and sauté for 4 minutes. Include the tomato puree, piquillo peppers, and paprika, and let simmer for 2 minutes. Add the broth, and bring the ingredients to boil for 6 minutes until slightly reduced.
4. Stir in the cauli rice, white wine, green beans, half of the parsley, and lay the chicken on top. Transfer the pan to the oven and continue cooking for 20-25 minutes. Let the paella sit to cool for 10 minutes before serving garnished with the remaining parsley and lemon wedges.

Per Serving
calories: 440 | fat: 28g | protein: 22g
carbs: 8g | net carbs: 6g | fiber: 2g

Chinese Flavor Chicken Legs

Prep time: 10 minutes | Cook time: 15 minutes | Serves 4

1 tablespoon sesame oil	2 tablespoons brown erythritol
4 chicken legs	¼ cup spicy tomato sauce
¼ cup Shaoxing wine	

1. Heat the sesame oil in a cast-iron skillet over medium-high flame. Now, sear chicken wings until they turn golden in color on all sides; reserve.
2. Then, in the same skillet, add a splash of wine to deglaze the pan.
3. Add in the remaining wine, brown erythritol, and spicy tomato sauce. Bring to a boil and immediately reduce the heat to medium-low.
4. Let it simmer for 5 to 10 minutes until the sauce coats the back of a spoon. Add the reserved chicken legs back to the skillet.
5. Cook for a further 3 minutes or until the chicken is well coated and heated through. Enjoy!

Per Serving
calories: 366 | fat: 14.6g | protein: 51.1g
carbs: 3.4g | net carbs: 2.4g | fiber: 1.0g

Itanlian Chicken Cacciatore

Prep time: 15 minutes | Cook time: 8 hours | Serves 6

3 tablespoons extra-virgin olive oil, divided	button mushrooms
2 pounds boneless chicken thighs	½ sweet onion, chopped
Salt, for seasoning	1 tablespoon minced garlic
Freshly ground black pepper, for seasoning	1 tablespoon dried oregano
1 (14-ounce / 397-g) can stewed tomatoes	1 teaspoon dried basil
2 cups chicken broth	pinch red pepper flakes
1 cup quartered	

1. Lightly grease the insert of the slow cooker with 1 tablespoon of the olive oil.
2. Lightly season the chicken thighs with salt and pepper.
3. In a large skillet over medium-high heat, heat the remaining 2 tablespoons of the olive oil. Add the chicken thighs and brown for about 8 minutes, turning once.
4. Transfer the chicken to the insert and add the tomatoes, broth, mushrooms, onion, garlic, oregano, basil, and red pepper flakes.
5. Cover and cook on low for 8 hours.
6. Serve warm.

Per Serving
calories: 425 | fat: 32g | protein: 27g
carbs: 8g | net carbs: 7g | fiber: 1g

Roasted Chicken Breasts with Capers

Prep time: 10 minutes | Cook time: 55 minutes | Serves 6

3 medium lemons, sliced	¼ cup almond flour
½ teaspoon salt	1 tablespoon capers, rinsed
2 teaspoons olive oil	1¼ cup chicken broth
3 chicken breasts, halved	1 teaspoon butter
Salt and black pepper to season	1½ tablespoon chopped fresh parsley
	Parsley for garnish

1. Preheat the oven to 350°F (180°C) and lay a piece of parchment paper on a baking sheet.
2. Lay the lemon slices on the baking sheet, drizzle with olive oil and sprinkle with salt. Roast in the oven for 25 minutes to brown the lemon rinds.
3. Cover the chicken with plastic wrap, place them on a flat surface, and gently pound with the rolling pin to flatten to about ½-inch thickness. Remove the plastic wraps and season with salt and pepper.
4. Next, dredge the chicken in the almond flour on each side, and shake off any excess flour. Set aside.
5. Heat the olive oil in a skillet over medium heat and fry the chicken on both sides to a golden brown, for about 8 minutes in total. Pour the chicken broth in, shake the skillet, and let the broth boil and reduce to a thick consistency, about 12 minutes.
6. Lightly stir in the capers, roasted lemon, pepper, butter, and parsley, and simmer on low heat for 10 minutes. Turn the heat off and serve the chicken with the sauce hot, an extra garnish of parsley with a creamy squash mash.

Per Serving
calories: 430 | fat: 23g | protein: 33g
carbs: 7g | net carbs: 3g | fiber: 4g

Parma Ham-Wrapped Stuffed Chicken

Prep time: 10 minutes | Cook time: 23 minutes | Serves 4

4 chicken breasts
1 tablespoon olive oil
3 cloves garlic, minced
3 shallots, finely chopped
1 tablespoon dried mixed herbs
8 slices Parma ham
8 ounces (227 g) cream cheese
2 lemons, zested
Salt, to taste

1. Preheat the oven to 350ºF (180ºC).
2. Heat the oil in a small skillet and sauté the garlic and shallots with a pinch of salt and lemon zest for 3 minutes; let it cool. After, stir the cream cheese and mixed herbs into the shallot mixture.
3. Score a pocket in each chicken breast, fill the holes with the cream cheese mixture and cover with the cut-out chicken. Wrap each breast with two Parma ham and secure the ends with a toothpick. Lay the chicken parcels on a greased baking sheet and cook in the oven for 20 minutes. Remove to rest for 4 minutes before serving with green salad and roasted tomatoes.

Per Serving
calories: 485 | fat: 35g | protein: 26g
carbs: 3g | net carbs: 2g | fiber: 1g

Ritzy Baked Chicken with Vegetable

Prep time: 10 minutes | Cook time: 43 minutes | Serves 6

3 cups cubed leftover chicken
3 cups spinach
2 cauliflower heads, cut into florets
3 cups water
3 eggs, lightly beaten
2 cups grated sharp cheddar cheese
1 cup pork rinds, crushed
½ cup unsweetened almond milk
1 tablespoon olive oil
3 cloves garlic, minced
Salt and black pepper to taste
Cooking spray

1. Preheat the oven to 350ºF (180ºC) and grease a baking dish with cooking spray. Set aside.
2. Pour the cauli florets and water in a pot; bring to boil over medium heat. Cover and steam the cauli florets for 8 minutes. Drain them through a colander and set aside.
3. Also, combine the cheddar cheese and pork rinds in a large bowl and mix in the chicken. Set aside.
4. Heat the olive oil in a skillet and cook the garlic and spinach until the spinach has wilted, about 5 minutes. Season with salt and black pepper, and add the spinach mixture and cauli florets to the chicken bowl.
5. Top with the eggs and almond milk, mix and transfer everything to the baking dish. Layer the top of the ingredients and place the dish in the oven to bake for 30 minutes.
6. By this time the edges and top must have browned nicely, then remove the chicken from the oven, let rest for 5 minutes, and serve. Garnish with steamed and seasoned green beans.

Per Serving
calories: 472 | fat: 26g | protein: 38g
carbs: 5g | net carbs: 3g | fiber: 2g

Double-Cheese Ranch Chicken

Prep time: 15 minutes | Cook time: 20 minutes | Serves 4

2 chicken breasts
2 tablespoons butter, melted
1 teaspoon salt
½ teaspoon garlic powder
½ teaspoon cayenne pepper
½ teaspoon black peppercorns, crushed
½ tablespoon ranch seasoning mix
4 ounces (113 g) Ricotta cheese, room temperature
½ cup Monterey-Jack cheese, grated
4 slices bacon, chopped
¼ cup scallions, chopped

1. Start by preheating your oven to 370ºF (188ºC).
2. Drizzle the chicken with melted butter. Rub the chicken with salt, garlic powder, cayenne pepper, black pepper, and ranch seasoning mix.
3. Heat a cast iron skillet over medium heat. Cook the chicken for 3 to 5 minutes per side. Transfer the chicken to a lightly greased baking dish.
4. Add cheese and bacon. Bake about 12 minutes. Top with scallions just before serving. Bon appétit!

Per Serving
calories: 290 | fat: 19.3g | protein: 25.1g
carbs: 2.5g | net carbs: 2.5g | fiber: 0g

Baked Chicken in Tomato Purée

Prep time: 15 minutes | Cook time: 1½ hours | Serves 4

8 chicken drumsticks
1½ tablespoon olive oil
1 medium white onion, diced
3 medium turnips, peeled and diced
2 green bell peppers, seeded, cut into chunks
2 cloves garlic, minced
¼ cup coconut flour
1 cup chicken broth
1 (28 ounce / 794-g) can sugar-free tomato purée
1 tablespoon dried Italian herbs
Salt and black pepper, to taste

1. Preheat oven to 400ºF (205ºC).
2. Heat the oil in a large skillet over medium heat, meanwhile season the drumsticks with salt and pepper, and fry in the oil to brown on both sides for 10 minutes. Remove to a baking dish. Sauté the onion, turnips, bell peppers, and garlic in the same oil and for 10 minutes with continuous stirring.
3. In a bowl, combine the broth, coconut flour, tomato purée, and Italian herbs together, and pour it over the vegetables in the pan. Stir and cook to thicken for 4 minutes. Pour the mixture on the chicken in the baking dish. Bake for around 1 hour. Remove from the oven and serve with steamed cauli rice.

Per Serving
calories: 515 | fat: 34g | protein: 51g
carbs: 15g | net carbs: 7g | fiber: 8g

Parmesan Spinach Stuffed Chicken

Prep time: 15 minutes | Cook time: 20 minutes | Serves 4

4 chicken breasts, boneless and skinless
½ cup mozzarella cheese
⅓ cup Parmesan cheese
6 ounces (170 g)
cream cheese
2 cups spinach, chopped
A pinch of nutmeg
½ teaspoon minced garlic

Breading:
2 eggs
⅓ cup almond flour
1 tablespoon olive oil
½ teaspoon parsley
⅓ cup Parmesan cheese
A pinch of onion powder

1. Pound the chicken until it doubles in size. Mix the cream cheese, spinach, mozzarella, nutmeg, salt, black pepper, and Parmesan cheese in a bowl. Divide the mixture between the chicken breasts and spread it out evenly. Wrap the chicken in a plastic wrap. Refrigerate for 15 minutes.
2. Heat the oil in a pan and preheat the oven to 370ºF (188ºC). Beat the eggs and combine all other breading ingredients in a bowl. Dip the chicken in egg first, then in the breading mixture.
3. Cook in the pan until browned. Place on a lined baking sheet and bake for 20 minutes.

Per Serving
calories: 491 | fat: 36g | protein: 38g
carbs: 6g | net carbs: 4g | fiber: 2g

Homemade Poulet en Papillote

Prep time: 10 minutes | Cook time: 25 minutes | Serves 4

4 chicken breasts, skinless, scored
1 tablespoon white wine
1 tablespoon olive oil, plus extra for drizzling
1 tablespoon butter
3 cups mixed mushrooms, teared up
2 cups water
3 cloves garlic, minced
4 sprigs thyme, chopped
3 lemons, juiced
Salt and black pepper, to taste
1 tablespoon Dijon mustard

1. Preheat the oven to 450ºF (235ºC).
2. In a bowl, evenly mix the chicken, mushrooms, garlic, thyme, lemon juice, salt, black pepper, and mustard. Make 4 large cuts of foil, fold them in half, and then fold them in half again. Tightly fold the two open edges together to create a bag.
3. Now, share the chicken mixture into each bag, top with the white wine, olive oil, and a tablespoon of butter. Seal the last open end securely making sure not to pierce the bag. Put the bag on a baking tray and bake the chicken in the middle of the oven for 25 minutes.

Per Serving
calories: 394 | fat: 13g | protein: 25g
carbs: 6g | net carbs: 5g | fiber: 1g

Hungarian Chicken Thighs

Prep time: 10 minutes | Cook time: 7 to 8 hours | Serves 4

1 tablespoon extra-virgin olive oil
2 pounds (907 g) boneless chicken thighs
½ cup chicken broth
Juice and zest of 1 lemon
2 teaspoons minced garlic
2 teaspoons paprika
¼ teaspoon salt
1 cup sour cream
1 tablespoon chopped parsley, for garnish

1. Lightly grease the insert of the slow cooker with the olive oil.
2. Place the chicken thighs in the insert.
3. In a small bowl, stir together the broth, lemon juice and zest, garlic, paprika, and salt.
4. Pour the broth mixture over the chicken.
5. Cover and cook on low for 7 to 8 hours.
6. Turn off the heat and stir in the sour cream.
7. Serve topped with the parsley.

Per Serving
calories: 404 | fat: 32g | protein: 23g
carbs: 4g | net carbs: 0g | fiber: 4g

Stir-Fried Chicken, Broccoli and Cashew

Prep time: 10 minutes | Cook time: 17 minutes | Serves 4

1 chicken breasts, cut into strips
1 tablespoon olive oil
1 tablespoon coconut aminos
1 teaspoon white wine vinegar
1 teaspoon erythritol
1 teaspoon xanthan gum
1 lemon, juiced
1 cup unsalted cashew nuts
2 cups broccoli florets
1 white onion, thinly sliced
Salt and black pepper to taste

1. In a bowl, mix the coconut aminos, vinegar, lemon juice, erythritol, and xanthan gum. Set aside.
2. Heat the oil in a wok and fry the cashew for 4 minutes until golden-brown. Remove to a paper towel lined plate. Sauté the onion in the same oil for 4 minutes until soft and browned; add to the cashew nuts.
3. Add the chicken to the wok and cook for 4 minutes; include the broccoli, salt, and black pepper. Stir-fry and pour the coconut aminos mixture in. Stir and cook the sauce for 4 minutes and pour in the cashews and onion. Stir once more, cook for 1 minute, and turn the heat off.
4. Serve the chicken stir-fry with some steamed cauli rice.

Per Serving
calories: 325 | fat: 21g | protein: 22g
carbs: 6g | net carbs: 4g | fiber: 2g

Chicken with Mayo-Avocado Sauce

Prep time: 10 minutes | Cook time: 12 minutes | Serves 4

For the Sauce:
1 avocado, pitted
½ cup mayonnaise
Salt to taste

For the Chicken:
1 tablespoon butter
4 chicken breasts
Pink salt and black pepper to taste
1 cup chopped cilantro leaves
½ cup chicken broth

1. Spoon the avocado, mayonnaise, and salt into a small food processor and puree until a smooth sauce is derived. Pour sauce into a jar and refrigerate while you make the chicken.
2. Melt butter in a large skillet, season chicken with salt and black pepper and fry for 4 minutes on each side to golden brown. Remove chicken to a plate.
3. Pour the broth in the same skillet and add the cilantro. Bring to simmer covered for 3 minutes and add the chicken. Cover and cook on low heat for 5 minutes until the liquid has reduced and chicken is fragrant. Dish chicken only into serving plates and spoon the mayoavocado sauce over.

Per Serving
calories: 398 | fat: 32g | protein:24 g
carbs: 9g | net carbs: 4g | fiber: 5g

Chicken with Cream of Mushroom Soup

Prep time: 10 minutes | Cook time: 15 minutes | Serves 2

1 tablespoon olive oil
1 yellow onion, chopped
2 garlic cloves, pressed
2 chicken breast, skinless and boneless, cut into bite-sized pieces
½ cup cream of mushroom soup

1. Heat the olive oil in a saucepan over medium-high heat. Once hot, sweat the yellow onion until tender and translucent about 3 minutes. Then, cook the garlic until aromatic or about 30 seconds.
2. Then, sear the chicken breast for 3 minutes, stirring frequently to ensure even cooking. Pour in the cream of mushroom soup and stir to combine.
3. Turn the heat to medium-low and let it simmer until the sauce has reduced by half or 6 to 8 minutes longer. Serve immediately.

Per Serving
calories: 336 | fat: 20.7g | protein: 30.7g
carbs: 4.2g | net carbs: 3.7g | fiber: 0.5g

Garlicky Sweet Chicken Skewers

Prep time: 10 minutes | Cook time: 10 minutes | Serves 4

For the Skewers:
1 tablespoon coconut aminos
1 tablespoon ginger-garlic paste
1 tablespoon Swerve
Chili pepper to taste
1 tablespoon olive oil
3 chicken breasts, cut into cubes

For the Dressing:
½ cup tahini
½ teaspoon garlic powder
Pink salt to taste
¼ cup warm water

1. In a small bowl, whisk the coconut aminos, ginger-garlic paste, Swerve, chili pepper, and olive oil.
2. Put the chicken in a zipper bag, pour the marinade over, seal and shake for an even coat. Marinate in the fridge for 2 hours.
3. Preheat a grill to 400°F and thread the chicken on skewers. Cook for 10 minutes in total with three to four turnings to be golden brown; remove to a plate. Mix the tahini, garlic powder, salt, and warm water in a bowl. Pour into serving jars.
4. Serve the chicken skewers and tahini dressing with cauli fried rice.

Per Serving
calories: 470 | fat: 25g | protein: 52g
carbs: 5g | net carbs: 2g | fiber: 3g

Braised Chicken and Veggies

Prep time: 10 minutes | Cook time: 21 minutes | Serves 4

1 tablespoon butter
1 pound (454 g) chicken thighs
Salt and black pepper, to taste
2 cloves garlic, minced
1 (14 ounce / 397-g) can whole tomatoes
1 eggplant, diced
10 fresh basil leaves, chopped, extra to garnish

1. Melt butter in a saucepan over medium heat, season the chicken with salt and black pepper and fry for 4 minutes on each side until golden brown. Remove to a plate.
2. Sauté the garlic in the butter for 2 minutes, pour in the tomatoes, and cook covered for 8 minutes. Add in the eggplant and basil. Cook for 4 minutes. Season the sauce with salt and black pepper, stir and add the chicken. Coat with sauce and simmer for 3 minutes.
3. Serve chicken with sauce on a bed of squash pasta. Garnish with extra basil.

Per Serving
calories: 330 | fat: 22g | protein: 21g
carbs: 13g | net carbs: 7g | fiber: 6g

Bacon-Wrapped Chicken with Asparagus

Prep time: 10 minutes | Cook time: 40 minutes | Serves 4

6 chicken breasts
Pink salt and black pepper to taste
8 bacon slices
1 tablespoon olive oil
1 pound (454 g) asparagus spears
1 tablespoon fresh lemon juice
Manchego cheese, for topping

1. Preheat the oven to 400ºF (205ºC).
2. Season chicken breasts with salt and black pepper, and wrap 2 bacon slices around each chicken breast. Arrange on a baking sheet that is lined with parchment paper, drizzle with oil and bake for 25-30 minutes until bacon is brown and crispy.
3. Preheat your grill to high heat.
4. Brush the asparagus spears with olive oil and season with salt. Grill for 8-10 minutes, frequently turning until slightly charred. Remove to a plate and drizzle with lemon juice. Grate over Manchego cheese so that it melts a little on contact with the hot asparagus and forms a cheesy dressing.

Per Serving
calories: 468 | fat: 38g | protein: 26g
carbs: 5g | net carbs: 2g | fiber: 3g

Parmesan Chicken Wings with Yogurt Sauce

Prep time: 10 minutes | Cook time: 20 minutes | Serves 6

For the Dipping Sauce:
1 cup plain yogurt
1 teaspoon fresh lemon juice
Salt and black pepper to taste

For the Wings:
2 pounds (907 g) chicken wings
Salt and black pepper to taste
Cooking spray
½ cup melted butter
½ cup Hot sauce
¼ cup grated Parmesan cheese

1. Mix the yogurt, lemon juice, salt, and black pepper in a bowl. Chill while making the chicken.
2. Preheat oven to 400ºF and season wings with salt and black pepper. Line them on a baking sheet and grease lightly with cooking spray. Bake for 20 minutes until golden brown. Mix butter, hot sauce, and Parmesan cheese in a bowl. Toss chicken in the sauce to evenly coat and plate. Serve with yogurt dipping sauce and celery strips.

Per Serving
calories: 371 | fat: 23g | protein: 36g
carbs: 3g | net carbs: 3g | fiber: 0g

Baked Cheesy Chicken and Spinach

Prep time: 10 minutes | Cook time: 35 minutes | Serves 6

6 chicken breasts, skinless and boneless
1 teaspoon mixed spice seasoning
Pink salt and black pepper to season
2 loose cups baby spinach
1 teaspoon olive oil
4 oz cream cheese, cubed
1¼ cups shredded mozzarella cheese
1 tablespoon water

1. Preheat oven to 370ºF (188ºC).
2. Season chicken with spice mix, salt, and black pepper. Pat with your hands to have the seasoning stick on the chicken. Put in the casserole dish and layer spinach over the chicken. Mix the oil with cream cheese, mozzarella, salt, and black pepper and stir in water a tablespoon at a time. Pour the mixture over the chicken and cover the pot with aluminium foil.
3. Bake for 20 minutes, remove foil and continue cooking for 15 minutes until a nice golden brown color is formed on top. Take out and allow sitting for 5 minutes. Serve warm with braised asparagus.

Per Serving
calories: 463 | fat: 18g | protein: 48g
carbs: 2g | net carbs: 2g | fiber: 0g

Lemony Chicken Skewers

Prep time: 10 minutes | Cook time: 12 minutes | Serves 4

3 chicken breasts, cut into cubes
1 tablespoon olive oil, divided
⅔ jar preserved lemon, flesh removed, drained
2 cloves garlic, minced
½ cup lemon juice
Salt and black pepper to taste
1 teaspoon rosemary leaves to garnish
2 to 4 lemon wedges to garnish

1. First, thread the chicken onto skewers and set aside.
2. In a wide bowl, mix half of the oil, garlic, salt, pepper, and lemon juice, and add the chicken skewers, and lemon rind. Cover the bowl and let the chicken marinate for at least 2 hours in the refrigerator.
3. When the marinating time is almost over, preheat a grill to 350ºF (180ºC), and remove the chicken onto the grill. Cook for 6 minutes on each side.
4. Remove and serve warm garnished with rosemary leaves and lemons wedges.

Per Serving
calories: 350 | fat: 11g | protein: 34g
carbs: 6g | net carbs: 4g | fiber: 2g

Paprika Chicken Wings

Prep time: 10 minutes | Cook time: 25 minutes | Serves 4

12 chicken wings, cut in half
1 tablespoon turmeric
1 tablespoon cumin
1 tablespoon fresh ginger, grated
1 tablespoon cilantro, chopped
1 tablespoon paprika
Salt and ground black pepper, to taste
1 tablespoon olive oil
Juice of ½ lime
1 cup thyme leaves
¾ cup cilantro, chopped
1 tablespoon water
1 jalapeño pepper

1. In a bowl, stir together 1 tablespoon ginger, cumin, paprika, salt, 1 tablespoon olive oil, black pepper, and turmeric. Place in the chicken wings pieces, toss to coat, and refrigerate for 20 minutes.
2. Heat the grill, place in the marinated wings, cook for 25 minutes, turning from time to time, remove and set to a serving plate.
3. Using a blender, combine thyme, remaining ginger, salt, jalapeno pepper, black pepper, lime juice, cilantro, remaining olive oil, and water, and blend well. Drizzle the chicken wings with the sauce to serve.

Per Serving
calories: 175 | fat: 7g | protein: 21g
carbs: 7g | net carbs: 4g | fiber: 3g

Oregano Chicken Breast

Prep time: 10 minutes | Cook time: 30 minutes | Serves 6

6 chicken breasts
4 cloves garlic, minced
½ cup oregano leaves, chopped
½ cup lemon juice
⅔ cup olive oil
¼ cup erythritol
Salt and black pepper, to taste
3 small chilies, minced

1. Preheat a grill to 350ºF (180ºC).
2. In a bowl, mix the garlic, oregano, lemon juice, olive oil, chilies and erythritol. Set aside.
3. While the spices incorporate in flavor, cover the chicken with plastic wraps, and use the rolling pin to pound to ½ -inch thickness. Remove the wrap, and brush the mixture on the chicken on both sides.
4. Place on the grill, cover the lid and cook for 15 minutes. Baste the chicken with more of the spice mixture, and continue cooking for 15 more minutes.

Per Serving
calories: 265 | fat: 9g | protein: 26g
carbs: 4g | net carbs: 3g | fiber: 1g

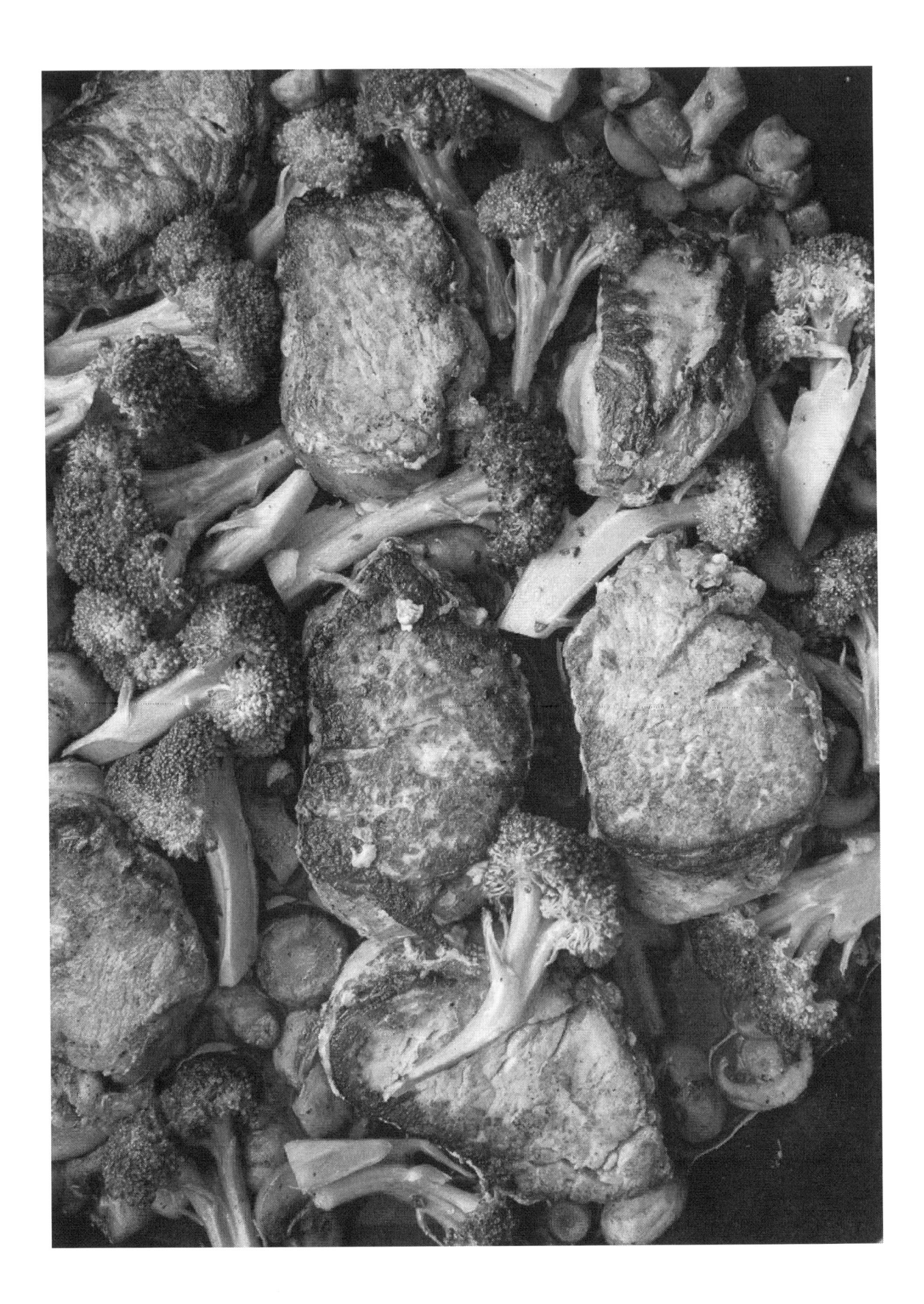

Chapter 9 Pork

Pork Paprikash

Prep time: 10 minutes | Cook time: 50 minutes | Serves 4

1 pound (454 g) pork stew meat, cut into bite-sized chunks
1 teaspoon Hungarian spice blend
2 bell peppers, deseeded and chopped
1 red onion, chopped
4 cups chicken bone broth

1. Heat up a medium-sized stockpot over a medium-high flame. Then, sear the pork for about 5 minutes, stirring periodically to ensure even cooking; add the Hungarian spice blend and reserve.
2. Cook the bell peppers and onion in the pan drippings until they have softened.
3. Pour in the chicken bone broth, stir and bring to a rapid boil. Add the reserved meat back to the stockpot. Immediately turn temperature to simmer. Let it simmer for 45 to 50 minutes.
4. Serve in individual bowls and enjoy!

Per Serving
calories: 271 | fat: 15.6g | protein: 25.4g
carbs: 5.5g | net carbs: 4.8g | fiber: 0.7g

Cream of Onion Pork Cutlets

Prep time: 10 minutes | Cook time: 10 minutes | Serves 4

2 tablespoons olive oil
4 pork cutlets
¼ cup cream of onion soup
½ teaspoon paprika
Sea salt and ground black pepper, to taste

1. Heat the olive oil in a sauté pan over moderate heat. Once hot, sear the pork cutlets for 5 to 6 minutes, turning once or twice to ensure even cooking.
2. Add in the cream of onion soup, paprika, salt, and black pepper. Cook for a further 3 minutes until heated through. The meat thermometer should register 145ºF (63ºC).
3. Serve in individual plates garnished with freshly snipped chives if desired. Enjoy!

Per Serving
calories: 396 | fat: 24.5g | protein: 40.2g
carbs: 0.9g | net carbs: 0.7g | fiber: 0.2g

Lemony Mustard Pork Roast

Prep time: 10 minutes | Cook time: 60 minutes | Serves 5

2 pounds (907 g) pork loin roast, trimmed
1½ tablespoons olive oil
1 tablespoon fresh lemon juice
1 tablespoon pork rub seasoning blend
1 tablespoon stone-ground mustard

1. Pat the pork loin roast dry.
2. Massage the pork loin roast with the olive oil. Then, sprinkle the lemon juice, pork rub seasoning blend, and mustard over all sides of the roast.
3. Prepare a grill for indirect heat. Grill the pork loin roast over indirect heat for about 1 hour. Let the grilled pork loin stand for 10 minutes before slicing and serving. Bon appétit!

Per Serving
calories: 385 | fat: 20.2g | protein: 48.0g
carbs: 0.1g | net carbs: 0g | fiber: 0.1g

Mediterranean Spiced Pork Roast

Prep time: 10 minutes | Cook time: 3 hours 50 minutes | Serves 4

2 pounds (907 g) pork shoulder
2 tablespoons coconut aminos
½ cup red wine
1 tablespoon Dijon mustard
1 tablespoon Mediterranean spice mix

1. Place the pork shoulder, coconut aminos, wine, mustard, and Mediterranean spice mix in a ceramic dish.
2. Cover and let it marinate in your refrigerator for 2 hours. Meanwhile, preheat your oven to 420ºF (216ºC).
3. Place the pork shoulder on a rack set into a roasting pan. Roast for 15 to 20 minutes; reduce the heat to 330ºF (166ºC).
4. Roast an additional 3 hours and 30 minutes, basting with the reserved marinade. Bon appétit!

Per Serving
calories: 610 | fat: 40.2g | protein: 57.0g
carbs: 0.7g | net carbs: 0.6g | fiber: 0.1g

Pork Cutlets with Juniper Berries

Prep time: 10 minutes | Cook time: 20 minutes | Serves 2

1 tablespoon lard, softened at room temperature
2 pork cutlets, 2-inch-thick
⅓ cup dry red wine
2 garlic cloves, sliced
½ teaspoon whole black peppercorns
4 tablespoons flaky salt
1 teaspoon juniper berries
½ teaspoon cayenne pepper

1. Melt the lard in a nonstick skillet over a moderate flame. Now, brown the pork cutlets for about 8 minutes, turning them over to ensure even cooking; reserve.
2. Add a splash of wine to deglaze the pan. Stir in the remaining ingredients and continue to cook until fragrant or for a minute or so.
3. Return the pork cutlets to the skillet, continue to cook until the sauce has thickened and everything is heated through about 10 minutes. Serve warm. Bon appétit!

Per Serving
calories: 370 | fat: 20.5g | protein: 40.2g
carbs: 1.2g | net carbs: 1.0g | fiber: 0.2g

Bolognese Pork Zoodles

Prep time: 10 minutes | Cook time: 25 minutes | Serves 3

3 teaspoons olive oil
¾ pound (340 g) ground pork
2 cloves garlic, pressed
2 medium-sized tomatoes, puréed
2 zucchini, spiralized

1. Heat the olive oil in a saucepan over medium-high heat. Once hot, sear the pork for 3 to 4 minutes or until no longer pink.
2. Stir in the garlic and cook for 30 seconds more or until fragrant.
3. Fold in the puréed tomatoes and bring to a boil; immediately turn the heat to medium-low and continue simmering an additional 20 minutes.
4. After that, fold in the zoodles and continue to cook for a further 1½ minutes until just al dente. Serve hot. Bon appétit!

Per Serving
calories: 358 | fat: 28.6g | protein: 20.2g
carbs: 4.0g | net carbs: 2.8g | fiber: 1.2g

Seared Pork Medallions

Prep time: 15 minutes | Cook time: 15 minutes | Serves 3

2 tablespoons olive oil
1 onion, sliced
2 garlic cloves, sliced
2 cups button mushrooms, sliced
3 pork medallions
Sea salt and ground black pepper, to taste
½ teaspoon paprika
1 tomato, sliced
1 bell pepper, deveined and sliced
¼ cup fresh parsley, chopped

1. Heat the olive oil in a frying pan over medium-high heat. Once hot, sauté the onion until tender and fragrant.
2. Stir in the garlic and mushrooms and continue to sauté an additional minute or so.
3. Add the pork medallions, salt, black pepper, paprika, tomato, and pepper to the frying pan; let it cook for 15 minutes or until heated through.
4. Garnish with fresh parsley and serve. Bon appétit!

Per Serving
calories: 365 | fat: 17.2g | protein: 45.0g
carbs: 4.5g | net carbs: 3.6g | fiber: 0.9g

White Wine Pork with Cabbage

Prep time: 15 minutes | Cook time: 1 hour 15 minutes | Serves 6

2 tablespoons olive oil
2 pounds (907 g) pork stew meat, cubed
Salt and black pepper, to taste
2 tablespoons butter
4 garlic cloves, minced
¾ cup vegetable stock
½ cup white wine
3 carrots, chopped
1 cabbage head, shredded
½ cup scallions, chopped
1 cup heavy cream

1. Set a pan over medium heat and warm butter and oil. Sear the pork until brown. Add garlic, scallions and carrots; sauté for 5 minutes. Pour in the cabbage, stock and wine, and bring to a boil. Reduce the heat and cook for 1 hour covered. Add in heavy cream as you stir for 1 minute, adjust seasonings and serve.

Per Serving
calories: 512 | fat: 32.6g | protein: 42.9g
carbs: 9.3g | net carbs: 5.9g | fiber: 3.4g

Pork Lettuce Wraps

Prep time: 10 minutes | Cook time: 14 minutes | Serves 6

2 pound (907 g) ground pork
1 tablespoon ginger-garlic paste
Pink salt and chili pepper, to taste
1 teaspoon butter
1 fresh head iceberg lettuce
2 sprigs green onion, chopped
1 red bell pepper, chopped
½ cucumber, finely chopped

1. Put the pork with ginger-garlic, salt, and chili pepper seasoning in a saucepan. Cook for 10
2. minutes over medium heat while breaking any lumps until the beef is no longer pink.
3. Drain liquid and add the butter, melt, and brown the meat for 4 minutes with continuous stirring. Pat the lettuce dry with paper towel and in each leaf spoon two to three tablespoons of pork, top with green onions, bell pepper, and cucumber. Serve with soy drizzling sauce.

Per Serving
calories: 311 | fat: 24g | protein: 19g
carbs: 3g | net carbs: 1g | fiber: 2g

Mustard Pork Meatballs

Prep time: 5 minutes | Cook time: 21 minutes | Serves 2

1 pound (454 g) ground pork
Salt and black pepper, to taste
1 tablespoon yellow mustard
½ cup almond flour
¼ cup mozzarella cheese, grated
¼ cup hot sauce
1 egg

1. Preheat oven to 400ºF (205ºC) and line a baking tray with parchment paper.
2. In a bowl, combine the pork, pepper, mustard, flour, mozzarella cheese, salt, and egg. Form meatballs and arrange them on the baking tray.
3. Cook for 16 minutes, then pour over the hot sauce and bake for 5 more minutes.
4. Serve warm.

Per Serving
calories: 518 | fat: 22g | protein: 60g
carbs: 2g | net carbs: 1g | fiber: 1g

BBQ Grilled Pork Spare Ribs

Prep time: 10 minutes | Cook time: 50 minutes | Serves 4

1 tablespoon erythritol
Salt and black pepper, to taste
1 tablespoon olive oil
1 teaspoon chipotle powder
1 teaspoon garlic powder
1 pound (454 g) pork spare ribs
1 tablespoon sugar-free BBQ sauce + extra for serving

1. Mix the erythritol, salt, pepper, oil, chipotle, and garlic powder. Brush on the meaty sides of the ribs, and wrap in foil. Sit for 30 minutes to marinate.
2. Preheat oven to 400ºF (205ºC), place wrapped ribs on a baking sheet, and cook for 40 minutes to be cooked through. Remove ribs and aluminum foil, brush with BBQ sauce, and brown under the broiler for 10 minutes on both sides. Slice and serve with extra BBQ sauce and lettuce tomato salad.

Per Serving
calories: 294 | fat: 18g | protein: 28g
carbs: 3g | net carbs: 3g | fiber: 0g

Spicy Pork and Capers with Olives

Prep time: 10 minutes | Cook time: 9 minutes | Serves 4

4 pork chops
1 tablespoon olive oil
1 garlic clove, minced
¼ tablespoon chili powder
¼ teaspoon cumin
Salt and black pepper, to taste
½ teaspoon hot pepper sauce
¼ cup capers
6 black olives, sliced

1. Preheat grill over medium heat. In a mixing bowl, combine olive oil, cumin, salt, hot pepper sauce, pepper, garlic and chili powder. Place in the pork chops, toss to coat, and refrigerate for 4 hours.
2. Arrange the pork on a preheated grill, cook for 7 minutes, turn, add in the capers, and cook for another 2 minutes. Place onto serving plates and sprinkle with olives to serve.

Per Serving
calories: 300 | fat: 14g | protein: 40g
carbs: 2g | net carbs: 1g | fiber: 1g

Pork Chops and Bacon

Prep time: 5 minutes | Cook time: 11 minutes | Serves 6

7 strips bacon, chopped
6 pork chops
Pink salt and black pepper to taste
5 sprigs fresh thyme
¼ cup chicken broth
½ cup heavy cream

1. Cook bacon in a large skillet over medium heat for 5 minutes to crispy. Remove with a slotted spoon onto a paper towel-lined plate to soak up excess fat. Season pork chops with salt and black pepper, and brown in the bacon grease for 4 minutes on each side. Remove to the bacon plate.
2. Stir the thyme, chicken broth, and heavy cream in the same skillet, and simmer for 5 minutes. Season with salt and black pepper. Put the chops and bacon in the skillet, and cook further for another 2 minutes. Serve chops and a generous ladle of sauce with cauli mash.

Per Serving
calories: 435 | fat: 37g | protein: 22g
carbs: 4g | net carbs: 3g | fiber: 1g

Pork with Raspberry Sauce

Prep time: 10 minutes | Cook time: 15 minutes | Serves 4

1 tablespoon olive oil
2 pound pork chops
Salt and black pepper to taste
2 cups raspberries
¼ cup water
1½ tablespoon Italian herb mix
1 tablespoon balsamic vinegar
1 teaspoon Worcestershire sauce

1. Heat oil in a skillet over medium heat, season the pork with salt and black pepper and cook for 5 minutes on each side. Put in serving plates, and reserve the pork drippings.
2. Mash raspberries with a fork in a bowl until jam-like. Pour into a saucepan, add water, and herb mix. Cook on low heat for 4 minutes. Stir in pork drippings, vinegar, and Worcestershire sauce. Simmer for 1 minute. Dish the pork chops, spoon sauce over, and serve with braised rapini.

Per Serving
calories: 413 | fat: 32g | protein: 26g
carbs: 5g | net carbs: 1g | fiber: 4g

Pork and Beef Meatballs

Prep time: 5 minutes | Cook time: 13 minutes | Serves 5

1 pound (454 g) ground pork
½ pound (227 g) ground beef
onion, chopped
garlic cloves, minced
1 teaspoon Hungarian spice blend

1. In a mixing bowl, thoroughly combine all ingredients until they are well incorporated. Form the mixture into meatballs with oiled hands. Place your meatballs on a tinfoil-lined baking sheet.
2. Bake in the preheated oven at 395ºF (202ºC) for 12 to 14 minutes or until they are golden brown.
3. Arrange on a nice serving platter and serve. Bon appétit!

Per Serving
calories: 377 | fat: 24g | protein: 36g
carbs: 2g | net carbs: 2g | fiber: 0g

Spicy Pork and Spanish Onion

Prep time: 10 minutes | Cook time: 10 minutes | Serves 2

1 tablespoon olive oil
2 pork cutlets
1 bell pepper, deveined and sliced
1 Spanish onion, chopped
2 garlic cloves, minced
½ teaspoon hot sauce
½ teaspoon mustard
½ teaspoon paprika
Coarse sea salt and ground black pepper, to taste

1. Heat the olive oil in a large saucepan over medium-high heat.
2. Then, fry the pork cutlets for 3 to 4 minutes until evenly golden and crispy on both sides.
3. Decrease the temperature to medium and add the bell pepper, Spanish onion, garlic, hot sauce, and mustard; continue cooking until the vegetables have softened, for a further 3 minutes.
4. Sprinkle with paprika, salt, and black pepper. Serve immediately and enjoy!

Per Serving
calories: 402 | fat: 24.2g | protein: 40.0g
carbs: 3.5g | net carbs: 2.7g | fiber: 0.8g

Creamy Dijon Pork Filet Mignon

Prep time: 10 minutes | Cook time: 10 minutes | Serves 6

2 teaspoons lard, at room temperature
2 pounds (907 g) pork filet mignon, cut into bite-sized chunks
Flaky salt and ground black pepper, to season
1 tablespoon Dijon mustard
1 cup double cream

1. Melt the lard in a saucepan over moderate heat; now, sear the filet mignon for 2 to 3 minutes per side. Season with salt and pepper to taste.
2. Fold in the Dijon mustard and cream. Reduce the heat to medium-low and continue to cook for a further 6 minutes or until the sauce has reduced slightly.
3. Serve in individual plates, garnished with cauli rice if desired. Enjoy!

Per Serving
calories: 302 | fat: 16.5g | protein: 34.1g
carbs: 2.2g | net carbs: 2.1g | fiber: 0.1g

Bacon and Pork Omelet

Prep time: 5 minutes | Cook time: 12 minutes | Serves 5

2 ounces (57 g) bacon, diced
1 pound (454 g) ground pork
1 shallot, chopped
1 teaspoon ginger-garlic paste
6 eggs, whisked

1. Heat up a nonstick skillet over a moderate flame. Now, cook the bacon until it releases easily from the bottom of the skillet.
2. Then, add in the ground pork and shallot and cook for 4 to 5 minutes or until the pork is no longer pink; discard the excess fat.
3. Fold in the ginger-garlic paste and whisked eggs; partially cover and let it cook on mediumlow temperature for 4 minutes. Flip your omelet and cook on the other side for 3 minutes longer.
4. Slide your omelet onto a plate and serve right now. Bon appétit!

Per Serving
calories: 393 | fat: 28g | protein: 31g
carbs: 1g | net carbs: 1g | fiber: 0g

Duo-Cheese Pork and Turkey Patties

Prep time: 15 minutes | Cook time: 15 minutes | Serves 6

1½ pounds (680 g) ground pork
½ pound (227 g) ground turkey
1 serrano pepper, deseeded and minced
2 garlic cloves, finely minced
½ cup onion, finely minced
1 cup Romano cheese, grated
½ cup Asiago cheese, shredded
1 teaspoon mustard seeds
½ teaspoon dried marjoram
½ teaspoon dried basil
1 teaspoon paprika
Sea salt and ground black pepper, to taste

1. Begin by preheating a gas grill to high.
2. Mix all of the above ingredients until everything is well incorporated. Form the mixture into 6 patties with oiled hands.
3. Place on the preheated grill and cook for 7 to 8 minutes on each side until slightly charred. Bon appétit!

Per Serving
calories: 514 | fat: 35.2g | protein: 44.2g
carbs: 2.5g | net carbs: 2.2g | fiber: 0.3g

Pork Steaks with Chimichurri Sauce

Prep time: 10 minutes | Cook time: 5 minutes | Serves 4

1 garlic clove, minced
½ teaspoon white wine vinegar
1 tablespoon parsley leaves, chopped
1 tablespoon cilantro leaves, chopped
1 tablespoon extra-virgin olive oil
16 ounces (454 g) pork loin steaks
Salt and black pepper to season
1 tablespoon sesame oil

1. To make the sauce: in a bowl, mix the parsley, cilantro and garlic. Add the vinegar, extra-virgin olive oil, and salt, and combine well.
2. Preheat a grill pan over medium heat. Rub the pork with sesame oil, and season with salt and pepper. Grill the meat for 4 to 5 minutes on each side until no longer pink in the center. Put the pork on a serving plate and spoon chimichurri sauce over, to serve.

Per Serving
calories: 326 | fat: 21g | protein: 32g
carbs: 2g | net carbs: 2g | fiber: 0g

Herbed Pork and Turkey Meatloaf

Prep time: 20 minutes | Cook time: 60 minutes | Serves 6

1 pound (454 g) ground pork
½ pound (227 g) ground turkey
¼ cup flax seed meal
2 eggs, beaten
2 cloves garlic, minced
½ cup scallions, chopped
Sea salt and ground black pepper, to season
1 teaspoon dried oregano
½ teaspoon dried basil
½ teaspoon dried marjoram
½ teaspoon dried rosemary
1 tablespoon fresh chives, chopped
3 ounces (85 g) tomato paste
1 tablespoon coconut aminos
1 tablespoon brown mustard

1. Begin by preheating your oven to 360ºF (182ºC). Now, spritz the sides and bottom of a loaf pan with nonstick cooking oil.
2. Thoroughly combine the ground meat with the flax seed meal, eggs, garlic, scallions, spices, and herbs.
3. Press the mixture into the prepared loaf pan. Bake in the preheated oven for 30 minutes
4. In a mixing bowl, whisk the tomato paste, coconut aminos, and mustard. Spread the mixture on top of the meatloaf.
5. Return to the oven; bake for a further 30 minutes or until internal temperature reaches 165ºF (74ºC). Bon appétit!

Per Serving
calories: 345 | fat: 23.2g | protein: 30.1g
carbs: 2.7g | net carbs: 1.7g | fiber: 1.0g

Olla Podrida

Prep time: 15 minutes | Cook time: 40 minutes | Serves 4

2 tablespoons olive oil
1½ pounds (680 g) pork ribs
1 yellow onion, chopped
2 garlic cloves, minced
2 Spanish peppers, chopped
1 Spanish Naga pepper, chopped
1 celery stalk, chopped
½ cup Marsala wine
8 ounces (227 g) button mushrooms, sliced
Sea salt and ground black pepper, to taste
1 teaspoon cayenne pepper
1 cup tomato purée
1 bay laurel

1. Heat 1 tablespoon of the olive oil in a stockpot over medium-high heat. Now, cook the pork ribs for 4 to 5 minutes per side or until brown; set aside.
2. Then, heat the remaining tablespoon of olive oil and sauté the onion, garlic, peppers, and celery for 5 minutes more or until tender and fragrant.
3. After that, add in a splash of red wine to scrape up the browned bits that stick to the bottom of the pot.
4. Add the mushrooms, salt, black pepper, cayenne pepper, tomatoes, and bay laurel to the stockpot.
5. When the mixture reaches boiling, turn the heat to a medium-low. Add the reserved pork back to the pot. Let it cook, partially covered, for 35 minutes. Serve warm and enjoy!

Per Serving
calories: 360 | fat: 19.1g | protein: 38.2g
carbs: 4.9g | net carbs: 3.2g | fiber: 1.7g

St. Louis Ribs

Prep time: 10 minutes | Cook time: 2 hours | Serves 5

2 pounds (907 g) St. Louis-style pork ribs
1 teaspoon cayenne pepper
Flaky salt and ground black pepper, to season
4 tablespoons sesame oil
2 tablespoons Swerve
1 tablespoon coconut aminos soy sauce
1 teaspoon oyster sauce
1 cup tomato sauce, no sugar added
1 teaspoon Chinese five-spice
2 garlic cloves, pressed

1. Season the pork ribs with the cayenne pepper, salt, and black pepper. Arrange them on a tinfoil-lined baking pan.
2. Cover with a piece of foil and bake in the preheated oven at 360ºF (182ºC) for 1 hour 30 minutes.
3. In the meantime, thoroughly combine the remaining ingredients for the glaze; whisk to combine well and brush the glaze over the pork ribs.
4. Continue to bake at 420ºF (216ºC) for 30 minutes longer. Bon appétit!

Per Serving
calories: 371 | fat: 21.1g | protein: 38.7g
carbs: 4.2g | net carbs: 3.0g | fiber: 1.2g

Pickle and Ham Stuffed Pork

Prep time: 20 minutes | Cook time: 35 minutes | Serves 4

Zest and juice from 2 limes
2 garlic cloves, minced
¾ cup olive oil
1 cup fresh cilantro, chopped
1 cup fresh mint, chopped
1 teaspoon dried oregano
Salt and black pepper, to taste
2 teaspoons cumin
4 pork loin steaks
2 pickles, chopped
4 ham slices
6 Swiss cheese slices
2 tablespoons mustard

Salad:
1 head red cabbage, shredded
2 tablespoons vinegar
3 tablespoons olive oil
Salt to taste

1. In a food processor, blitz the lime zest, oil, oregano, black pepper, cumin, cilantro, lime juice, garlic, mint, and salt. Rub the steaks with the mixture and toss well to coat; set aside for some hours in the fridge.
2. Arrange the steaks on a working surface, split the pickles, mustard, cheese, and ham on them, roll, and secure with toothpicks. Heat a pan over medium heat, add in the pork rolls, cook each side for 2 minutes and remove to a baking sheet. Bake in the oven at 350ºF (180ºC) for 25 minutes. Prepare the red cabbage salad by mixing all salad ingredients and serve with the meat.

Per Serving
calories: 412 | fat: 37.1g | protein: 25.8g
carbs: 8.1g | net carbs: 3.1g | fiber: 5.0g

BBQ Pork Ribs

Prep time: 15 minutes | Cook time: 7 hours 5 minutes | Serves 6

3 racks pork ribs, silver lining removed
2 cups sugar-free BBQ sauce
2 tablespoons erythritol
2 teaspoons chili powder
2 teaspoons cumin powder
2 teaspoons onion powder
2 teaspoons smoked paprika
2 teaspoons garlic powder
Salt and black pepper to taste
1 teaspoon mustard powder

1. Preheat a smoker to 400ºF (205ºC) using mesquite wood to create flavor in the smoker.
2. In a bowl, mix the erythritol, chili powder, cumin powder, black pepper, onion powder, smoked paprika, garlic powder, salt, and mustard powder. Rub the ribs and let marinate for 30 minutes.
3. Place on the grill grate, and cook at reduced heat of 225ºF (107ºC) for 4 hours. Flip the ribs after and continue cooking for 4 hours. Brush the ribs with BBQ sauce on both sides and sear them in increased heat for 3 minutes per side. Remove and let sit for 4 minutes before slicing. Serve with red cabbage coleslaw.

Per Serving
calories: 581 | fat: 36.5g | protein: 44.6g
carbs: 1.8g | net carbs: 0g | fiber: 1.8g

Chili Con Carne

Prep time: 15 minutes | Cook time: 45 minutes | Serves 4

2 ounces (57 g) bacon, diced
1 red onion, chopped
1 pound (454 g) ground pork
1 teaspoon ground cumin
2 cloves garlic, minced
1 teaspoon chipotle powder
Kosher salt and ground black pepper, to taste
½ cup beef broth
2 ripe tomatoes, crushed

1. Heat up a medium stockpot over a moderate flame. Cook the bacon until crisp; reserve.
2. Cook the onion and ground pork in the bacon grease. Cook until the ground pork is no longer pink and the onion just begins to brown.
3. Stir in the ground cumin and garlic and continue to sauté for 30 seconds more or until aromatic.
4. Add the chipotle powder, salt, black pepper, broth, and tomatoes to the pot. Cook, partially covered, for 45 minutes or until heated through.
5. You can add ¼ cup of water during the cooking, as needed. Serve with the reserved bacon and other favorite toppings. Enjoy!

Per Serving
calories: 390 | fat: 29.8g | protein: 22.3g
carbs: 5.2g | net carbs: 3.7g | fiber: 1.5g

Tangy-Garlicky Pork Chops

Prep time: 10 minutes | Cook time: 15 minutes | Serves 4

1 pound (454 g) boneless center-cut pork chops, pounded to ¼ inch thick
Sea salt, for seasoning
Freshly ground black pepper, for seasoning
¼ cup good-quality olive oil, divided
¼ cup finely chopped fresh cilantro
1 tablespoon minced garlic
Juice of 1 lime

1. Marinate the pork. Pat the pork chops dry and season them lightly with salt and pepper. Place them in a large bowl, add 2 tablespoons of the olive oil, and the cilantro, garlic, and lime juice. Toss to coat the chops. Cover the bowl and marinate the chops at room temperature for 30 minutes.
2. Cook the pork. In a large skillet over medium-high heat, warm the remaining 2 tablespoons of olive oil. Add the pork chops in a single layer and fry them, turning them once, until they're just cooked through and still juicy, 6 to 7 minutes per side.
3. Serve. Divide the chops between four plates and serve them immediately.

Per Serving
calories: 249 | fat: 16g | protein: 25g
carbs: 2g | net carbs: 2g | fiber: 0g

Paprika Pork Loin Shoulder

Prep time: 10 minutes | Cook time: 20 minutes | Serves 4

2 teaspoons olive oil
1 pound (454 g) pork loin shoulder, cut into bite-sized cubes
4 cloves garlic, minced
¼ cup red wine
½ teaspoon paprika
Sea salt and ground black pepper, to season
1 tablespoon hot sauce

1. Heat the olive oil in a saucepan over a moderate flame. Once hot, sear the pork for 5 to 6 minutes, stirring continuously to ensure even cooking; reserve.
2. Now, sauté the garlic for 30 to 40 seconds or until just tender and aromatic.
3. Add a splash of wine and stir, scraping the browned bits from the bottom of the saucepan. Add in the paprika, salt, pepper, and hot sauce; add the pork back to the saucepan.
4. Turn the heat to simmer. Partially cover and simmer approximately 13 minutes until the sauce has thickened. Bon appétit!

Per Serving
calories: 301 | fat: 18.0g | protein: 30.2g
carbs: 2.5g | net carbs: 2.2g | fiber: 0.3g

Pork and Yellow Squash Traybake

Prep time: 15 minutes | Cook time: 31 minutes | Serves 4

1 pound (454 g) ground pork
1 large yellow squash, thinly sliced
Salt and black pepper to taste
1 garlic clove, minced
2 red onions, chopped
1 cup broccoli, chopped
1 (15 ounce / 425-g) can diced tomatoes
½ cup pork rinds, crushed
¼ cup parsley, chopped
2 cups cottage cheese
1 tablespoon olive oil
⅓ cup chicken broth

1. Heat the olive oil in a skillet over medium heat, add the pork, season it with salt and pepper, and cook for 3 minutes or until no longer pink. Stir occasionally while breaking any lumps apart.
2. Add the garlic, half of the red onions, broccoli, and 2 tablespoons of pork rinds. Continue cooking for 3 minutes. Stir in the tomatoes, half of the parsley, and chicken broth. Cook further for 3 minutes.
3. Mix the remaining parsley and cottage cheese and set aside. Sprinkle the bottom of a baking dish with 1 tablespoon of pork rinds; top with half of the squash and a season of salt, ⅔ of the pork mixture, and the cheese mixture. Repeat the layering process a second time to exhaust the ingredients.
4. Cover the baking dish with foil and put in the oven to bake for 20 minutes at 380°F (193°C). Remove the foil and brown the top of the casserole with the broiler side of the oven for 2 minutes.
5. Serve immediately.

Per Serving
calories: 531 | fat: 35g | protein: 49g
carbs: 10g | net carbs: 3g | fiber: 7g

Creamy Pepper Loin Steaks

Prep time: 15 minutes | Cook time: 10 minutes | Serves 2

1 teaspoon lard, at room temperature
2 pork loin steaks
½ cup beef bone broth
2 bell peppers, deseeded and chopped
1 shallot, chopped
1 garlic clove, minced
Sea salt, to season
½ teaspoon cayenne pepper
¼ teaspoon paprika
1 teaspoon Italian seasoning mix
¼ cup Greek yogurt

1. Melt the lard in a cast-iron skillet over moderate heat. Once hot, cook the pork loin steaks until slightly browned or approximately 5 minutes per side; reserve.
2. Add a splash of the beef bone broth to deglaze the pan. Now, cook the bell peppers, shallot, and garlic until tender and aromatic. Season with salt, cayenne pepper, paprika, and Italian seasoning mix.
3. After that, decrease the temperature to medium-low, add the Greek yogurt to the skillet and let it simmer for 2 minutes more or until heated through. Serve immediately.

Per Serving
calories: 450 | fat: 19.1g | protein: 62.2g
carbs: 6.0g | net carbs: 4.9g | fiber: 1.1g

Pork Ragout

Prep time: 15 minutes | Cook time: 35 minutes | Serves 2

1 teaspoon lard, melted at room temperature
¾ pound (340 g) pork butt, cut into bite-sized cubes
1 red bell pepper, deveined and chopped
1 poblano pepper, deveined and chopped
2 cloves garlic, pressed
½ cup leeks, chopped
Sea salt and ground black pepper, to season
½ teaspoon mustard seeds
¼ teaspoon ground allspice
¼ teaspoon celery seeds
1 cup roasted vegetable broth
2 vine-ripe tomatoes, puréed

1. Melt the lard in a stockpot over moderate heat. Once hot, cook the pork cubes for 4 to 6 minutes, stirring occasionally to ensure even cooking.
2. Then, stir in the vegetables and continue cooking until they are tender and fragrant. Add in the salt, black pepper, mustard seeds, allspice, celery seeds, roasted vegetable broth, and tomatoes.
3. Reduce the heat to simmer. Let it simmer for 30 minutes longer or until everything is heated through.
4. Ladle into individual bowls and serve hot. Bon appétit!

Per Serving
calories: 390 | fat: 24.2g | protein: 33.0g
carbs: 5.3g | net carbs: 4.1g | fiber: 1.2g

Roasted Pork Shoulder

Prep time: 20 minutes | Cook time: 60 minutes | Serves 2

1 pound (454 g) pork shoulder
4 tablespoons red wine
1 teaspoon stone ground mustard
1 tablespoon coconut aminos
1 tablespoon lemon juice
1 tablespoon sesame oil
2 sprigs rosemary
1 teaspoon sage
1 shallot, peeled and chopped
½ celery stalk, chopped
½ head garlic, peeled and separated into cloves
Sea salt and freshly cracked black pepper, to season

1. Place the pork shoulder, red wine, mustard, coconut aminos, lemon juice, sesame oil, rosemary, and sage in a ceramic dish; cover and let it marinate in your refrigerator at least 3 hours.
2. Discard the marinade and place the pork shoulder in a lightly greased baking dish. Scatter the vegetables around the pork shoulder and sprinkle with salt and black pepper.
3. Roast in the preheated oven at 390ºF (199ºC) for 15 minutes.
4. Now, reduce the temperature to 310ºF (154ºC) and continue baking an additional 40 to 45 minutes. Baste the meat with the reserved marinade once or twice.
5. Place on cooling racks before carving and serving. Bon appétit!

Per Serving
calories: 500 | fat: 35.4g | protein: 40.1g
carbs: 2.6g | net carbs: 2.1g | fiber: 0.5g

Pork Chops and Brussel Sprouts

Prep time: 10 minutes | Cook time: 16 minutes | Serves 6

1 tablespoon lemon juice
3 cloves garlic, pureed
Salt and black pepper to taste
1 tablespoon olive oil
6 pork loin chops
1 tablespoon butter
1 pound (454 g) Brussel sprouts, halved
1 tablespoon white wine

1. Preheat grill to 400ºF (205ºC), and mix the lemon juice, garlic, salt, pepper, and oil in a bowl.
2. Brush the pork with mixture, place onto a baking sheet, and cook for 6 minutes on each side until browned. Share into 6 plates, and make the side dish.
3. Melt butter in a small wok, or pan and cook in Brussel sprouts for 5 minutes until tender.
4. Drizzle with white wine, sprinkle with salt and black pepper, and cook for another 5 minutes. Ladle Brussel sprouts to the side of the chops, and serve with a hot sauce.

Per Serving
calories: 400 | fat: 22g | protein: 36g
carbs: 7g | net carbs: 4g | fiber: 3g

Pork Chops with Greek Salsa

Prep time: 15 minutes | Cook time: 15 minutes | Serves 4

¼ cup good-quality olive oil, divided
1 tablespoon red wine vinegar
3 teaspoons chopped fresh oregano, divided
1 teaspoon minced garlic
4 (4-ounce / 113-g) boneless center-cut loin pork chops
½ cup halved cherry tomatoes
½ yellow bell pepper, diced
½ English cucumber, chopped
¼ red onion, chopped
1 tablespoon balsamic vinegar
Sea salt, for seasoning
Freshly ground black pepper, for seasoning

1. Marinate the pork. In a medium bowl, stir together 3 tablespoons of the olive oil, the vinegar, 2 teaspoons of the oregano, and the garlic. Add the pork chops to the bowl, turning them to get them coated with the marinade. Cover the bowl and place it in the refrigerator for 30 minutes.
2. Make the salsa. While the pork is marinating, in a medium bowl, stir together the remaining 1 tablespoon of olive oil, the tomatoes, yellow bell pepper, cucumber, red onion, vinegar, and the remaining 1 teaspoon of oregano. Season the salsa with salt and pepper. Set the bowl aside.
3. Grill the pork chops. Heat a grill to medium-high heat. Remove the pork chops from the marinade and grill them until just cooked through, 6 to 8 minutes per side.
4. Serve. Rest the pork for 5 minutes. Divide the pork between four plates and serve them with a generous scoop of the salsa.

Per Serving
calories: 277 | fat: 17g | protein: 25g
carbs: 4g | net carbs: 3g | fiber: 1g

Hearty Pork Stew Meat

Prep time: 10 minutes | Cook time: 1 hour | Serves 5

2 tablespoons olive oil
2 pounds pork stew meat
1 yellow onion, chopped
1 garlic cloves, minced
¼ cup dry sherry wine
4 cups chicken bone broth
1 cup tomatoes, pureed
1 bay laurel
Sea salt and ground black pepper, to taste
1 tablespoon fresh cilantro, chopped

1. Heat the olive oil in a soup pot over a moderate flame. Sear the pork for about 5 minutes, stirring continuously to ensure even cooking; reserve.
2. Cook the yellow onion in the pan drippings until just tender and translucent. Stir in the garlic and continue to sauté for a further 30 seconds.
3. Pour in a splash of dry sherry to deglaze the pan.
4. Pour in the chicken bone broth and bring to a boil. Stir in the tomatoes and bay laurel. Season with salt and pepper to taste. Turn the heat to medium-low and continue to cook 10 minutes longer.
5. Add the reserved pork back to the pot, partially cover, and continue to simmer for 45 minutes longer. Garnish with cilantro and serve hot. Bon appétit!

Per Serving
calories: 332 | fat: 15g | protein: 41g
carbs: 4g | net carbs: 3g | fiber: 1g

Spicy Pork Meatballs with Seeds

Prep time: 15 minutes | Cook time: 20 minutes | Serves 2

1 tablespoon ground flax seeds
2 ounces (57 g) bacon rinds
½ pound (227 g) ground pork
1 garlic clove, minced
½ cup scallions, chopped
Sea salt and cayenne pepper, to taste
½ teaspoon smoked paprika
¼ teaspoon ground cumin
¼ teaspoon mustard seeds
½ teaspoon fennel seeds
½ teaspoon chili pepper flakes
2 tablespoons olive oil

1. In a mixing bowl, thoroughly combine all ingredients, except for the olive oil, until well combined. Form the mixture into balls and set aside.
2. Heat the olive oil in a nonstick skillet and fry the meatballs for about 15 minutes or until cooked through.
3. Serve with marinara sauce if desired. Bon appétit!

Per Serving
calories: 558 | fat: 50.0g | protein: 0.6g carbs: 2.2g | net carbs: 1.4g | fiber: 0.8g

Tangy Pork Rib Roast

Prep time: 10 minutes | Cook time: 1 hour | Serves 6

¼ cup good-quality olive oil
Zest and juice of 1 lemon
Zest and juice of 1 lemon
4 rosemary sprigs, lightly crushed
4 thyme sprigs, lightly crushed
1 (4-bone) pork rib roast, about 2½ pounds
6 garlic cloves, peeled
Sea salt, for seasoning
Freshly ground black pepper, for seasoning

1. Make the marinade. In a large bowl, combine the olive oil, lemon zest, lemon juice, lemon zest, lemon juice, rosemary sprigs, and thyme sprigs.
2. Marinate the roast. Use a small knife to make six 1-inch-deep slits in the fatty side of the roast. Stuff the garlic cloves in the slits. Put the roast in the bowl with the marinade and turn it to coat it well with the marinade. Cover the bowl and refrigerate it overnight, turning the roast in the marinade several times.
3. Preheat the oven. Set the oven temperature to 350ºF (180ºC).
4. Roast the pork. Remove the pork from the marinade and season it with salt and pepper, then put it in a baking dish and let it come to room temperature. Roast the pork until it's cooked through (145- to 160-ºF / 63- to 71-ºC internal temperature), about 1 hour. Throw out any leftover marinade.
5. Serve. Let the pork rest for 10 minutes, then cut it into slices and arrange the slices on a platter. Serve it warm.

Per Serving
calories: 403 | fat: 30g | protein: 30g carbs: 1g | net carbs: 1g | fiber: 0g

Pulled Boston Butt

Prep time: 15 minutes | Cook time: 5 minutes | Serves 2

1 teaspoon lard, melted at room temperature
¾ pork Boston butt, sliced
2 garlic cloves, pressed
½ teaspoon red pepper flakes, crushed
½ teaspoon black peppercorns, freshly cracked
Sea salt, to taste
2 bell peppers, deveined and sliced
1 tablespoon fresh mint leaves, snipped
4 tablespoons cream cheese

1. Melt the lard in a cast-iron skillet over a moderate flame. Once hot, brown the pork for 2 minutes per side until caramelized and crispy on the edges.
2. Reduce the temperature to medium-low and continue cooking another 4 minutes, turning over periodically. Shred the pork with two forks and return to the skillet.
3. Add the garlic, red pepper, black peppercorns, salt, and bell pepper and continue cooking for a further 2 minutes or until the peppers are just tender and fragrant.
4. Serve with fresh mint and a dollop of cream cheese. Enjoy!

Per Serving
calories: 371 | fat: 21.8g | protein: 35.0g carbs: 5.0g | net carbs: 4.0g | fiber: 1.0g

Pork and Butternut Squash Stew

Prep time: 15 minutes | Cook time: 45 minutes | Serves 6

1 cup butternut squash
2 pounds (907 g) pork, chopped
1 tablespoon peanut butter
1 tablespoon peanuts, chopped
1 garlic clove, minced
½ cup onion, chopped
½ cup white wine
1 tablespoon olive oil
1 teaspoon lemon juice
¼ cup sweetener, granulated
¼ teaspoon cardamom
¼ teaspoon all spice
2 cups chicken stock

1. Heat olive oil in a large pot. Add onions and sauté for 3 minutes until translucent. Add garlic, and cook for 30 more seconds. Add the pork, and cook until browned, about 5-6 minutes, stirring periodically. Pour in the wine, and cook for one minute. Throw in the remaining ingredients, except for the lemon juice and peanuts. Add two cups of water, bring the mixture to a boil, and cook for 5 minutes.
2. Reduce the heat to low, cover the pot, and let cook for about 30 minutes. Adjust seasoning.
3. Stir in the lemon juice before serving. Ladle into serving bowls, and serve topped with peanuts, and enjoy.

Per Serving
calories: 545 | fat: 33g | protein: 46g
carbs: 7g | net carbs: 4g | fiber: 3g

Herbed Pork Chops with Cranberry Sauce

Prep time: 20 minutes | Cook time: 2²/₃ hours | Serves 2

4 pork chops
½ teaspoon garlic powder
Salt and black pepper to taste
1 teaspoon fresh basil, chopped
A drizzle of olive oil
½ onion, chopped
½ cup white wine
Juice of ½ lemon
1 bay leaf
1 cup chicken stock
Fresh parsley, chopped, for serving
1 cup cranberries
½ teaspoon fresh rosemary, chopped
½ cup xylitol
½ cup water
½ teaspoon harissa paste sriracha sauce

1. Preheat oven to 360ºF (182ºC). In a bowl, combine the pork chops with basil, salt, garlic powder, and black pepper. Heat a pan with a drizzle of oil over medium heat, place in the pork, and cook until browned, about 4-5 minutes; set aside.
2. Stir in the onion and cook for 2 minutes. Place in the bay leaf and wine, and cook for 4 minutes. Pour in lemon juice, and chicken stock, and simmer for 5 minutes. Return the pork and cook for 10 minutes. Cover the pan and place it in the oven for 2 hours.
3. Set a pan over medium-high heat, add in the cranberries, rosemary, sriracha sauce, water and xylitol, and bring to a simmer for 15 minutes. Remove the pork chops from the oven and discard the bay leaf. Pour the sauce over the pork and serve sprinkled with parsley.

Per Serving
calories: 450 | fat: 24g | protein: 42g
carbs: 10g | net carbs: 7g | fiber: 3g

Pork Medallions

Prep time: 15 minutes | Cook time: 15 minutes | Serves 2

1 ounce (28 g) bacon, diced
2 pork medallions
2 garlic cloves, sliced
1 red onion, chopped
1 jalapeño pepper, deseeded and chopped
1 tablespoon apple cider vinegar
½ cup chicken bone broth
⅓ pound (136 g) red cabbage, shredded
1 bay leaf
1 sprig rosemary
1 sprig thyme
Kosher salt and ground black pepper, to taste

1. Heat a Dutch pot over medium-high heat. Once hot, cook the bacon until it is crisp or about 3 minutes; reserve.
2. Now, cook the pork medallions in the bacon grease until they are browned on both sides.
3. Add the remaining ingredients and reduce the heat to medium-low. Let it cook for 13 minutes more, gently stirring periodically to ensure even cooking.
4. Taste and adjust the seasonings. Serve in individual bowls topped with the reserved fried bacon. Bon appétit!

Per Serving
calories: 529 | fat: 31.7g | protein: 51.1g
carbs: 6.2g | net carbs: 3.7g | fiber: 2.5g

Roasted Stuffed Pork Loin Steak

Prep time: 15 minutes | Cook time: 30 minutes | Serves 4

1 tablespoon olive oil	to taste
Zest and juice from 1 lime	1 teaspoon cumin
1 garlic clove, minced	2 pork loin steaks
1 tablespoon fresh cilantro, chopped	1 pickle, chopped
1 tablespoon fresh mint, chopped	2 ounces (57 g) smoked ham, sliced
Salt and black pepper,	2 ounces (57 g) Gruyere cheese sliced
	1 tablespoon mustard

1. Start with making the marinade: combine the lime zest, oil, black pepper, cumin, cilantro, lime juice, garlic, mint and salt, in a food processor. Place the steaks in the marinade, and toss well to coat; set aside for some hours in the fridge.
2. Arrange the steaks on a working surface, split the pickles, mustard, cheese, and ham on them, roll, and secure with toothpicks. Heat a pan over medium heat, add in the pork rolls, cook each side for 2 minutes and remove to a baking sheet. Bake in the oven at 350ºF (180ºC) for 25 minutes.
3. Serve immediately.

Per Serving
calories: 433 | fat: 38g | protein: 30g
carbs: 5g | net carbs: 4g | fiber: 1g

Parmesan Bacon-Stuffed Pork Roll

Prep time: 15 minutes | Cook time: 30 minutes | Serves 4

1 tablespoon olive oil	1 garlic clove, minced
4 ounces (113 g) bacon, sliced	1 tablespoon Parmesan cheese, grated
1 tablespoon fresh parsley, chopped	5 ounces (142 g) canned diced tomatoes
4 pork chops, boneless and flatten	Salt and black pepper to taste
1 cup ricotta cheese	½ teaspoon herbes de Provence
1 tablespoon pine nuts	
1 spring onion, chopped	

1. Put the pork chops on a flat surface. Set the bacon slices on top, then divide the ricotta cheese, pine nuts, and Parmesan cheese. Roll each pork piece and secure with a toothpick.
2. Set a pan over medium heat and warm oil. Cook the pork rolls until browned, and remove to a plate.
3. Add in the spring onion and garlic, and cook for 5 minutes. Place in the stock and cook for 3 minutes. Get rid of the toothpicks from the rolls and return them to the pan. Stir in the black pepper, salt, tomatoes and herbes de Provence. Bring to a boil, set heat to medium-low, and cook for 20 minutes while covered. Sprinkle with parsley to serve.

Per Serving
calories: 568 | fat: 38g | protein: 51g
carbs: 6g | net carbs: 3g | fiber: 2g

Pork Chops with Veggies

Prep time: 10 minutes | Cook time: 12 minutes | Serves 4

1 tablespoon olive oil	1 tablespoon white wine
1 tablespoon lemon juice	Salt and black pepper to taste
1 garlic clove, pureed	¼ teaspoon cumin
4 pork loin chops	¼ teaspoon ground nutmeg
⅓ head cabbage, shredded	1 tablespoon parsley
1 tomato, chopped	

1. In a bowl, mix the lemon juice, garlic, salt, pepper and olive oil. Brush the pork with the mixture.
2. Preheat grill to high heat. Grill the pork for 2 to 3 minutes on each side until cooked through.
3. Remove to serving plates. Warm the remaining olive oil in a pan and cook in cabbage for 5 minutes.
4. Drizzle with white wine, sprinkle with cumin, nutmeg, salt and pepper. Add in the tomatoes, cook for another 5 minutes, stirring occasionally. Ladle the sautéed cabbage to the side of the chops and serve sprinkled with parsley.

Per Serving
calories: 382 | fat: 21g | protein: 41g
carbs: 6g | net carbs: 4g | fiber: 2g

Pork and Veggies Burgers

Prep time: 10 minutes | Cook time: 5 minutes | Serves 6

2 pound (907 g) ground pork
Pink salt and chili pepper, to taste
1 tablespoon olive oil
1 tablespoon butter
1 white onion, sliced into rings
1 tablespoon balsamic vinegar
3 drops liquid stevia
6 low carb burger buns, halved
2 firm tomatoes, sliced into rings

1. Combine the pork, salt and chili pepper in a bowl, and mold out 6 patties.
2. Heat the olive oil in a skillet over medium heat, and fry the patties for 4 to 5 minutes on each side until golden brown on the outside. Remove onto a plate, and sit for 3 minutes.
3. Melt butter in a skillet over medium heat, sauté onions for 2 minutes, and stir in the balsamic vinegar and liquid stevia. Cook for 30 seconds stirring once, or twice until caramelized. In each bun, place a patty, top with some onion rings and 2 tomato rings.
4. Serve the burgers with cheddar cheese dip.

Per Serving
calories: 315 | fat: 23g | protein: 16g
carbs: 7g | net carbs: 6g | fiber: 1g

Pork Kofte with Cauliflower Mash

Prep time: 15 minutes | Cook time: 30 minutes | Serves 4

1 pound (454 g) ground pork
1 tablespoon olive oil
1 tablespoon pork rinds, crushed
1 garlic clove, minced
1 shallot, chopped
1 small egg
⅓ teaspoon paprika
Salt and black pepper to taste
1 tablespoon parsley, chopped
½ cup tomato purée, sugar-free
½ teaspoon oregano
⅓ cup Italian blend kinds of cheeses
1 tablespoon basil, chopped to garnish

1. In a bowl, mix the ground pork, shallot, pork rinds, garlic, egg, paprika, oregano, parsley, salt, and black pepper, just until combined. Form balls of the mixture and place them in an oiled baking pan; drizzle with olive oil. Bake in the oven for 18 minutes at 390ºF (199ºC).
2. Pour the tomato purée all over the meatballs. Sprinkle with the Italian blend cheeses, and put it back in the oven to bake for 10 to 15 minutes until the cheese melts. Once ready, take out the pan and garnish with basil. Delicious when served with cauliflower mash.

Per Serving
calories: 458 | fat: 30g | protein: 34g
carbs: 8g | net carbs: 6g | fiber: 2g

Tomato purée Pork Chops

Prep time: 10 minutes | Cook time: 37 minutes | Serves 4

4 pork chops
½ tablespoon fresh basil, chopped
1 garlic clove, minced
1 tablespoon olive oil
7 ounces (198 g) canned diced tomatoes
½ tablespoon tomato purée
Salt and black pepper, to taste
½ red chili, finely chopped

1. Season the pork with salt and black pepper. Set a pan over medium heat and warm oil, place in the pork chops, cook for 3 minutes, turn and cook for another 3 minutes; remove to a bowl. Add in the garlic and cook for 30 seconds.
2. Stir in the tomato purée, tomatoes, and chili; bring to a boil, and reduce heat to medium-low. Place in the pork chops, cover the pan and simmer everything for 30 minutes. Remove the pork chops to plates and sprinkle with fresh oregano to serve.

Per Serving
calories: 372 | fat: 21g | protein: 40g
carbs: 3g | net carbs: 2g | fiber: 1g

Baked Cheesy Pork and Veggies

Prep time: 10 minutes | Cook time: 40 minutes | Serves 4

1 pound (454 g) ground pork
1 onion, chopped
1 garlic clove, minced
½ green beans, chopped
Salt and black pepper to taste
1 zucchini, sliced
¼ cup heavy cream
5 eggs
½ cup Monterey Jack cheese, grated

1. In a bowl, mix onion, green beans, ground pork, garlic, black pepper and salt. Layer the meat mixture on the bottom of a small greased baking dish. Spread zucchini slices on top.
2. In a separate bowl, combine cheese, eggs and heavy cream. Top with this creamy mixture and bake for 40 minutes at 360°F (182°C), until the edges and top become brown.
3. Serve immediately.

Per Serving
calories: 335 | fat: 21g | protein: 28g
carbs: 4g | net carbs: 4g | fiber: 0g

Pork and Mashed Cauliflower Crust

Prep time: 15 minutes | Cook time: 1 hour | Serves 8

Crust:
1 egg
¼ cup butter
2 cups almond flour
¼ teaspoon xanthan gum
¼ cup mozzarella, shredded
A pinch of salt

Filling:
2 pounds (907 g) ground pork
⅓ cup onion, pureed
¾ teaspoon allspice
1 cup cauliflower, mashed
1 tablespoon ground sage
1 tablespoon butter

1. Preheat your oven to 350°F (180°C). Whisk together all of the crust ingredients in a bowl. Make two balls out of the mixture, and refrigerate for 10 minutes.
2. Melt the butter in a pan over medium heat and add the ground pork. Cook for about 10minutes, stirring occasionally. Remove to a bowl. Add in the other ingredients and mix to combine.
3. Roll out the tart crusts and place one at the bottom of a greased baking pan. Spread the filling over the crust. Top with the other coat. Bake for 50 minutes, then serve.

Per Serving
calories: 444 | fat: 19g | protein: 40g
carbs: 6g | net carbs: 4g | fiber: 2g

Texas Pulled Boston Butt

Prep time: 15 minutes | Cook time: 3 hours | Serves 4

Kosher salt, to season
1 teaspoon paprika
½ teaspoon oregano
½ teaspoon rosemary
1 teaspoon mustard seeds
½ teaspoon chipotle powder
1 teaspoon black peppercorns, whole
3 tablespoons apple cider vinegar
1 cup tomato sauce
1½ pounds (680 g) Boston butt

1. Thoroughly combine all ingredients, except for the Boston butt, in a big casserole dish. Now, place Boston butt on top skin-side up.
2. Bake in the preheated oven at 300°F (150°C) for about 3 hours, checking and turning every 30 minutes.
3. Cut the skin off and shred the pork with two forks; discard any fatty bits.
4. Serve with coleslaw and the bowl of cooking juices on the side for dipping. Bon appétit!

Per Serving
calories: 340 | fat: 21.1g | protein: 30.7g
carbs: 4.3g | net carbs: 3.2g | fiber: 1.1g

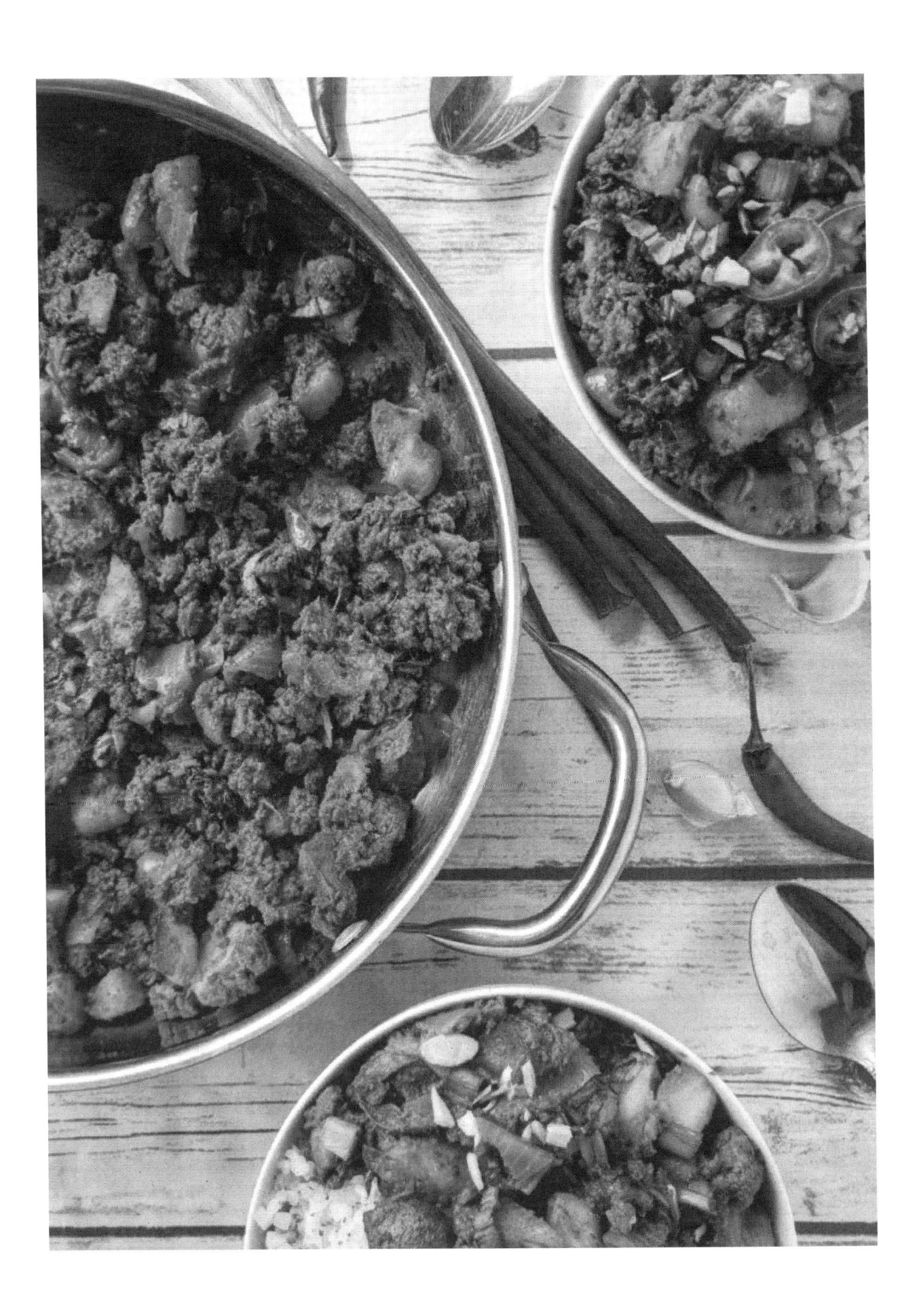

Chapter 10 Beef and Lamb

King Size Beef Burgers

Prep time: 5 minutes | Cook time: 18 minutes | Serves 4

2 tablespoons olive oil
1 pound (454 g) ground beef
2 green onions, chopped
1 garlic clove, minced
1 tablespoon thyme
2 tablespoons almond flour
2 tablespoons beef broth
½ tablespoon chopped parsley
½ tablespoon Worcestershire sauce

1. Grease a baking dish with the olive oil. Combine all ingredients except for the parsley in a bowl. Mix well with your hands and make 2 patties out of the mixture. Arrange on a lined baking sheet. Bake at 370ºF (188ºC), for about 18 minutes, until nice and crispy. Serve sprinkled with parsley.

Per Serving

calories: 371 | fat: 30g | protein: 20g carbs: 5g | net carbs: 4g | fiber: 1g

Zoodles with Beef Bolognese Sauce

Prep time: 10 minutes | Cook time: 25 to 27 minutes | Serves 4

2 cups zoodles
1 pound (454 g) ground beef
2 garlic cloves
1 onion, chopped
1 teaspoon oregano
1 teaspoon sage
1 teaspoon rosemary
7 ounces (198 g) canned chopped tomatoes
2 tablespoons olive oil

1. Cook the zoodles in warm olive oil over medium heat for 3-4 minutes and remove to a serving plate. To the same pan, add onion and garlic and cook for 3 minutes. Add beef and cook until browned, about 4-5 minutes. Stir in the herbs and tomatoes. Cook for 15 minutes and serve over the zoodles.

Per Serving

calories: 371 | fat: 30g | protein: 20g carbs: 5g | net carbs: 3g | fiber: 2g

Ground Beef and Cauliflower Curry

Prep time: 5 minutes | Cook time: 21 minutes | Serves 6

1 tablespoon olive oil
1½ pounds (680 g) ground beef
1 tablespoon ginger-garlic paste
1 teaspoon garam masala
1 (7-ounce / 198-g) can whole tomatoes
1 small head cauliflower, cut into florets
Pink salt and chili pepper, to taste
¼ cup water

1. Heat oil in a saucepan over medium heat, add in beef, ginger-garlic paste and season with garam masala. Cook for 5 minutes while breaking any lumps. Stir in tomatoes and cauliflower, season with salt and chili pepper, and cook for 6 minutes. Add the water and bring to a boil over medium heat for 10 minutes, or until the liquid has reduced by half.
2. Adjust taste with salt. Serve with shirataki rice.

Per Serving

calories: 255 | fat: 17g | protein: 23g carbs: 4g | net carbs: 2g | fiber: 2g

Simple Beef Burgers

Prep time: 15 minutes | Cook time: 20 minutes | Serves 6

2 pounds (907 g) ground beef
1 tablespoon onion flakes
¾ cup almond flour
¼ cup beef broth
1 tablespoon chopped parsley
1 tablespoon Worcestershire sauce

1. Combine all ingredients in a bowl. Mix well with your hands and make 6 patties out of the mixture. Arrange on a lined baking sheet. Bake at 370ºF (188ºC), for about 18 minutes, until nice and crispy.

Per Serving

calories: 355 | fat: 28.1g | protein: 27.1g carbs: 3.2g | net carbs: 2.6g | fiber: 0.6g

Texas Chili

Prep time: 20 minutes | Cook time: 7 to 8 hours | Serves 4

¼ cup extra-virgin olive oil
1½ pounds (680 g) beef sirloin, cut into 1-inch chunks
1 sweet onion, chopped
2 green bell peppers, chopped
1 jalapeño pepper, seeded, finely chopped
2 teaspoons minced garlic
1 (28-ounce / 794-g) can diced tomatoes
1 cup beef broth
3 tablespoons chili powder
½ teaspoon ground cumin
¼ teaspoon ground coriander
1 cup sour cream, for garnish
1 avocado, diced, for garnish
1 tablespoon cilantro, chopped, for garnish

1. Lightly grease the insert of the slow cooker with 1 tablespoon of the olive oil.
2. In a large skillet over medium-high heat, heat the remaining 2 tablespoons of the olive oil. Add the beef and sauté until it is cooked through, about 8 minutes.
3. Add the onion, bell peppers, jalapeño pepper, and garlic, and sauté for an additional 4 minutes.
4. Transfer the beef mixture to the insert and stir in the tomatoes, broth, chili powder, cumin, and coriander.
5. Cover and cook on low for 7 to 8 hours.
6. Serve topped with the sour cream, avocado, and cilantro.

Per Serving
calories: 488 | fat: 38.1g | protein: 25.9g
carbs: 17.1g | net carbs: 10.2g | fiber: 6.9g

Chipotle Beef Spare Ribs

Prep time: 15 minutes | Cook time: 50 minutes | Serves 4

2 tablespoons erythritol
Pink salt and black pepper to taste
1 tablespoon olive oil
3 teaspoons chipotle powder
1 teaspoon garlic powder
1 pound (454 g) beef spare ribs
4 tablespoons sugar-free BBQ sauce plus extra for serving

1. Mix the erythritol, salt, pepper, oil, chipotle, and garlic powder. Brush on the meaty sides of the ribs and wrap in foil. Sit for 30 minutes to marinate.
2. Preheat oven to 400ºF (205ºC), place wrapped ribs on a baking sheet, and cook for 40 minutes to be cooked through. Remove ribs and aluminium foil, brush with BBQ sauce, and brown under the broiler for 10 minutes on both sides. Slice and serve with extra BBQ sauce and lettuce tomato salad.

Per Serving
calories: 396 | fat: 32.8g | protein: 20.9g
carbs: 3.7g | net carbs: 3.0g | fiber: 0.7g

Zucchini and Beef Lasagna

Prep time: 15 minutes | Cook time: 45 minutes | Serves 4

1 pound (454 g) ground beef
2 large zucchinis, sliced lengthwise
3 cloves garlic
1 medium white onion, finely chopped
3 tomatoes, chopped
Salt and black pepper to taste
2 teaspoons sweet paprika
1 teaspoon dried thyme
1 teaspoon dried basil
1 cup shredded Mozzarella cheese
1 tablespoon olive oil
Cooking spray

1. Preheat the oven to 370ºF (188ºC) and lightly grease a baking dish with cooking spray.
2. Heat the olive oil in a skillet and cook the beef for 4 minutes while breaking any lumps as you stir. Top with onion, garlic, tomatoes, salt, paprika, and pepper. Stir and continue cooking for 5 minutes.
3. Then, lay ⅓ of the zucchini slices in the baking dish. Top with ⅓ of the beef mixture and repeat the layering process two more times with the same quantities. Season with basil and thyme.
4. Finally, sprinkle the Mozzarella cheese on top and tuck the baking dish in the oven. Bake for 35 minutes. Remove the lasagna and let it rest for 10 minutes before serving.

Per Serving
calories: 346 | fat: 17.9g | protein: 40.2g
carbs: 5.5g | net carbs: 2.8g | fiber: 2.7g

Beef and Broccoli Casserole

Prep time: 15 minutes | Cook time: 4 hours | Serves 6

1 tablespoon olive oil
2 pounds (907 g) ground beef
1 head broccoli, cut into florets
Salt and black pepper, to taste
2 teaspoons mustard
2 teaspoons Worcestershire sauce
28 ounces (794 g) canned diced tomatoes
2 cups Mozzarella cheese, grated
16 ounces (454 g) tomato sauce
2 tablespoons fresh parsley, chopped
1 teaspoon dried oregano

1. Apply black pepper and salt to the broccoli florets, set them into a bowl, drizzle over the olive oil, and toss well to coat completely. In a separate bowl, combine the beef with Worcestershire sauce, salt, mustard, and black pepper, and stir well. Press on the slow cooker's bottom.
2. Scatter in the broccoli, add the tomatoes, parsley, Mozzarella, oregano, and tomato sauce.
3. Cook for 4 hours on low; covered. Split the casserole among bowls and enjoy while hot.

Per Serving
calories: 435 | fat: 21.1g | protein: 50.9g
carbs: 13.5g | net carbs: 5.5g | fiber: 8.0g

Balsamic Mushroom Beef Meatloaf

Prep time: 15 minutes | Cook time: 1 hour 5 minutes | Serves 12

Meatloaf:
3 pounds (1.4 kg) ground beef
½ cup chopped onions
½ cup almond flour
2 garlic cloves, minced
1 cup sliced mushrooms
3 eggs
¼ teaspoon ground black pepper
2 tablespoons chopped parsley
¼ cup chopped bell peppers
⅓ cup grated Parmesan cheese
1 teaspoon balsamic vinegar
1 teaspoon salt

Glaze:
2 cups balsamic vinegar
1 tablespoon Swerve
2 tablespoons sugar-free ketchup

1. Combine all meatloaf ingredients in a large bowl. Press this mixture into 2 greased loaf pans. Bake at 370ºF (188ºC) for about 30 minutes.
2. Meanwhile, make the glaze by combining all ingredients in a saucepan over medium heat. Simmer for 20 minutes, until the glaze is thickened. Pour ¼ cup of the glaze over the meatloaf. Save the extra for future use.
3. Put the meatloaf back in the oven and cook for 20 more minutes.

Per Serving
calories: 295 | fat: 18.9g | protein: 23.1g
carbs: 6.5g | net carbs: 6.1g | fiber: 0.4g

Beef and Veggie Stuffed Butternut Squash

Prep time: 15 minutes | Cook time: 60 minutes | Serves 4

2 pounds (907 g) butternut squash, pricked with a fork
Salt and black pepper, to taste
3 garlic cloves, minced
1 onion, chopped
1 button mushroom, sliced
28 ounces (794 g) canned diced tomatoes
1 teaspoon dried oregano
¼ teaspoon cayenne pepper
½ teaspoon dried thyme
1 pound (454 g) ground beef
1 green bell pepper, chopped

1. Lay the butternut squash on a lined baking sheet, set in the oven at 400ºF (205ºC), and bake for 40 minutes. After, cut in half, set aside to let cool, deseed, scoop out most of the flesh and let sit. Heat a greased pan over medium heat, add in the garlic, mushrooms, onion, and beef, and cook until the meat browns.
2. Stir in the green pepper, salt, thyme, tomatoes, oregano, black pepper, and cayenne, and cook for 10 minutes; stir in the flesh. Stuff the squash halves with the beef mixture, and bake in the oven for 10 minutes. Split into plates and enjoy.

Per Serving
calories: 405 | fat: 14.5g | protein: 33.8g
carbs: 20.7g | net carbs: 12.3g | fiber: 8.4g

Lemony Beef Rib Roast

Prep time: 15 minutes | Cook time: 35 minutes | Serves 6

5 pounds (2.3 kg) beef rib roast, on the bone
3 heads garlic, cut in half
3 tablespoons olive oil
6 shallots, peeled and halved
2 lemons, zested and juiced
3 tablespoons mustard seeds
3 tablespoons Swerve
Salt and black pepper to taste
3 tablespoons thyme leaves

1. Preheat oven to 450°F (235°C). Place garlic heads and shallots in a roasting dish, toss with olive oil, and bake for 15 minutes. Pour lemon juice on them. Score shallow crisscrosses patterns on the meat and set aside.
2. Mix Swerve, mustard seeds, thyme, salt, pepper, and lemon zest to make a rub; and apply it all over the beef. Place the beef on the shallots and garlic; cook in the oven for 15 minutes. Reduce the heat to 400°F (205°C), cover the dish with foil, and continue cooking for 5 minutes.
3. Once ready, remove the dish, and let sit covered for 15 minutes before slicing.

Per Serving
calories: 555 | fat: 38.5g | protein: 58.3g
carbs: 7.7g | net carbs: 2.4g | fiber: 5.3g

Mexican Beef and Tomato Chili

Prep time: 20 minutes | Cook time: 40 minutes | Serves 4

1 onion, chopped
2 tablespoons olive oil
2 pounds (907 g) ground beef
15 ounces (425 g) canned tomatoes with green chilies, chopped
3 ounces (85 g) tomato paste
½ cup pickled jalapeños, chopped
1 teaspoon chipotle chili paste
4 tablespoons garlic, minced
3 celery stalks, chopped
2 tablespoons coconut aminos
Salt and black pepper, to taste
A pinch of cayenne pepper
2 tablespoons cumin
1 teaspoon onion powder
1 teaspoon garlic powder
1 bay leaf
1 teaspoon chopped cilantro

1. Heat oil in a pan over medium heat, add in the onion, celery, garlic, beef, black pepper, and salt; cook until the meat browns. Stir in jalapeños, tomato paste, canned tomatoes with green chilies, salt, garlic powder, bay leaf, onion powder, cayenne, coconut aminos, chipotle chili paste, and cumin, and cook for 30 minutes while covered. Remove and discard bay leaf. Serve in bowls sprinkled with cilantro.

Per Serving
calories: 435 | fat: 25.9g | protein: 16.9g
carbs: 7.9g | net carbs: 5.1g | fiber: 2.8g

Lamb Curry

Prep time: 15 minutes | Cook time: 7 to 8 hours | Serves 6

3 tablespoons extra-virgin olive oil, divided
1½ pounds (680 g) lamb shoulder chops
Salt, for seasoning
Freshly ground black pepper, for seasoning
3 cups coconut milk
½ sweet onion, sliced
¼ cup curry powder
1 tablespoon grated fresh ginger
2 teaspoons minced garlic
1 carrot, diced
2 tablespoons chopped cilantro, for garnish

1. Lightly grease the insert of the slow cooker with 1 tablespoon of the olive oil.
2. In a large skillet over medium-high heat, heat the remaining 2 tablespoons of the olive oil.
3. Season the lamb with salt and pepper. Add the lamb to the skillet and brown for 6 minutes, turning once. Transfer to the insert.
4. In a medium bowl, stir together the coconut milk, onion, curry, ginger, and garlic.
5. Add the mixture to the lamb along with the carrot.
6. Cover and cook on low for 7 to 8 hours.
7. Serve topped with the cilantro.

Per Serving
calories: 491 | fat: 41.2g | protein: 25.9g
carbs: 10.1g | net carbs: 5.2g | fiber: 4.9g

Italian Sausage and Okra Stew

Prep time: 20 minutes | Cook time: 30 minutes | Serves 6

1 pound (454 g) Italian sausage, sliced
1 red bell pepper, seeded and chopped
2 onions, chopped
Salt and black pepper, to taste
1 cup fresh parsley, chopped
6 green onions, chopped
¼ cup avocado oil
1 cup beef stock
4 garlic cloves
24 ounces (680 g) canned diced tomatoes
16 ounces (454 g) okra, trimmed and sliced
6 ounces (170 g) tomato sauce
2 tablespoons coconut aminos
1 tablespoon hot sauce

1. Set a pot over medium heat and warm oil, place in the sausages, and cook for 2 minutes. Stir in the onions, green onions, garlic, black pepper, bell pepper, and salt, and cook for 5 minutes.
2. Add in the hot sauce, stock, tomatoes, coconut aminos, okra, and tomato sauce, bring to a simmer and cook for 15 minutes. Adjust the seasoning with salt and black pepper. Share into serving bowls and sprinkle with fresh parsley to serve.

Per Serving
calories: 315 | fat: 25.1g | protein: 16.1g
carbs: 16.8g | net carbs: 6.9g | fiber: 8.9g

Beef, Pancetta, and Mushroom Bourguignon

Prep time: 15 minutes | Cook time: 60 minutes | Serves 4

3 tablespoons coconut oil
1 tablespoon dried parsley flakes
1 cup red wine
1 teaspoon dried thyme
Salt and black pepper, to taste
1 bay leaf
⅓ cup coconut flour
2 pounds (907 g) beef, cubed
12 small white onions
4 pancetta slices, chopped
2 garlic cloves, minced
½ pound (227 g) mushrooms, chopped

1. In a bowl, combine the wine with bay leaf, olive oil, thyme, pepper, parsley, salt, and the beef cubes; set aside for 3 hours. Drain the meat, and reserve the marinade. Toss the flour over the meat to coat.
2. Heat a pan over medium heat, stir in the pancetta, and cook until slightly browned. Place in the onions and garlic, and cook for 3 minutes. Stir-fry in the meat and mushrooms for 4-5 minutes.
3. Pour in the marinade and 1 cup of water; cover and cook for 50 minutes. Season to taste and serve.

Per Serving
calories: 434 | fat: 25.9g | protein: 44.8g
carbs: 11.5g | net carbs: 6.9g | fiber: 4.6g

Beef and Onion Stuffed Zucchinis

Prep time: 5 minutes | Cook time: 21 minutes | Serves 4

4 zucchinis
2 tablespoons olive oil
1½ pounds (680 g) ground beef
1 medium red onion, chopped
2 tablespoons pimiento rojo, chopped
Pink salt and black pepper, to taste
1 cup yellow Cheddar cheese, grated

1. Preheat oven to 350°F (180°C).
2. Lay the zucchinis on a flat surface, trim off the ends, and cut in half lengthwise. Scoop out pulp from each half with a spoon to make shells. Chop the flesh.
3. Heat oil in a skillet; add the ground beef, red onion, pimiento, and zucchini pulp, and season with salt and black pepper. Cook for 6 minutes while stirring to break up lumps until beef is no longer pink. Spoon the beef into the boats, and sprinkle with Cheddar cheese.
4. Place on a greased baking sheet, and cook to melt the cheese for 15 minutes until zucchini boats are tender. Take out, cool for 2 minutes, and serve warm with a mixed green salad.

Per Serving
calories: 535 | fat: 40g | protein: 42g
carbs: 4g | net carbs: 3g | fiber: 1g

Veggie Cauliflower Rice with Beef Steak

Prep time: 5 minutes | Cook time: 9 minutes | Serves 4

2 cups cauliflower rice
3 cups mixed vegetables
3 tablespoons butter
1 pound (454 g) beef skirt steak
Salt and black pepper, to taste
4 fresh eggs
Hot sauce (sugar-free) for topping (optional)

1. Mix the cauliflower rice with mixed vegetables in a bowl, sprinkle with a little water, and steam in the microwave for 1 minute to tender. Share into 4 serving bowls.
2. Melt the butter in a skillet, season the beef with salt and pepper, and brown in the butter for 5 minutes on each side. Use a perforated spoon to ladle the meat onto the vegetables.
3. Wipe out the skillet and return to medium heat, crack in an egg, season with salt and pepper, and cook until the egg white has set, but the yolk is still runny, for 3 minutes. Remove egg onto the vegetable bowl, and fry the remaining 3 eggs. Add to the other bowls. Drizzle the beef bowl with hot sauce (if desired) and serve.

Per Serving
calories: 791 | fat: 47g | protein: 65g
carbs: 22g | net carbs: 14g | fiber: 8g

Beef and Pimiento in Zucchini Boats

Prep time: 10 minutes | Cook time: 25 minutes | Serves 4

4 zucchinis
2 tablespoons olive oil
1½ pounds (680 g) ground beef
1 medium red onion, chopped
2 tablespoons chopped pimiento
Pink salt and black pepper to taste
1 cup grated yellow Cheddar cheese

1. Preheat oven to 350ºF (180ºC).
2. Lay the zucchinis on a flat surface, trim off the ends and cut in half lengthwise. Scoop out the pulp from each half with a spoon to make shells. Chop the pulp.
3. Heat oil in a skillet; add the ground beef, red onion, pimiento, and zucchini pulp, and season with salt and black pepper. Cook for 6 minutes while stirring to break up lumps until beef is no longer pink. Turn the heat off. Spoon the beef into the boats and sprinkle with Cheddar cheese.
4. Place on a greased baking sheet and cook to melt the cheese for 15 minutes until zucchini boats are tender. Take out, cool for 2 minutes, and serve warm with a mixed green salad.

Per Serving
calories: 334 | fat: 24.0g | protein: 17.9g
carbs: 7.6g | net carbs: 6.9g | fiber: 0.7g

Mascarpone Beef Balls with Cilantro

Prep time: 15 minutes | Cook time: 33 minutes | Serves 4

1 garlic clove, minced
1 pound (454 g) ground beef
1 small onion, chopped
1 jalapeño pepper, chopped
2 teaspoons cilantro
½ teaspoon allspice
1 teaspoon cumin
Salt and black pepper, to taste
1 tablespoon butter plus 1½ tablespoon, melted
½ cup mascarpone cheese, at room temperature
¼ teaspoon turmeric
¼ teaspoon baking powder
1 cup flax meal
¼ cup coconut flour

1. Purée onion with garlic, jalapeño pepper, and ¼ cup water in a blender. Set a pan over medium heat, add in 1 tablespoon butter and cook the beef for 3 minutes. Stir in the onion mixture, and cook for 2 minutes. Stir in cilantro, salt, cumin, turmeric, allspice, and black pepper, and cook for 3 minutes.
2. In a bowl, combine coconut flour, flax meal, and baking powder. In a separate bowl, combine the melted butter with the mascarpone cheese. Combine the 2 mixtures to obtain a dough. Form balls from this mixture, set them on a parchment paper, and roll each into a circle.
3. Split the beef mix on one-half of the dough circles, cover with the other half, seal edges, and lay on a lined sheet. Bake for 25 minutes in the oven at 350ºF (180ºC).

Per Serving
calories: 668 | fat: 44g | protein: 32g
carbs: 17g | net carbs: 13g | fiber: 4g

Spicy Beef Brisket Roast

Prep time: 15 minutes | Cook time: 60 minutes | Serves 4

2 pounds (907 g) beef brisket	A pinch of cayenne pepper
½ teaspoon celery salt	½ teaspoon garlic powder
1 teaspoon chili powder	½ cup beef stock
1 tablespoon avocado oil	1 tablespoon garlic, minced
1 tablespoon sweet paprika	¼ teaspoon dry mustard

1. Preheat oven to 340°F (171°C). In a bowl, combine the paprika with dry mustard, chili powder, salt, garlic powder, cayenne pepper, and celery salt. Rub the meat with this mixture.
2. Set a pan over medium heat and warm avocado oil, place in the beef, and sear until brown. Remove to a baking dish. Pour in the stock, add garlic and bake for 60 minutes.
3. Set the beef to a cutting board, leave to cool before slicing and splitting in serving plates.
4. Take the juices from the baking dish and strain, sprinkle over the meat, and enjoy.

Per Serving
calories: 481 | fat: 23.6g | protein: 54.8g
carbs: 4.2g | net carbs: 3.3g | fiber: 0.9g

Thai Beef Steak with Mushrooms

Prep time: 15 minutes | Cook time: 25 minutes | Serves 6

1 cup beef stock	1 pound (454 g) beef steak, cut into strips
4 tablespoons butter	Salt and black pepper, to taste
¼ teaspoon garlic powder	1 cup shiitake mushrooms, sliced
¼ teaspoon onion powder	3 green onions, chopped
1 tablespoon coconut aminos	1 tablespoon thai red curry paste
1½ teaspoons lemon pepper	

1. Melt butter in a pan over medium heat, add in the beef, season with garlic powder, black pepper, salt, and onion powder and cook for 4 minutes. Mix in the mushrooms and stir-fry for 5 minutes.
2. Pour in the stock, coconut aminos, lemon pepper, and thai curry paste and cook for 15 minutes. Serve sprinkled with the green onions.

Per Serving
calories: 225 | fat: 15.1g | protein: 18.9g
carbs: 4.1g | net carbs: 2.9g | fiber: 1.2g

Juicy Beef with Thyme and Rosemary

Prep time: 15 minutes | Cook time: 17 minutes | Serves 4

2 garlic cloves, minced	½ cup heavy cream
2 tablespoons butter	½ cup beef stock
2 tablespoons olive oil	1 tablespoon mustard
1 tablespoon fresh rosemary, chopped	2 teaspoons coconut aminos
1 pound (454 g) beef rump steak, sliced	2 teaspoons lemon juice
Salt and black pepper, to taste	1 teaspoon xylitol
	A sprig of rosemary
1 shallot, chopped	A sprig of thyme

1. Set a pan to medium heat, warm in a tablespoon of olive oil and stir in the shallot; cook for 3 minutes. Stir in the stock, coconut aminos, xylitol, thyme sprig, cream, mustard and rosemary sprig, and cook for 8 minutes. Stir in butter, lemon juice, pepper and salt. Get rid of the rosemary and thyme. Set aside.
2. In a bowl, combine the remaining oil with black pepper, garlic, rosemary, and salt. Toss in the beef to coat, and set aside for some minutes.
3. Heat a pan over medium-high heat, place in the beef steak, cook for 6 minutes, flipping halfway through; set aside and keep warm. Plate the beef slices, sprinkle over the sauce, and enjoy.

Per Serving
calories: 339 | fat: 25g | protein: 26g
carbs: 3g | net carbs: 2g | fiber: 1g

Pinwheel Beef and Spinach Steaks

Prep time: 10 minutes | Cook time: 35 minutes | Serves 6

1½ pounds (680 g) beef flank steak
Salt and black pepper to taste
1 cup crumbled Feta cheese
½ loose cup baby spinach
1 jalapeño pepper, chopped
¼ cup chopped basil leaves

1. Preheat oven to 400ºF (205ºC) and grease a baking sheet with cooking spray.
2. Wrap the steak in plastic wrap, place on a flat surface, and gently run a rolling pin over to flatten. Take off the wraps. Sprinkle with half of the Feta cheese, top with spinach, jalapeño, basil leaves, and the remaining cheese. Roll the steak over on the stuffing and secure with toothpicks.
3. Place in the baking sheet and cook for 30 minutes, flipping once until nicely browned on the outside and the cheese melted within. Cool for 3 minutes, slice into pinwheels and serve with sautéed veggies.

Per Serving
calories: 491 | fat: 41.0g | protein: 28.0g
carbs: 2.1g | net carbs: 2.0g | fiber: 0.1g

Beef and Mushroom Cheeseburgers

Prep time: 5 minutes | Cook time: 11 to 13 minutes | Serves 4

2 tablespoons olive oil
1 pound (454 g) ground beef
½ teaspoon fresh parsley, chopped
½ teaspoon Worcestershire sauce
Salt and black pepper, to taste
2 slices Mozzarella cheese
2 portobello mushroom caps

1. In a bowl, mix the beef, parsley, Worcestershire sauce, salt and black pepper with your hands until evenly combined. Make medium-sized patties out of the mixture.
2. Preheat a grill to 400ºF (205ºC) and coat the mushroom caps with olive oil, salt and black pepper.
3. Lay portobello caps, rounded side up and burger patties onto the hot grill pan and cook for 5 minutes. Turn the mushroom caps and continue cooking for 1 minute.
4. Lay a Mozzarella slice on top of each patty. Continue cooking until the mushroom caps are softened, 4-5 minutes. Flip the patties and top with cheese. Cook for another 2-3 minutes until the cheese melts onto the meat. Remove the patties and sandwich into two mushroom caps each.

Per Serving
calories: 397 | fat: 32g | protein: 24g
carbs: 2g | net carbs: 1g | fiber: 1g

Beef Meatloaf with Balsamic Glaze

Prep time: 15 minutes | Cook time: 50 minutes | Serves 4

Meatloaf:
1 pound (454 g) ground beef
½ onion, chopped
1 tablespoon almond milk
1 tablespoon almond flour
1 garlic clove, minced
1 cup sliced mushrooms
1 small egg
Salt and black pepper, to taste
1 tablespoon parsley, chopped
⅓ cup Parmesan cheese, grated

Glaze:
⅓ cup balsamic vinegar
¼ tablespoon xylitol
¼ teaspoon garlic powder
¼ teaspoon onion powder
1 tablespoon plus ¼ teaspoon tomato purée

1. Grease a loaf pan with cooking spray and set aside. Preheat oven to 390ºF (199ºC). Combine all meatloaf ingredients in a large bowl. Press this mixture into the prepared loaf pan. Bake for about 30 minutes.
2. To make the glaze, whisk all ingredients in a bowl. Pour the glaze over the meatloaf. Put the meatloaf back in the oven and cook for 20 more minutes. Let meatloaf sit for 10 minutes before slicing.

Per Serving
calories: 377 | fat: 26g | protein: 24g
carbs: 10g | net carbs: 9g | fiber: 1g

Lamb Chops with Fennel and Zucchini

Prep time: 10 minutes | Cook time: 6 hours | Serves 4

¼ cup extra-virgin olive oil, divided
1 pound (454 g) boneless lamb chops, about ½-inch thick
Salt, for seasoning
Freshly ground black pepper, for seasoning
½ sweet onion, sliced
½ fennel bulb, cut into 2-inch chunks
1 zucchini, cut into 1-inch chunks
¼ cup chicken broth
2 tablespoons chopped fresh basil, for garnish

1. Lightly grease the insert of the slow cooker with 1 tablespoon of the olive oil.
2. Season the lamb with salt and pepper.
3. In a medium bowl, toss together the onion, fennel, and zucchini with the remaining 3 tablespoons of the olive oil and then place half of the vegetables in the insert.
4. Place the lamb on top of the vegetables, cover with the remaining vegetables, and add the broth.
5. Cover and cook on low for 6 hours.
6. Serve topped with the basil.

Per Serving
calories: 430 | fat: 36.9g | protein: 20.9g
carbs: 5.0g | net carbs: 3.0g | fiber: 2.0g

Balsamic Glazed Meatloaf

Prep time: 15 minutes | Cook time: 1 hour 10 minutes | Serves 12

3 pounds (1.4 kg) ground beef
½ cup onion, chopped
½ cup almond flour
2 garlic cloves, minced
1 cup mushrooms, sliced
3 eggs
Salt and black pepper, to taste
2 tablespoons parsley, chopped
¼ cup bell peppers, chopped
⅓ cup Parmesan cheese, grated
1 teaspoon balsamic vinegar
Glaze:
2 cups balsamic vinegar
1 tablespoon sweetener
2 tablespoons tomato purée

1. Combine all of the meatloaf ingredients in a large bowl. Press the mixture into greased loaf pan. Bake at 375°F (190°C) for about 30 minutes.
2. Make the glaze by combining all of the ingredients in a saucepan over medium heat.
3. Simmer for 20 minutes, until the glaze is thickened. Pour ¼ cup of the glaze over the meatloaf. Save the extra for future use. Put the meatloaf back in the oven, and cook for 20 more minutes.

Per Serving
calories: 375 | fat: 25g | protein: 23g
carbs: 13g | net carbs: 12g | fiber: 1g

Beef Steaks with Mushrooms and Bacon

Prep time: 10 minutes | Cook time: 40 minutes | Serves 4

2 ounces (57 g) bacon, chopped
1 cup mushrooms, sliced
1 garlic clove, chopped
1 shallot, chopped
1 cup heavy cream
1 pound (454 g) beef steaks
1 teaspoon ground nutmeg
¼ cup coconut oil
Salt and black pepper, to taste
1 tablespoon parsley, chopped

1. In a frying pan over medium heat, cook the bacon for 2-3 minutes and set aside. In the same pan, warm the oil, add in the onions, garlic and mushrooms, and cook for 4 minutes.
2. Stir in the beef, season with salt, black pepper and nutmeg, and sear until browned, about 2 minutes per side.
3. Preheat oven to 360°F (182°C) and insert the pan in the oven to bake for 25 minutes. Remove the beef steaks to a bowl and cover with foil.
4. Place the pan over medium heat, pour in the heavy cream over the mushroom mixture, add in the reserved bacon and cook for 5 minutes; remove from heat. Spread the bacon/mushroom sauce over beef steaks, sprinkle with parsley and serve.

Per Serving
calories: 447 | fat: 37g | protein: 27g
carbs: 3g | net carbs: 2g | fiber: 1g

Beef Ragout with Green Beans

Prep time: 15 minutes | Cook time: 1 hour 48 minutes | Serves 4

2 tablespoons olive oil
1 pound (454 g) chuck steak, cubed
Salt and black pepper, to taste
2 tablespoons almond flour
4 green onions, diced
½ cup dry white wine
1 yellow bell pepper, diced
1 cup green beans, chopped
2 teaspoons Worcestershire sauce
4 ounces (113 g) tomato purée
3 teaspoons smoked paprika
1 cup beef broth
Parsley leaves, for garnish

1. Dredge the meat in the almond flour and set aside.
2. Place a large skillet over medium heat, add 1 tablespoon of oil to heat and then sauté the green onion, green beans, and bell pepper for 3 minutes. Stir in the paprika and the remaining olive oil.
3. Add the beef and cook for 10 minutes while turning them halfway. Stir in white wine, let it reduce by half, about 3 minutes, and add Worcestershire sauce, tomato purée, and beef broth.
4. Let the mixture boil for 2 minutes, then reduce the heat to lowest and let simmer for 1½ hours; stirring now and then. Adjust the taste and dish the ragout. Serve garnished with parsley leaves.

Per Serving
calories: 302 | fat: 17g | protein: 27g
carbs: 12g | net carbs: 9g | fiber: 3g

Beef Chuck Roast with Mushrooms

Prep time: 15 minutes | Cook time: 3 hours 10 minutes | Serves 6

2 pounds (907 g) beef chuck roast, cubed
2 tablespoons olive oil
14.5 ounces (411 g) canned diced tomatoes
2 carrots, chopped
Salt and black pepper, to taste
½ pound (227 g) mushrooms, sliced
2 celery stalks, chopped
2 yellow onions, chopped
1 cup beef stock
1 tablespoon fresh thyme, chopped
½ teaspoon dry mustard
3 tablespoons almond flour

1. Set an ovenproof pot over medium heat, warm olive oil and brown the beef on each side for a few minutes. Stir in the tomatoes, onions, salt, pepper, mustard, carrots, mushrooms, celery, and stock.
2. In a bowl, combine 1 cup water with flour. Place this to the pot, stir then set in the oven, and bake for 3 hours at 325ºF (163ºC) stirring at intervals of 30 minutes. Scatter the fresh thyme over and serve warm.

Per Serving
calories: 326 | fat: 18.1g | protein: 28.1g
carbs: 10.4g | net carbs: 6.9g | fiber: 3.5g

Veal, Mushroom, and Green Bean Stew

Prep time: 15 minutes | Cook time: 1 hour 55 minutes | Serves 6

2 tablespoons olive oil
3 pounds (1.4 kg) veal shoulder, cubed
1 onion, chopped
1 garlic clove, minced
Salt and black pepper, to taste
1 cup water
1½ cups red wine
12 ounces (340 g) canned tomato sauce
1 carrot, chopped
1 cup mushrooms, chopped
½ cup green beans
2 teaspoons dried oregano

1. Set a pot over medium heat and warm the oil. Brown the veal for 5-6 minutes. Stir in the onion, and garlic, and cook for 3 minutes. Place in the wine, oregano, carrot, black pepper, salt, tomato sauce, water, and mushrooms, bring to a boil, reduce the heat to low. Cook for 1 hour and 45 minutes, then add in the green beans and cook for 5 minutes. Adjust the seasoning and split among serving bowls to serve.

Per Serving
calories: 416 | fat: 21.1g | protein: 44.2g
carbs: 7.3g | net carbs: 5.1g | fiber: 2.2g

Bacon and Beef Stew

Prep time: 15 minutes | Cook time: 1 hour 10 minutes | Serves 6

8 ounces (227 g) bacon, chopped
4 pounds (1.8 kg) beef meat for stew, cubed
4 garlic cloves, minced
2 brown onions, chopped
2 tablespoons olive oil
4 tablespoons red vinegar
4 cups beef stock
2 tablespoons tomato purée
2 cinnamon sticks
3 lemon peel strips
½ cup fresh parsley, chopped
4 thyme sprigs
2 tablespoons butter
Salt and black pepper, to taste

1. Set a saucepan over medium heat and warm oil, add in the garlic, bacon, and onion, and cook for 5 minutes. Stir in the beef, and cook until slightly brown. Pour in the vinegar, black pepper, butter, lemon peel strips, stock, salt, tomato purée, cinnamon sticks and thyme; stir for 3 minutes.
2. Cook for 1 hour while covered. Get rid of the thyme, lemon peel, and cinnamon sticks. Split into serving bowls and sprinkle with parsley to serve.

Per Serving
calories: 591 | fat: 36.1g | protein: 63.1g
carbs: 8.1g | net carbs: 5.6g | fiber: 2.5g

Pork Rind Crusted Beef Meatballs

Prep time: 10 minutes | Cook time: 40 minutes | Serves 5

½ cup pork rinds, crushed
1 egg
Salt and black pepper, to taste
1½ pounds (680 g) ground beef
10 ounces (283 g) canned onion soup
1 tablespoon almond flour
¼ cup free-sugar ketchup
3 teaspoons Worcestershire sauce
½ teaspoon dry mustard
¼ cup water

1. In a bowl, combine ⅓ cup of the onion soup with the beef, pepper, pork rinds, egg, and salt. Heat a pan over medium heat, shape the mixture into 12 meatballs. Brown in the pan for 12 minutes on both sides.
2. In a separate bowl, combine the rest of the soup with the almond flour, dry mustard, ketchup, Worcestershire sauce, and water. Pour this over the beef meatballs, cover the pan, and cook for 20 minutes as you stir occasionally. Split among serving bowls and serve.

Per Serving
calories: 333 | fat: 18.1g | protein: 24.9g
carbs: 7.4g | net carbs: 6.9g | fiber: 0.5g

Asian-Flavored Beef and Broccoli

Prep time: 10 minutes | Cook time: 24 minutes | Serves 4

½ cup coconut milk
2 tablespoons coconut oil
¼ teaspoon garlic powder
¼ teaspoon onion powder
½ tablespoon coconut aminos
1 pound (454 g) beef steak, cut into strips
Salt and black pepper, to taste
1 head broccoli, cut into florets
½ tablespoon Thai green curry paste
1 teaspoon ginger paste
1 tablespoon cilantro, chopped
½ tablespoon sesame seeds

1. Warm coconut oil in a pan over medium heat, add in beef, season with garlic powder, pepper, salt, ginger paste, and onion powder and cook for 4 minutes. Mix in the broccoli and stir-fry for 5 minutes.
2. Pour in the coconut milk, coconut aminos, and Thai curry paste and cook for 15 minutes.
3. Serve sprinkled with cilantro and sesame seeds.

Per Serving
calories: 350 | fat: 22g | protein: 30g
carbs: 13g | net carbs: 8g | fiber: 5g

Creole Beef Tripe Stew with Onions

Prep time: 5 minutes | Cook time: 22 minutes | Serves 6

1½ pounds (680 g) beef tripe
4 cups coconut milk
Pink salt
2 teaspoons Creole seasoning
3 tablespoons olive oil
2 onions, sliced
3 tomatoes, diced

1. Put tripe in a bowl, and cover with coconut milk. Refrigerate for 3 hours to extract bitterness and gamey taste. Remove from coconut milk, pat dry with paper towels, and season with salt and creole seasoning.
2. Heat 2 tablespoons of oil in a skillet over medium heat and brown the tripe on both sides for 6 minutes in total. Remove, and set aside. Add the remaining oil, and sauté onions for 3 minutes. Include the tomatoes and cook for 10 minutes. Put the tripe in the sauce, and cook for 3 minutes.

Per Serving
calories: 284 | fat: 16g | protein: 20g
carbs: 14g | net carbs: 12g | fiber: 2g

Cauliflower and Tomato Beef Curry

Prep time: 10 minutes | Cook time: 21 minutes | Serves 6

1 tablespoon olive oil
1½ pounds (680 g) ground beef
1 tablespoon ginger-garlic paste
1 teaspoon garam masala
1 (7-ounce / 198-g) can whole tomatoes
1 head cauliflower, cut into florets
Pink salt and chili pepper to taste
¼ cup water

1. Heat oil in a saucepan over medium heat, add the beef, ginger-garlic paste and season with garam masala. Cook for 5 minutes while breaking any lumps.
2. Stir in the tomatoes and cauliflower, season with salt and chili pepper, and cook covered for 6 minutes. Add the water and bring to a boil over medium heat for 10 minutes or until the water has reduced by half. Adjust taste with salt. Spoon the curry into serving bowls and serve with shirataki rice.

Per Serving
calories: 373 | fat: 32.8g | protein: 21.9g
carbs: 4.0g | net carbs: 2.2g | fiber: 2.8g

Grilled Ribeye Steaks with Green Beans

Prep time: 5 minutes | Cook time: 12 to 13 minutes | Serves 4

4 ribeye steaks
2 tablespoons unsalted butter
1 teaspoon olive oil
½ cup green beans, sliced
Salt and ground pepper, to taste
1 tablespoon fresh thyme, chopped
1 tablespoon fresh rosemary, chopped
1 tablespoon fresh parsley, chopped

1. Brush the steaks with olive oil and season with salt and pepper. Preheat a grill pan over high heat and cook the steaks for about 4 minutes per side; set aside. Steam the green beans for 3-4 minutes until tender. Season with salt. Melt the butter in the pan and stir-fry the herbs for 1 minute; then mix in the green beans. Transfer over the steaks and serve.

Per Serving
calories: 516 | fat: 33g | protein: 49g
carbs: 6g | net carbs: 5g | fiber: 1g

Mozzarella Beef Gratin

Prep time: 15 minutes | Cook time: 25 minutes | Serves 4

2 tablespoons olive oil
1 onion, chopped
1 pound (454 g) ground beef
2 garlic cloves, minced
Salt and black pepper, to taste
1 cup Mozzarella cheese, shredded
1 cup fontina cheese, shredded
1 (14-ounce / 397-g) canned tomatoes, chopped
2 tablespoons sesame seeds, toasted
20 dill pickle slices

1. Preheat the oven to 390ºF (199ºC). Heat olive oil in a pan over medium heat, place in the beef, garlic, salt, onion, and black pepper, and cook for 5 minutes. Remove and set to a baking dish, stir in half of the tomatoes and Mozzarella cheese. Lay the pickle slices on top, spread over the fontina cheese and sesame seeds, and place in the oven to bake for 20 minutes.

Per Serving
calories: 620 | fat: 49g | protein: 36g
carbs: 9g | net carbs: 6g | fiber: 3g

Beef Sausage Casserole with Okra

Prep time: 15 minutes | Cook time: 25 minutes | Serves 4

1 cup okra, trimmed
1 tablespoon olive oil
1 celery stalk, chopped
¼ cup almond flour
1 egg
1 pound (454 g) beef sausage, chopped
Salt and black pepper, to taste
½ tablespoon dried parsley
¼ teaspoon red pepper flakes
¼ cup Parmesan cheese, grated
2 green onions, chopped
½ teaspoon garlic powder
¼ teaspoon dried oregano
½ cup ricotta cheese
½ cup marinara sauce, sugar-free
1 cup Cheddar cheese, shredded

1. In a bowl, combine the sausage, pepper, pepper flakes, oregano, egg, Parmesan cheese, green onions, almond flour, salt, parsley, celery, and garlic powder. Form balls, lay them on a lined baking sheet, place in the oven at 390°F (199°C), and bake for 15 minutes.
2. Remove the balls from the oven and cover with half of the marinara sauce and okra. Pour ricotta cheese all over followed by the rest of the marinara sauce. Scatter the Cheddar cheese and bake in the oven for 10 minutes. Allow the meatballs casserole to cool before serving.

Per Serving
calories: 611 | fat: 44g | protein: 36g
carbs: 14g | net carbs: 12g | fiber: 2g

Caribbean Beef with Peppers

Prep time: 15 minutes | Cook time: 1 hour 5 minutes | Serves 8

2 onions, chopped
2 tablespoons avocado oil
2 pounds (907 g) beef stew meat, cubed
2 red bell peppers, seeded and chopped
1 habanero pepper, chopped
4 green chilies, chopped
14.5 ounces (411 g) canned diced tomatoes
2 tablespoons fresh cilantro, chopped
4 garlic cloves, minced
½ cup vegetable broth
Salt and black pepper, to taste
1½ teaspoons cumin
½ cup black olives, chopped
1 teaspoon dried oregano

1. Set a pan over medium heat and warm avocado oil. Brown the beef on all sides; remove and set aside. Stir-fry in the red bell peppers, green chilies, oregano, garlic, habanero pepper, onions, and cumin, for about 5-6 minutes. Pour in the tomatoes and broth, and cook for 1 hour. Stir in the olives, adjust the seasonings and serve in bowls sprinkled with fresh cilantro.

Per Serving
calories: 304 | fat: 14.1g | protein: 25.1g
carbs: 10.9g | net carbs: 7.9g | fiber: 3.0g

Beef Stew with Black Olives

Prep time: 15 minutes | Cook time: 1 hour 5 minutes | Serves 4

1 onion, chopped
2 tablespoons olive oil
1 teaspoon ginger paste
1 teaspoon coconut aminos
1 pound (454 g) beef stew meat, cubed
1 red bell pepper, seeded and chopped
½ scotch bonnet pepper, chopped
2 green chilies, chopped
1 cup tomatoes, chopped
1 tablespoon fresh cilantro, chopped
1 garlic clove, minced
¼ cup vegetable broth
Salt and black pepper, to taste
¼ cup black olives, chopped
1 teaspoon jerk seasoning

1. Brown the beef on all sides in warm olive oil over medium heat; remove and set aside. Stir-fry in the red bell peppers, green chilies, jerk seasoning, garlic, scotch bonnet pepper, onion, ginger paste, and coconut aminos, for about 5-6 minutes. Pour in the tomatoes and broth, and cook for 1 hour.
2. Stir in the olives, adjust the seasonings and serve sprinkled with fresh cilantro.

Per Serving
calories: 254 | fat: 12g | protein: 27g
carbs: 11g | net carbs: 9g | fiber: 2g

Onion Sauced Beef Meatballs

Prep time: 15 minutes | Cook time: 30 minutes | Serves 5

2 pounds (907 g) ground beef
Salt and black pepper, to taste
½ teaspoon garlic powder
1¼ tablespoons coconut aminos
1 cup beef stock
¾ cup almond flour

1 tablespoon fresh parsley, chopped
1 tablespoon dried onion flakes
1 onion, sliced
2 tablespoons butter
¼ cup sour cream

1. In a bowl, combine the beef with salt, garlic powder, almond flour, onion flakes, parsley, 1 tablespoon coconut aminos, black pepper, ¼ cup of beef stock. Form 6 patties, place them on a baking sheet, put in the oven at 370ºF (188ºC), and bake for 18 minutes.
2. Set a pan with the butter over medium heat, stir in the onion, and cook for 3 minutes. Stir in the remaining beef stock, sour cream, and remaining coconut aminos, and bring to a simmer. Remove from heat, adjust the seasonings. Serve the meatballs topped with onion sauce.

Per Serving
calories: 434 | fat: 22.9g | protein: 32.1g | carbs: 6.9g | net carbs: 6.1g | fiber: 0.8g

Butternut Squash and Beef Stew

Prep time: 15 minutes | Cook time: 35 minutes | Serves 4

3 teaspoons olive oil
1 pound (454 g) ground beef
1 cup beef stock
14 ounces (397 g) canned tomatoes with juice
1 tablespoon stevia
1 pound (454 g) butternut squash, chopped

1 tablespoon Worcestershire sauce
2 bay leaves
Salt and black pepper, to taste
1 onion, chopped
1 teaspoon dried sage
1 tablespoon garlic, minced

1. Set a pan over medium heat and heat olive oil, stir in the onion, garlic, and beef, and cook for 10 minutes. Add in butternut squash, Worcestershire sauce, bay leaves, stevia, beef stock, canned tomatoes, and sage, and bring to a boil. Reduce heat, and simmer for 30 minutes.
2. Remove and discard the bay leaves and adjust the seasonings. Split into bowls and enjoy.

Per Serving
calories: 342 | fat: 17.1g | protein: 31.9g | carbs: 11.6g | net carbs: 7.4g | fiber: 4.2g

Flank Steak and Kale Roll

Prep time: 10 minutes | Cook time: 30 minutes | Serves 4

1 pound (454 g) flank steak
Salt and black pepper, to taste
½ cup ricotta cheese, crumbled

½ cup baby kale, chopped
1 serrano pepper, chopped
1 tablespoon basil leaves, chopped

1. Wrap the steak in plastic wraps, place on a flat surface, and gently run a rolling pin over to flatten. Take off the wraps. Sprinkle with half of the ricotta cheese, top with kale, serrano pepper, and the remaining cheese. Roll the steak over on the stuffing and secure with toothpicks.
2. Place in the greased baking sheet and cook for 30 minutes at 390ºF (199ºC), flipping once until nicely browned on the outside and the cheese melted within. Cool for 3 minutes, slice and serve with basil.

Per Serving
calories: 211 | fat: 10g | protein: 28g | carbs: 1g | net carbs: 1g | fiber: 0g

Creamy Reuben Soup with Sauerkraut

Prep time: 10 minutes | Cook time: 20 minutes | Serves 6

1 onion, diced
7 cups beef stock
1 teaspoon caraway seeds
2 celery stalks, diced
2 garlic cloves, minced
¾ teaspoon black pepper
2 cups heavy cream
1 cup sauerkraut
1 pound (454 g) corned beef, chopped
3 tablespoons butter
1½ cups Swiss cheese
Salt and black pepper, to taste

1. Melt the butter in a large pot. Add onions and celery, and fry for 3 minutes until tender. Add garlic, and cook for another minute.
2. Pour the broth over and stir in sauerkraut, salt, caraway seeds, and add a pinch of pepper. Bring to a boil. Reduce the heat to low, and add the corned beef. Cook for about 15 minutes.
3. Adjust the seasoning. Stir in heavy cream and cheese, and cook for 1 minute.

Per Serving

calories: 567 | fat: 46g | protein: 29g | carbs: 12g | net carbs: 9g | fiber: 3g

Beef Brisket with Red Wine

Prep time: 10 minutes | Cook time: 2 hours | Serves 4

1 tablespoon olive oil
1 pound (454 g) brisket
1 red onion, quartered
2 stalks celery, cut into chunks
1 garlic clove, minced
Salt and black pepper, to taste
1 bay leaf
1 tablespoon fresh thyme, chopped
1 cup red wine

1. Season the brisket with salt and pepper. Brown the meat on both sides in warm olive oil over medium heat for 6-8 minutes. Transfer to a deep casserole dish.
2. In the dish, arrange the onion, garlic, celery, and bay leaf around the brisket and pour the wine all over it. Cover the pot and cook the ingredients in the oven for 2 hours at 370ºF (188ºC). When ready, remove the casserole. Transfer the beef to a chopping board and cut it into thick slices. Serve the beef and vegetables with a drizzle of the sauce.

Per Serving

calories: 203 | fat: 9g | protein: 25g | carbs: 3g | net carbs: 2g | fiber: 1g

Basil Feta Flank Steak Pinwheels

Prep time: 5 minutes | Cook time: 15 minutes | Serves 6

1½ pounds (680 g) beef flank steak
Salt and black pepper, to season
⅔ cup feta cheese, crumbled
½ loose cup baby spinach
1 jalapeño pepper, chopped
¼ cup basil leaves, chopped

1. Preheat oven to 400ºF (205ºC). Grease a baking sheet with cooking spray.
2. Wrap the steak in plastic wrap, place on a flat surface, and gently run a rolling pin over to flatten. Take off the wraps. Sprinkle with half of the feta cheese, top with spinach, jalapeño, basil leaves, and the remaining cheese. Carefully roll the steak over on the stuffing and secure with toothpicks.
3. Place in the greased baking sheet, and cook for 15 minutes, flipping once until nicely browned on the outside and the cheese melted within. Cool for 3 minutes, slice into pinwheels, and serve.

Per Serving

calories: 199 | fat: 9g | protein: 27g | carbs: 1g | net carbs: 1g | fiber: 0g

Beef Chuck Roast with Veggies

Prep time: 15 minutes | Cook time: 1 hour 35 minutes | Serves 4

2 tablespoons olive oil
1 pound (454 g) beef chuck roast, cubed
1 cup canned diced tomatoes
Salt and black pepper, to taste
½ pound (227 g) mushrooms, sliced
1 celery stalk, chopped
1 bell pepper, sliced
1 onion, chopped
1 bay leaf
½ cup beef stock
1 tablespoon fresh rosemary, chopped
½ teaspoon dry mustard
1 tablespoon almond flour

1. Preheat oven to 350°F (180°C). Set a pot over medium heat, warm olive oil and brown the beef on each side for 4-5 minutes. Stir in tomatoes, onion, mustard, mushrooms, bell pepper, celery, and stock. Season with salt and pepper.
2. In a bowl, combine ½ cup of water with flour and stir in the pot. Transfer to a baking dish and bake for 90 minutes, stirring at intervals of 30 minutes. Scatter the rosemary over and serve warm.

Per Serving
calories: 329 | fat: 17g | protein: 34g | carbs: 8g | net carbs: 4g | fiber: 4g

Beef Casserole with Cauliflower

Prep time: 10 minutes | Cook time: 24 minutes | Serves 4

2 tablespoons olive oil
1 pound (454 g) ground beef
Salt and black pepper, to taste
½ cup cauliflower rice
1 tablespoon parsley, chopped
½ teaspoon dried oregano
1 cup kohlrabi, chopped
1 (5-ounce / 142-g) can diced tomatoes
¼ cup water
½ cup Mozzarella cheese, shredded

1. Put beef in a pot and season with salt and pepper; cook over medium heat for 6 minutes until no longer pink. Add cauliflower rice, kohlrabi, tomatoes, and water. Stir and bring to boil for 5 minutes to thicken the sauce. Spoon the beef mixture into the baking dish and spread evenly. Sprinkle with cheese and bake in the oven for 15 minutes at 380°F (193°C) until cheese has melted and it's golden brown. Remove and cool for 4 minutes, and serve sprinkled with parsley.

Per Serving
calories: 409 | fat: 33g | protein: 24g | carbs: 5g | net carbs: 3g | fiber: 2g

Beef Lasagna with Zucchinis

Prep time: 15 minutes | Cook time: 44 minutes | Serves 4

2 tablespoons olive oil
½ red chili, chopped
1 pound (454 g) ground beef
3 large zucchinis, sliced lengthwise
2 garlic cloves, minced
1 shallot, chopped
1 cup tomato purée
Salt and black pepper, to taste
2 teaspoons sweet paprika
1 teaspoon dried thyme
1 teaspoon dried basil
1 cup Mozzarella cheese, shredded
1 cup chicken broth

1. Heat the oil in a skillet and cook the beef for 4 minutes while breaking any lumps as you stir. Top with shallot, garlic, chili, tomatoes, salt, paprika and black pepper. Stir and cook for 5 more minutes.

2. Lay ⅓ of the zucchinis slices in a greased baking dish. Top with ⅓ of the beef mixture and repeat the layering process two more times with the same quantities. Season with basil and thyme. Pour in the chicken broth. Sprinkle the Mozzarella cheese on top and tuck the baking dish in the oven. Bake for 35 minutes at 380°F (193°C). Remove the lasagna and let it rest for 10 minutes before serving.

Per Serving
calories: 412 | fat: 30g | protein: 30g | carbs: 6g | net carbs: 4g | fiber: 2g

Juicy Beef Meatballs with Parsley

Prep time: 10 minutes | Cook time: 21 minutes | Serves 4

1 pound (454 g) ground beef
Salt and black pepper, to taste
½ teaspoon garlic powder
1¼ tablespoons coconut aminos
1 cup beef stock
¾ cup almond flour
1 tablespoon fresh parsley, chopped
1 onion, sliced
2 tablespoons butter
1 tablespoon olive oil
¼ cup sour cream

1. Preheat the oven to 390°F (199°C) and grease a baking dish. In a bowl, combine beef with salt, garlic powder, almond flour, parsley, 1 tablespoon of coconut aminos, black pepper, ¼ cup of beef stock. Form patties and place on the baking sheet. Bake for 18 minutes.
2. Set a pan with the butter and olive oil over medium heat, stir in the onion, and cook for 3 minutes. Stir in the remaining beef stock, sour cream, and remaining coconut aminos, and bring to a simmer. Adjust the seasoning with black pepper and salt. Serve the meatballs topped with onion sauce.

Per Serving
calories: 519 | fat: 36g | protein: 24g | carbs: 18g | net carbs: 16g | fiber: 2g

Beef and Cauliflower Rice Casserole

Prep time: 5 minutes | Cook time: 26 minutes | Serves 6

2 pounds (907 g) ground beef
Pink salt and black pepper, to taste
1 cup cauliflower rice
2 cups cabbage, chopped
1 (14-ounce / 397-g) can diced tomatoes
¼ cup water
1 cup Colby Jack cheese, shredded

1. Preheat oven to 375°F (190°C) and grease a baking dish with cooking spray.
2. Put beef in a pot and season with salt and pepper and cook over medium heat for 6 minutes until no longer pink. Drain grease. Add cauliflower rice, cabbage, tomatoes, and water. Stir and bring to boil covered for 5 minutes to thicken the sauce. Adjust taste with salt and black pepper.
3. Spoon the beef mixture into the baking dish. Sprinkle with cheese, and bake in the oven for 15 minutes until cheese has melted and golden brown. Remove, cool for 4 minutes, and serve.

Per Serving
calories: 501 | fat: 38g | protein: 33g | carbs: 6g | net carbs: 3g | fiber: 3g

Russian Beef and Dill Pickle Gratin

Prep time: 15 minutes | Cook time: 40 minutes | Serves 5

2 teaspoons onion flakes
2 pounds (907 g) ground beef
2 garlic cloves, minced
Salt and black pepper, to taste
1 cup Mozzarella cheese, shredded
2 cups Fontina cheese, shredded
1 cup Russian dressing
2 tablespoons sesame seeds, toasted
20 dill pickle slices
1 iceberg lettuce head, torn

1. Set a pan over medium heat, place in beef, garlic, salt, onion flakes, and pepper, and cook for 5 minutes. Remove to a baking dish, stir in Russian dressing, Mozzarella, and spread 1 cup of the Fontina cheese.
2. Lay the pickle slices on top, spread over the remaining Fontina cheese and sesame seeds, place in the oven at 350°F (180°C), and bake for 20 minutes. Arrange the lettuce on a serving platter and top with the gratin.

Per Serving
calories: 585 | fat: 48.1g | protein: 40.9g | carbs: 8.5g | net carbs: 5.2g | fiber: 3.3g

Beef Tripe with Onions and Tomatoes

Prep time: 10 minutes | Cook time: 25 minutes | Serves 6

1½ pounds (680 g) beef tripe
4 cups buttermilk
Salt to taste
2 teaspoons creole seasoning
3 tablespoons olive oil
2 large onions, sliced
3 tomatoes, diced

1. Put the tripe in a bowl and cover with buttermilk. Refrigerate for 3 hours to extract bitterness and gamey taste. Remove from buttermilk, pat dry with a paper towel, and season with salt and creole seasoning.
2. Heat 2 tablespoons of oil in a skillet over medium heat and brown the tripe on both sides for 6 minutes in total. Set aside. Add the remaining oil and sauté the onions for 3 minutes until soft. Include the tomatoes and cook for 10 minutes. Pour in a few tablespoons of water if necessary. Put the tripe in the sauce and cook for 3 minutes. Adjust taste with salt and serve with low carb rice.

Per Serving
calories: 341 | fat: 26.9g | protein: 21.9g | carbs: 2.7g | net carbs: 1.0g | fiber: 1.7g

Skirt Steak with Green Beans

Prep time: 5 minutes | Cook time: 13 minutes | Serves 4

3 cups green beans, chopped
2 cups cauliflower rice
2 tablespoons butter
1 tablespoon olive oil
1 pound (454 g) skirt steak
Salt and black pepper. to taste
4 fresh eggs
Hot sauce (sugar-free) for topping (optional)

1. Put cauliflower rice and green beans in a bowl, sprinkle with a little water, and steam in the microwave for 90 seconds. Share into bowls. Warm butter and olive oil in a skillet, season the beef with salt and pepper, and brown for 5 minutes on each side. Ladle the meat onto the vegetables.

2. Wipe out the skillet and return to medium heat, crack in an egg, season with salt and pepper and cook until the egg white has set, but the yolk is still runny, for 3 minutes. Remove egg onto the vegetable bowl and fry the remaining 3 eggs. Add to the other bowls. Drizzle with hot sauce (if desired) and serve.

Per Serving

calories: 409 | fat: 25g | protein: 40g | carbs: 8g | net carbs: 5g | fiber: 3g

Herbed Veggie and Beef Stew

Prep time: 10 minutes | Cook time: 25 minutes | Serves 4

1 pound (454 g)ground beef
2 tablespoons olive oil
1 onion, chopped
2 garlic cloves, minced
14 ounces (397 g) canned diced tomatoes
1 tablespoon dried rosemary
1 tablespoon dried sage
1 tablespoon dried oregano
1 tablespoon dried basil
1 tablespoon dried marjoram
Salt and black pepper, to taste
2 carrots, sliced
2 celery stalks, chopped
1 cup vegetable broth

1. Set a pan over medium heat, add in the olive oil, onion, celery, and garlic, and sauté for 5 minutes. Place in the beef, and cook for 6 minutes. Stir in the tomatoes, carrots, broth, black pepper, oregano, marjoram, basil, rosemary, salt, and sage, and simmer for 15 minutes. Serve and enjoy!

Per Serving

calories: 254 | fat: 13.1g | protein: 29.9g | carbs: 10.1g | net carbs: 5.1g | fiber: 5.0g

Beef and Fennel Provençal

Prep time: 10 minutes | Cook time: 45 minutes | Serves 4

12 ounces (340 g) beef steak racks
2 fennel bulbs, sliced
Salt and black pepper, to taste
3 tablespoons olive oil
½ cup apple cider vinegar
1 teaspoon herbs de Provence
1 tablespoon Swerve

1. In a bowl, mix the fennel with 2 tablespoons of oil, Swerve, and vinegar, toss to coat well, and set to a baking dish. Season with herbs de Provence, pepper and salt, and cook in the oven at 400ºF (205ºC) for 15 minutes.
2. Sprinkle black pepper and salt to the beef, place into an oiled pan over medium heat, and cook for a couple of minutes. Place the beef to the baking dish with the fennel, and bake for 20 minutes. Split everything among plates and enjoy.

Per Serving

calories: 231 | fat: 11.4g | protein: 19.1g | carbs: 8.7g | net carbs: 5.1g | fiber: 3.6g

Italian Veal Cutlets with Pecorino

Prep time: 15 minutes | Cook time: 1 hour 5 minutes | Serves 6

6 veal cutlets
½ cup Pecorino cheese, grated
6 provolone cheese slices
Salt and black pepper, to taste
4 cups tomato sauce
A pinch of garlic salt
2 tablespoons butter
2 tablespoons coconut oil, melted
1 teaspoon Italian seasoning

1. Season the veal cutlets with garlic salt, black pepper, and salt. Set a pan over medium heat and warm oil and butter, place in the veal, and cook until browned on all sides. Spread half of the tomato sauce on the bottom of a baking dish that is coated with some cooking spray.
2. Place in the veal cutlets then spread with Italian seasoning and sprinkle over the remaining sauce. Set in the oven at 360ºF (182ºC), and bake for 40 minutes. Scatter with the provolone cheese, then sprinkle with Pecorino cheese, and bake for another 5 minutes until the cheese is golden and melted. Serve.

Per Serving
calories: 363 | fat: 21.1g | protein: 26.1g | carbs: 8.4g | net carbs: 5.9g | fiber: 2.5g

Grilled Beef Skewers with Fresh Salad

Prep time: 10 minutes | Cook time: 13 minutes | Serves 4

1 pound (454 g) sirloin steak, boneless, cubed
¼ cup ranch dressing
1 red onion, sliced
½ tablespoon white wine vinegar
1 tablespoon extra-virgin olive oil
2 ripe tomatoes, sliced
2 tablespoons fresh parsley, chopped
1 cucumber, sliced
Salt, to taste

1. Thread the beef cubes on the skewers, about 4-5 cubes per skewer. Brush half of the ranch dressing on the skewers (all around). Preheat grill to 400ºF (205ºC) and place the skewers on the grill grate to cook for 6 minutes. Turn the skewers once and cook further for 6 minutes.
2. Brush the remaining ranch dressing on the meat and cook them for 1 more minute on each side.
3. In a salad bowl mix together red onion, tomatoes, and cucumber, sprinkle with salt, vinegar, and extra-virgin olive oil; toss to combine. Top the salad with skewers and scatter the parsley all over.

Per Serving
calories: 357 | fat: 23g | protein: 25g | carbs: 12g | net carbs: 10g | fiber: 2g

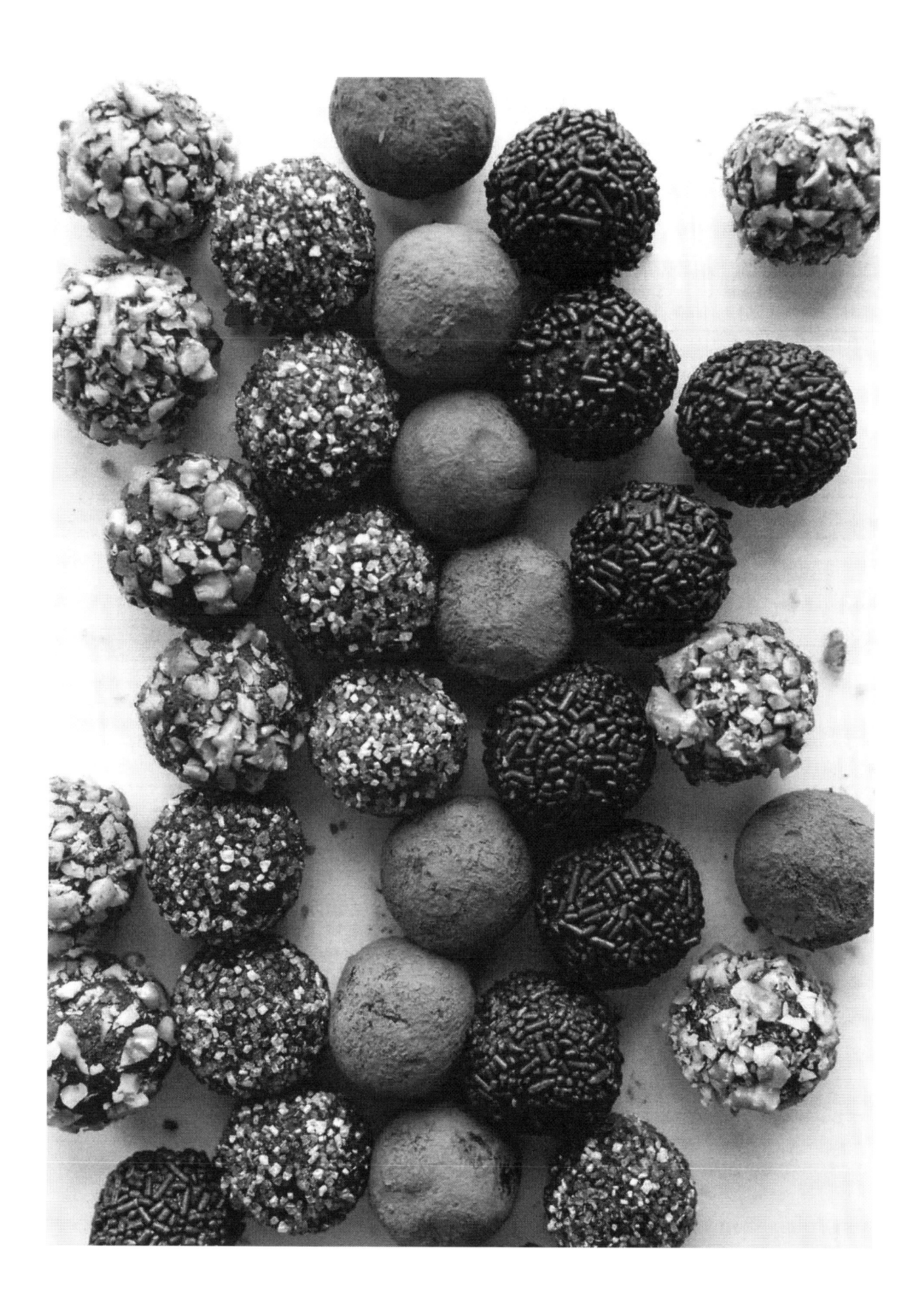

Chapter 11 Desserts

Creamy Strawberry Shake

Prep time: 10 minutes | Cook time: 0 minutes | Serves 2

¾ cup heavy (whipping) cream
2 ounces (57 g) cream cheese, at room temperature
1 tablespoon Swerve natural sweetener
¼ teaspoon vanilla extract
6 strawberries, sliced
6 ice cubes

1. In a food processor (or blender), combine the heavy cream, cream cheese, sweetener, and vanilla. Mix on high to fully combine.
2. Add the strawberries and ice, and blend until smooth.
3. Pour into two tall glasses and serve.

Per Serving
calories: 407 | fat: 42g | protein: 4g
carbs: 13g | net carbs: 6g | fiber: 7g

Chocolate-Coconut Shake

Prep time: 10 minutes | Cook time: 0 minutes | Serves 2

¾ cup heavy (whipping) cream
4 ounces (113 g) coconut milk
1 tablespoon Swerve natural sweetener
¼ teaspoon vanilla extract
2 tablespoons unsweetened cocoa powder

1. Pour the cream into a medium cold metal bowl, and with your hand mixer and cold beaters, beat the cream just until it forms peaks.
2. Slowly pour in the coconut milk, and gently stir it into the cream. Add the sweetener, vanilla, and cocoa powder, and beat until fully combined.
3. Pour into two tall glasses, and chill in the freezer for 1 hour before serving. I usually stir the shakes twice during this time.

Per Serving
calories: 444 | fat: 47g | protein: 4g
carbs: 15g | net carbs: 7g | fiber: 8g

Vanilla Chocolate Pudding

Prep time: 5 minutes | Cook time: 15 minutes | Serves 4

2 cups heavy whipping cream
2 ounces (57 g) unsweetened baking chocolate, coarsely chopped
1 teaspoon vanilla extract
6 large egg yolks
⅓ cup granulated erythritol–monk fruit blend

1. In the medium saucepan, heat the heavy cream over low heat for 2 to 3 minutes, until warm. Stir in the chocolate and vanilla and heat for about 3 minutes, stirring occasionally, until the chocolate has melted. Set aside to cool.
2. In a medium bowl, whisk the egg yolks and erythritol–monk fruit blend for about 2 minutes, or until the mixture is a pale yellow.
3. Once the heavy cream mixture has cooled to room temperature, 15 to 20 minutes, pour one-quarter of it into the egg mixture and whisk until well combined. Add the remaining three-quarters of the cream mixture and whisk until combined.
4. Pour the cream and egg mixture back into the saucepan. Cook over low heat, stirring constantly for 3 to 5 minutes, until the mixture begins to thicken. You'll know the pudding is thick enough when it coats the back of a spoon without dripping.
5. Pour the pudding through the sieve into another medium bowl. Put a sheet of plastic wrap directly onto the surface of the pudding to prevent a skin from forming. Completely cool the pudding in the refrigerator, about 1 to 2 hours.
6. Serve in small shallow bowls or in individual ramekins. Store leftovers in an airtight container for up to 5 days in the refrigerator.

Per Serving (½ Cup)
calories: 586 | fat: 57.8g | protein: 8.9g
carbs: 7.9g | net carbs: 5.9g | fiber: 2.0g

Chocolate Almond Bark

Prep time: 10 minutes | Cook time: 0 minutes | Makes 15 pieces

¾ cup coconut oil
¼ cup confectioners' erythritol–monk fruit blend; less sweet: 3 tablespoons
3 tablespoons dark cocoa powder
½ cup slivered almonds
¾ teaspoon almond extract

1. Line the baking pan with parchment paper and set aside.
2. In the microwave-safe bowl, melt the coconut oil in the microwave in 10-second intervals.
3. In the medium bowl, whisk together the melted coconut oil, confectioners' erythritol–monk fruit blend, and cocoa powder until fully combined. Stir in the slivered almonds and almond extract.
4. Pour the mixture into the prepared baking pan and spread evenly. Put the pan in the freezer for about 20 minutes, or until the chocolate bark is solid.
5. Once the chocolate bark is solid, break apart into 15 roughly even pieces to serve.
6. Store the chocolate bark in an airtight container in the freezer. Allow to slightly thaw about 5 minutes before eating. Thaw only what you will be eating.

Per Serving (1 Pieces)
calories: 118 | fat: 13.0g | protein: 1.0g carbs: 1.0g | net carbs: 0g | fiber: 1.0g

Fresh Strawberry Cheesecake Mousse

Prep time: 10 minutes | Cook time: 0 minutes | Serves 2

4 ounces (113 g) cream cheese, at room temperature
1 tablespoon heavy (whipping) cream
1 teaspoon Swerve natural sweetener or 1 drop liquid stevia
1 teaspoon vanilla extract
4 fresh strawberries, sliced

1. Break up the cream cheese block into smaller pieces and distribute evenly in a food processor (or blender). Add the cream, sweetener, and vanilla.
2. Mix together on high. I usually stop and stir twice and scrape down the sides of the bowl with a small rubber scraper to make sure everything is mixed well.
3. Add the strawberries to the food processor, and mix until combined.
4. Divide the strawberry cheesecake mixture between two small dishes, and chill for 1 hour before serving.

Per Serving
calories: 221 | fat: 21g | protein: 4g carbs: 11g | net carbs: 4g | fiber: 7g

Chocolate Truffles

Prep time: 10 minutes | Cook time: 5 minutes | Makes 16 truffles

¼ cup full-fat coconut milk
5 ounces (142 g) sugar-free dark chocolate, finely chopped
1 tablespoon solid coconut oil, at room temperature
¼ cup unsweetened cocoa powder, for coating

1. Line the baking sheet with parchment paper and set aside.
2. In the small saucepan, heat the coconut milk over medium heat for about 3 minutes, until hot. Stir in the chocolate and let sit in the coconut milk until beginning to melt. When most of the chocolate has softened, stir carefully with a whisk until all of the chocolate is melted and the texture is smooth and glossy. Add the coconut oil and stir gently until combined.
3. Transfer the mixture to the medium airtight container and refrigerate until firm and set, about 30 minutes.
4. Using a small cookie scoop or spoon, scoop out the truffles, about 1 inch in diameter each, and shape lightly in your hands. Move quickly, and only lightly touch the chocolate or it will begin to melt in your hands.
5. Roll the truffles in the cocoa powder and place on the lined baking sheet. Refrigerate for another 10 minutes to set before serving.
6. Store leftovers in an airtight container in the refrigerator for up to 3 days or freeze for up to 3 weeks.

Per Serving (1 Truffle)
calories: 75 | fat: 6.0g | protein: 2.0g carbs: 3.0g | net carbs: 1.0g | fiber: 2.0g

Salted Vanilla Caramels

Prep time: 5 minutes | Cook time: 15 minutes | Makes 24

2 tablespoons unsalted butter, at room temperature
1 cup allulose
¼ teaspoon sea salt
¼ cup heavy whipping cream
½ teaspoon vanilla extract

1. Line the baking pan with wax paper and set aside.
2. In a small saucepan, brown the butter over medium heat for about 3 minutes, making sure to stir often while the butter browns. Add the allulose and stir until well combined. Simmer for about 7 minutes, until melted, then stir in the salt. Once it starts to bubble, add the heavy cream and vanilla and stir constantly, making sure it doesn't boil over. Once combined, reduce the heat and allow to gently simmer for about 3 minutes, until reduced slightly.
3. Remove the caramel sauce from the heat and pour it evenly into the prepared baking pan. Put into the refrigerator for a couple of hours or overnight, until cool and hardened.
4. Cut the caramel into 24 pieces and serve.
5. To store, wrap each candy in wax paper, twisting the sides closed. Put the candies in an airtight container in the refrigerator for up to 5 days. With refrigeration, the candies will become very firm but will soften at room temperature.

Per Serving
calories: 5 | fat: 0.8g | protein: 0g
carbs: 0g | net carbs: 0g | fiber: 0g

Chocolate Fudge

Prep time: 10 minutes | Cook time: 5 minutes | Makes 24 bars

8 tablespoons (1 stick) unsalted butter, at room temperature
4 ounces (113 g) unsweetened baking chocolate, coarsely chopped
1 cup confectioners' erythritol–monk fruit blend; less sweet: ½ cup
8 ounces (227 g) full-fat cream cheese, at room temperature
¼ cup dark cocoa powder
1 teaspoon vanilla extract
1½ teaspoons peppermint extract

1. Line the baking pan with parchment paper.
2. In the microwave-safe bowl, melt the butter and baking chocolate in the microwave in 30-second intervals, then set aside.
3. In the large mixing bowl, using an electric mixer on medium high, mix the confectioners' erythritol–monk fruit blend, cream cheese, cocoa powder, vanilla, and peppermint extract until well combined, stopping and scraping the bowl once or twice, as needed. Add the melted chocolate mixture and mix until fully incorporated.
4. Evenly spread the batter into the prepared baking pan. Put the baking pan in the freezer for about 30 minutes, or until the fudge firms. Cut the fudge into 24 squares and serve.
5. Store the fudge in an airtight container in the refrigerator for up to 5 days or freeze for up to 3 weeks.

Per Serving
calories: 100 | fat: 10.1g | protein: 0.8g
carbs: 1.9g | net carbs: 1.0g | fiber: 0.9g

Cheesecake Fat Bomb with Berries

Prep time: 10 minutes | Cook time: 0 minutes | Serves 2

4 ounces (113 g) cream cheese, at room temperature
4 tablespoons butter, at room temperature
2 teaspoons Swerve natural sweetener or 2 drops liquid stevia
1 teaspoon vanilla extract
¼ cup berries, fresh or frozen

1. In a medium bowl, use a hand mixer to beat the cream cheese, butter, sweetener, and vanilla.
2. In a small bowl, mash the berries thoroughly. Fold the berries into the cream-cheese mixture using a rubber scraper.
3. Spoon the cream-cheese mixture into fat bomb molds.
4. Freeze for at least 2 hours, unmold them, and eat! Leftover fat bombs can be stored in the freezer in a zip-top bag for up to 3 months. It's nice to have some in your freezer for when you are craving a sweet treat.

Per Serving
calories: 414 | fat: 43g | protein: 4g
carbs: 9g | net carbs: 4g | fiber: 5g

Bacon Fudge

Prep time: 10 minutes | Cook time: 40 minutes | Makes 24 bars

½ cup granulated erythritol–monk fruit blend
6 bacon slices
8 tablespoons (1 stick) unsalted butter, at room temperature
4 ounces (113 g) unsweetened baking chocolate, coarsely chopped
1 cup confectioners' erythritol–monk fruit blend; less sweet: ½ cup
8 ounces (227 g) full-fat cream cheese, at room temperature
¼ cup dark cocoa powder
1 teaspoon vanilla extract
1 cup chopped pistachios

1. Preheat the oven to 350ºF (180ºC). Line the baking sheet with aluminum foil. Line the baking pan with parchment paper and set aside.
2. In the shallow mixing bowl, put the granulated erythritol–monk fruit blend and dip the bacon slices into it to evenly coat both sides. Place the coated bacon on the prepared baking sheet and bake for 30 to 40 minutes, or until fully cooked. Once cooled, break into smaller pieces and set aside.
3. In the small microwave-safe bowl, melt the butter and baking chocolate in the microwave in 30-second intervals, then set aside.
4. In the medium mixing bowl, using an electric mixer on medium high, mix the confectioners' erythritol–monk fruit blend, cream cheese, dark cocoa powder, and vanilla until well combined, stopping and scraping the bowl once or twice, as needed. Add the melted chocolate mixture and combine until fully incorporated. Fold in three-quarters of the candied bacon and the chopped pistachios.
5. Spread the batter into the prepared baking pan. Sprinkle the remaining candied bacon on top of the fudge.
6. Put the baking pan in the freezer for about 30 minutes or until the fudge firms. Cut the fudge into 24 squares and serve.
7. Store the fudge in the refrigerator for up to 5 days or freeze for up to 3 weeks.

Per Serving (1 Piece)
calories: 142 | fat: 13.0g | protein: 3.0g
carbs: 4.0g | net carbs: 2.0g | fiber: 2.0g

Classic Flan

Prep time: 5 minutes | Cook time: 45 minutes | Serves 6

2 tablespoons unsalted butter, at room temperature
1 cup allulose
3 large eggs
2 large egg yolks
½ cup granulated erythritol–monk fruit blend
2¾ cups heavy whipping cream
2 teaspoons vanilla extract
¼ teaspoon salt

1. Preheat the oven to 350ºF (180ºC). Position the rack in the center of oven.
2. In the small saucepan, brown the butter over medium heat, stirring constantly using a silicone spatula. The butter will begin to foam and bubble after 2 to 4 minutes and you should begin to see browned bits on the bottom of the pan. At this point, remove from the heat and continue to stir until the butter begins to lightly brown. Add the allulose and continue stirring over low heat for 3 to 5 minutes, until the sweetener completely dissolves and is a golden amber color.
3. Pour the sauce into the bottom of each ramekin, being sure to wiggle the dish side to side so the sauce covers the sides and bottom of the ramekins. Put the ramekins in the baking pan and set aside.
4. In the large bowl, whisk the whole eggs, egg yolks, and erythritol–monk fruit blend until combined. Gently whisk in the heavy cream, vanilla, and salt, avoiding creating a foam by whisking too vigorously.
5. Pour the custard through the sieve into the prepared ramekins. Add enough hot water to the baking pan to come halfway up the sides of the ramekins.
6. Bake for 30 minutes, or until the centers of the flans are gently set. Transfer the flans to the cooling rack to cool for 15 to 20 minutes.
7. Once cooled, cover the flans and put them in the refrigerator to chill overnight or for at least 8 hours. When ready to serve, put a plate over the top of the ramekins and flip them over to release the flans. You made need to wiggle the dish a little to ease them out. Serve and enjoy.
8. Store leftovers in an airtight container in the refrigerator for up to 3 days.

Per Serving
calories: 469 | fat: 47.9g | protein: 6.0g
carbs: 4.0g | net carbs: 4.0g | fiber: 0g

Almond Fat Bombs with Chocolate Chips

Prep time: 5 minutes | Cook time: 0 minutes | Makes 18

8 ounces (227 g) full-fat cream cheese, at room temperature	erythritol–monk fruit blend; less sweet: ¼ cup
8 tablespoons (1 stick) unsalted butter, at room temperature	1 teaspoon vanilla extract
¾ cup almond flour	¼ teaspoon sea salt
½ cup granulated	¼ cup chocolate chips

1. Line the baking sheet with parchment paper and set aside.
2. In the medium bowl, using an electric mixer on high, blend the cream cheese and butter, stopping and scraping the bowl once or twice, as needed. Add the almond flour, erythritol–monk fruit blend, vanilla, and salt and mix until fully incorporated. Fold in the chocolate chips.
3. Refrigerate the mixture for 1 hour until firm (like ice cream). Using a small cookie scoop or spoon, scoop the fat bombs into 1 tablespoon-size mounds and place onto the baking sheet. Put the baking sheet back into the refrigerator for about 15 minutes to allow the fat bombs to firm before serving.
4. To store, put in an airtight container in the refrigerator for up to 10 days or in the freezer for up to 3 weeks.

Per Serving (1 Piece)
calories: 125 | fat: 12.0g | protein: 2.0g
carbs: 2.0g | net carbs: 1.0g | fiber: 1.0g

Pecan Pralines

Prep time: 5 minutes | Cook time: 15 minutes | Makes 18 clusters

4 tablespoons (½ stick) unsalted butter, at room temperature	blend
	1½ cups pecan halves
¼ cup granulated erythritol–monk fruit	½ teaspoon salt
	2 tablespoons heavy whipping cream

1. Line the baking sheet with parchment paper and set aside.
2. In the skillet, melt the butter over medium-high heat. Using the silicone spatula, stir in the erythritol–monk fruit blend and combine well, making sure to dissolve the sugar in the butter. Stir in the pecan halves and salt.
3. Once the pecans are completely covered in the glaze, add the heavy cream and quickly stir. When the heavy cream bubbles and evaporates, remove from the heat immediately. Quickly spoon the clusters of 4 to 5 pecan halves each onto the prepared baking sheet and allow to fully cool and set, 15 to 20 minutes, before enjoying.
4. Store leftovers in an airtight container on the counter or in the refrigerator for up 5 days.

Per Serving (1 Cluster)
calories: 86 | fat: 9.0g | protein: 1.0g
carbs: 1.0g | net carbs: 0g | fiber: 1.0g

Panna Cotta

Prep time: 10 minutes | Cook time: 20 minutes | Serves 4

Unsalted butter, for greasing	erythritol–monk fruit blend; less sweet: 3 tablespoons
2 tablespoons unflavored gelatin	½ teaspoon vanilla extract
3 tablespoons cold water	½ teaspoon espresso instant powder
2 cups heavy whipping cream	⅛ teaspoon salt
⅓ cup granulated	

1. Grease the silicone molds with butter and set aside.
2. In the small mixing bowl, dissolve the gelatin in the cold water and set aside.
3. In the medium saucepan, boil the heavy cream on medium heat. Lower the heat and simmer for about 4 minutes, until the cream begins to thicken.
4. Add the erythritol–monk fruit blend, vanilla, espresso powder, and salt. Continue to stir to combine all the ingredients. Remove from the heat and add the dissolved gelatin. Stir until the gelatin is well incorporated.
5. Pour the mixture into the molds and allow it to cool at room temperature for about 30 minutes. After cooling, cover the molds with plastic wrap and put them in the refrigerator for at least 4 hours before taking the panna cotta out of the molds. Serve cold.
6. Store leftovers in an airtight container in the refrigerator for up to 3 days.

Per Serving
calories: 451 | fat: 46.8g | protein: 6.0g
carbs: 2.9g | net carbs: 2.9g | fiber: 0g

Cinnamon Crusted Almonds

Prep time: 5 minutes | Cook time: 45 minutes | Makes 2½ cups

2½ cups whole raw almonds
2 tablespoons unsalted butter, melted
1 large egg white
½ teaspoon vanilla extract
¼ cup brown or golden erythritol–monk fruit blend; less sweet: 2 tablespoons
1 teaspoon ground cinnamon
¼ teaspoon sea salt

1. Preheat the oven to 275ºF (135ºC). Line the baking sheet with parchment paper and set aside.
2. In a large bowl, toss the almonds in the melted butter.
3. In another large bowl, using an electric mixer on medium high, lightly beat the egg white for about 1 minute, until frothy. Add the vanilla to the egg white and mix until just combined. Add the almonds and stir until well coated.
4. In the small bowl, combine the brown erythritol–monk fruit blend, cinnamon, and salt and sprinkle over the nut mixture. Toss to coat and spread evenly on the prepared baking sheet.
5. Bake for 45 minutes, stirring occasionally, until golden.
6. Allow to cool fully, 15 to 20 minutes, before eating.
7. Store in an airtight container at room temperature for up to 1 week.

Per Serving
calories: 385 | fat: 33.9g | protein: 13.0g
carbs: 13.0g | net carbs: 4.9g | fiber: 8.1g

Strawberries Coated with Chocolate Chips

Prep time: 10 minutes | Cook time: 5 minutes | Makes 15

5 ounces (142 g) sugar-free dark chocolate chips
1 tablespoon vegetable shortening
or lard
15 medium whole strawberries, fresh or frozen

1. Line the baking sheet with parchment paper and set aside.
2. In the microwave-safe bowl, combine the chocolate and shortening. Melt in the microwave in 30-second intervals, stirring in between.
3. Dip the strawberries into the melted chocolate mixture and place them on the prepared baking sheet.
4. Put the strawberries in the freezer for 10 to 15 minutes to set before serving.
5. Store leftovers in an airtight container in the refrigerator for up to 3 days.

Per Serving (3 Strawberries)
calories: 216 | fat: 18.0g | protein: 4.0g
carbs: 11.0g | net carbs: 6.0g | fiber: 5.0g

Meringues

Prep time: 20 minutes | Cook time: 2 hours | Makes 30

4 large egg whites
¼ teaspoon cream of tartar
¼ teaspoon sea salt
½ cup granulated erythritol-monk fruit blend
¼ cup powdered erythritol-monk fruit blend
½ teaspoon vanilla extract

1. Preheat the oven to 200ºF (93ºC). Line the baking sheet with parchment paper and set aside.
2. In the large bowl, using an electric mixer on medium, beat the egg whites, cream of tartar, and salt for 1 to 2 minutes, until foamy and the egg whites just begin to turn opaque.
3. Continue to whip the egg whites, adding in the granulated and powdered erythritol–monk fruit blend about 1 teaspoon at a time and scraping the bowl once or twice.
4. Once all the erythritol–monk fruit blend has been added, increase the mixer speed to high and whip for 5 to 7 minutes, until the meringue is glossy and very stiff. Using a rubber spatula, gently fold in the vanilla.
5. Scoop the meringue into the pastry bag fitted with a French star tip and pipe 2-inch-diameter kisses onto the prepared baking sheet. Alternatively, spoon the meringue onto the sheet for a more organic shape.
6. Bake for 2 hours, or until crisp and lightly browned. Allow to cool completely on the cooling rack before serving. Leftovers can be stored in an airtight, nonporous container at room temperature for about 1 week.

Per Serving (3 Meringues)
calories: 8 | fat: 0g | protein: 2.0g
carbs: 0g | net carbs: 0g | fiber: 0g

Cream Cheese Fat Bombs

Prep time: 10 minutes | Cook time: 0 minutes | Makes 30 bombs

8 ounces (227 g) full-fat cream cheese, at room temperature
8 tablespoons (1 stick) unsalted butter, at room temperature
3 tablespoons confectioners' erythritol–monk fruit blend
3 tablespoons coconut oil
½ teaspoon vanilla extract

1. In the large mixing bowl, using an electric mixer on high, beat the cream cheese and butter for 2 to 3 minutes, until light and fluffy, stopping and scraping the bowl once or twice, as needed. Add the confectioners' erythritol–monk fruit blend, coconut oil, and vanilla and mix until well combined.
2. Scoop the mixture into a pastry bag and pipe into the molds or cupcake liners. Put the molds in the freezer for 1 hour to firm. Pop out the fat bombs to serve.
3. Store in an airtight container in the freezer for up to 3 weeks.

Per Serving (1 Piece)
calories: 66 | fat: 6.9g | protein: 0g
carbs: 0g | net carbs: 0g | fiber: 0g

Lime and Coconut Panna Cotta

Prep time: 10 minutes | Cook time: 10 minutes | Serves 4

Coconut oil, for greasing
2 tablespoons unflavored gelatin
3 tablespoons cold water
1 (13.5-ounce / 383-g) can full-fat coconut milk
⅓ cup granulated erythritol–monk fruit blend; less sweet: 3 tablespoons
1 teaspoon grated lime zest
1 tablespoon freshly squeezed lime juice
½ teaspoon vanilla extract
⅛ teaspoon salt

1. Grease the molds with coconut oil and set aside.
2. In the small bowl, soften the gelatin powder in the cold water and set aside.
3. In the medium saucepan, heat the coconut milk over medium heat until boiling. Reduce the heat and simmer for a couple of minutes, until the cream begins to thicken. While stirring, add the erythritol–monk fruit blend, lime zest, lime juice, vanilla, and salt. Continue to stir to combine all the ingredients. Remove from the heat and add the dissolved gelatin. Stir until the gelatin is dissolved.
4. Pour the mixture into the prepared molds and allow them to cool at room temperature for about 30 minutes. Cover with plastic wrap and put in the refrigerator for at least 4 hours before unmolding.
5. To remove the panna cotta from the molds, dip the molds in a bowl of hot water to help loosen. Serve cold.
6. Store leftovers in an airtight container or covered with plastic wrap in the refrigerator for up to 3 days.

Per Serving
calories: 211 | fat: 21.0g | protein: 5.1g
carbs: 2.9g | net carbs: 2.9g | fiber: 0g

Posset

Prep time: 5 minutes | Cook time: 10 minutes | Serves 4

2½ cups heavy whipping cream
½ cup granulated erythritol–monk fruit blend
¼ cup freshly squeezed lemon juice
2 tablespoons freshly squeezed lime juice
½ teaspoon orange extract
¼ teaspoon sea salt
¼ cup blueberries, for garnish (optional)

1. In the small saucepan, cook the heavy cream and erythritol–monk fruit blend over medium heat for 6 minutes, or until the sweetener has dissolved. Stir constantly so the mixture does not boil over.
2. Remove the cream mixture from the heat and stir in the lemon juice, lime juice, orange extract, and salt.
3. Pour the mixture into the ramekins and cover with plastic wrap.
4. Chill for at least 6 hours or overnight to allow the mixture to fully set before serving. Garnish with the blueberries (if using).
5. Store leftovers in an airtight container for up to 5 days in the refrigerator.

Per Serving
calories: 520 | fat: 54.8g | protein: 3.0g
carbs: 6.0g | net carbs: 6.0g | fiber: 0g

Peanut Butter and Chocolate Fat Bombs

Prep time: 5 minutes | Cook time: 5 minutes | Makes 24 bombs

½ cup no-sugar-added peanut butter
½ cup coconut oil
¼ cup unsweetened cocoa powder
⅓ cup confectioners' erythritol–monk fruit blend; less sweet: 2½ tablespoons
¼ teaspoon sea salt

1. In the small microwave-safe bowl, melt the peanut butter, coconut oil, and cocoa powder in the microwave in 30-second intervals, mixing in between. Once the peanut butter mixture is completely melted, stir in the confectioners' erythritol–monk fruit blend and salt.
2. Pour the mixture into the silicone molds and put in the freezer for about 30 minutes, or until they are completely set.
3. Remove the bombs from the silicone molds to serve.
4. To store, transfer to an airtight container and put in the freezer for up to 3 weeks.

Per Serving (1 Piece)
calories: 70 | fat: 7.1g | protein: 1.0g
carbs: 1.9g | net carbs: 1.9g | fiber: 0g

Simple Peanut Butter Fat Bomb

Prep time: 10 minutes | Cook time: 1 minute | Serves 2

1 tablespoon butter, at room temperature
1 tablespoon coconut oil
2 tablespoons all-natural peanut butter or almond butter
2 teaspoons Swerve natural sweetener or 2 drops liquid stevia

1. In a microwave-safe medium bowl, melt the butter, coconut oil, and peanut butter in the microwave for 1 minute on 50 percent power. Mix in the sweetener.
2. Pour the mixture into fat bomb molds.
3. Freeze for 30 minutes, unmold them, and eat! Keep some extras in your freezer so you can eat them anytime you are craving a sweet treat.

Per Serving
calories: 196 | fat: 20g | protein: 3g
carbs: 8g | net carbs: 3g | fiber: 5g

Coffee-Coconut Ice Pops

Prep time: 5 minutes | Cook time: 0 minutes | Serves 4

2 cups brewed coffee, cold
¾ cup coconut cream
2 teaspoons Swerve natural sweetener or 2 drops liquid stevia
2 tablespoons sugar-free chocolate chips

1. In a food processor (or blender), mix together the coffee, coconut cream, and sweetener until thoroughly blended.
2. Pour into ice pop molds, and drop a few chocolate chips into each mold.
3. Freeze for at least 2 hours before serving.

Per Serving
calories: 105 | fat: 10g | protein: 1g
carbs: 7g | net carbs: 2g | fiber: 5g

Cheesy Lemonade Fat Bomb

Prep time: 10 minutes | Cook time: 0 minutes | Serves 2

½ lemon
4 ounces (113 g) cream cheese, at room temperature
2 ounces (57 g) butter, at room temperature
2 teaspoons Swerve natural sweetener or 2 drops liquid stevia
Pinch pink Himalayan salt

1. Zest the lemon half with a very fine grater into a small bowl. Squeeze the juice from the lemon half into the bowl with the zest.
2. In a medium bowl, combine the cream cheese and butter. Add the sweetener, lemon zest and juice, and pink Himalayan salt. Using a hand mixer, beat until fully combined.
3. Spoon the mixture into the fat bomb molds. (I use small silicone cupcake molds. If you don't have molds, you can use cupcake paper liners that fit into the cups of a muffin tin.)
4. Freeze for at least 2 hours, unmold, and eat! Keep extras in your freezer in a zip-top bag so you and your loved ones can have them anytime you are craving a sweet treat. They will keep in the freezer for up to 3 months.

Per Serving
calories: 404 | fat: 43g | protein: 4g
carbs: 8g | net carbs: 4g | fiber: 4g

Baked Cheesecake Bites

Prep time: 10 minutes | Cook time: 30 minutes | Serves 4

4 ounces (113 g) cream cheese, at room temperature
¼ cup sour cream
2 large eggs
⅓ cup Swerve natural sweetener
¼ teaspoon vanilla extract

1. Preheat the oven to 350ºF (180ºC).
2. In a medium mixing bowl, use a hand mixer to beat the cream cheese, sour cream, eggs, sweetener, and vanilla until well mixed.
3. Place silicone liners (or cupcake paper liners) in the cups of a muffin tin.
4. Pour the cheesecake batter into the liners, and bake for 30 minutes.
5. Refrigerate until completely cooled before serving, about 3 hours. Store extra cheesecake bites in a zip-top bag in the freezer for up to 3 months.

Per Serving
calories: 169 | fat: 15g | protein: 5g
carbs: 18g | net carbs: 2g | fiber: 16g

Pumpkin Cheesecake Bites

Prep time: 10 minutes | Cook time: 30 minutes | Serves 4

4 ounces (113 g) pumpkin purée
4 ounces (113 g) cream cheese, at room temperature
2 large eggs
⅓ cup Swerve natural sweetener
2 teaspoons pumpkin pie spice

1. Preheat the oven to 350ºF (180ºC).
2. In a medium mixing bowl, use a hand mixer to mix the pumpkin purée, cream cheese, eggs, sweetener, and pumpkin pie spice until thoroughly combined.
3. Place silicone liners (or cupcake paper liners) into the cups of a muffin tin.
4. Pour the batter into the liners, and bake for 30 minutes.
5. Refrigerate until completely cooled before serving, about 3 hours. Put leftover cheesecake bites in a zip-top plastic bag and store in the freezer for up to 3 months.

Per Serving
calories: 156 | fat: 12g | protein: 5g
carbs: 21g | net carbs: 4g | fiber: 17g

Chocolate Pecan-Berry Mascarpone Bowl

Prep time: 5 minutes | Cook time: 0 minutes | Serves 2

1 cup chopped pecans
1 teaspoon Swerve natural sweetener or 1 drop liquid stevia
¼ cup mascarpone
30 Lily's dark-chocolate chips
6 strawberries, sliced

1. Divide the pecans between two dessert bowls.
2. In a small bowl, mix the sweetener into the mascarpone cheese. Top the nuts with a dollop of the sweetened mascarpone.
3. Sprinkle in the chocolate chips, top each dish with the strawberries, and serve.

Per Serving
calories: 462 | fat: 47g | protein: 6g
carbs: 15g | net carbs: 6g | fiber: 9g

Blackberry Cobbler with Almonds

Prep time: 15 minutes | Cook time: 3 to 4 hours | Serves 10

For the Filling:
1 tablespoon coconut oil
6 cups blackberries
½ cup granulated erythritol
1 teaspoon ground cinnamon

For the Topping:
2 cups ground almonds
½ cup granulated erythritol
1 tablespoon baking powder
½ teaspoon salt
1 cup heavy (whipping) cream
½ cup butter, melted

1. Lightly grease the insert of a 4-quart slow cooker with the coconut oil.
2. Add the blackberries, erythritol, and cinnamon to the insert. Mix to combine.
3. In a large bowl, stir together the almonds, erythritol, baking powder, and salt. Add the heavy cream and butter and stir until a thick batter forms.
4. Drop the batter by the tablespoon on top of the blackberries.
5. Cover and cook on low for 3 to 4 hours.
6. Serve warm.

Per Serving
calories: 281 | fat: 31g | protein: 8g
carbs: 10g | net carbs: 4g | fiber: 6g

Crispy Strawberry Chocolate Bark

Prep time: 10 minutes | Cook time: 1 minute | Serves 2

½ (2.8-ounce / 79-g) keto-friendly chocolate bar
1 tablespoon heavy (whipping) cream
2 tablespoons salted almonds
1 fresh strawberry, sliced

1. Line a baking sheet with parchment paper.
2. Break up the chocolate bar half into small pieces, and put them in a microwave-safe bowl with the cream.
3. Heat in the microwave for 45 seconds at 50 percent power. Stir the chocolate, and cook for 20 seconds more at 50 percent power. Stir again, making sure the mixture is fully melted and combined. If not, microwave for another 20 seconds.
4. Pour the chocolate mixture onto the parchment paper and spread it in a thin, uniform layer.
5. Sprinkle on the almonds, then add the strawberry slices.
6. Refrigerate until hardened, about 2 hours.
7. Once the bark is nice and hard, break it up into smaller pieces to nibble on. Yum!
8. The bark will keep for up to 4 days in a sealed container in the refrigerator.

Per Serving
calories: 111 | fat: 10g | protein: 3g
carbs: 9g | net carbs: 4g | fiber: 5g

Almond-Sour Cream Cheesecake

Prep time: 15 minutes | Cook time: 5 to 6 hours | Serves 10

¼ cup butter, melted, divided
1 cup ground almonds
¾ cup plus 1 tablespoon granulated erythritol, divided
¼ teaspoon ground cinnamon
12 ounces (340 g) cream cheese, at room temperature
2 eggs
2 teaspoons pure vanilla extract
1 cup sour cream

1. Lightly grease a 7-inch springform pan with 1 tablespoon of the butter.
2. In a small bowl, stir together the almonds, 1 tablespoon of the erythritol, and cinnamon until blended.
3. Add the remaining 3 tablespoons of the butter and stir until coarse crumbs form.
4. Press the crust mixture into the springform pan along the bottom and about 2 inches up the sides.
5. In a large bowl, using a handheld mixer, beat together the cream cheese, eggs, vanilla, and remaining ¾ cup of the erythritol. Beat the sour cream into the cream-cheese mixture until smooth.
6. Spoon the batter into the springform pan and smooth out the top.
7. Place a wire rack in the insert of the slow cooker and place the springform pan on top.
8. Cover and cook on low for 5 to 6 hours, or until the cheesecake doesn't jiggle when shaken.
9. Cool completely before removing from pan.
10. Chill the cheesecake completely before serving, and store leftovers in the refrigerator.

Per Serving
calories: 279 | fat: 25g | protein: 8g
carbs: 4g | net carbs: 3g | fiber: 1g

Keto Peanut Butter Cookies

Prep time: 5 minutes | Cook time: 10 minutes | Makes 15 cookies

1 cup natural crunchy peanut butter
½ cup Swerve natural sweetener
1 egg

1. Preheat the oven to 350ºF (180ºC). Line a baking sheet with a silicone baking mat or parchment paper.
2. In a medium bowl, use a hand mixer to mix together the peanut butter, sweetener, and egg.
3. Roll up the batter into small balls about 1 inch in diameter.
4. Spread out the cookie-dough balls on the prepared pan. Press each dough ball down with the tines of a fork, then repeat to make a crisscross pattern.
5. Bake for about 12 minutes, or until golden.
6. Let the cookies cool for 10 minutes on the lined pan before serving. If you try to move them too soon, they will crumble.
7. Store leftover cookies covered in the refrigerator for up to 5 days.

Per Serving (1 cookie)
calories: 98 | fat: 8g | protein: 4g
carbs: 10g | net carbs: 3g | fiber: 7g

Slow Cooker Chocolate Pot De Crème

Prep time: 10 minutes | Cook time: 3 hours | Serves 6

6 egg yolks
2 cups heavy (whipping) cream
⅓ cup cocoa powder
1 tablespoon pure vanilla extract
½ teaspoon liquid stevia
Whipped coconut cream, for garnish (optional)
Shaved dark chocolate, for garnish (optional)

1. In a medium bowl, whisk together the yolks, heavy cream, cocoa powder, vanilla, and stevia.
2. Pour the mixture into a 1½-quart baking dish and place the dish in the insert of the slow cooker.
3. Pour in enough water to reach halfway up the sides of the baking dish.
4. Cover and cook on low for 3 hours.
5. Remove the baking dish from the insert and cool to room temperature on a wire rack.
6. Chill the dessert completely in the refrigerator and serve, garnished with the whipped coconut cream and shaved dark chocolate (if desired).

Per Serving
calories: 198 | fat: 18g | protein: 5g
carbs: 4g | net carbs: 3g | fiber: 1g

Lemon Custard

Prep time: 10 minutes | Cook time: 3 hours | Serves 4

5 egg yolks
¼ cup freshly squeezed lemon juice
1 tablespoon lemon zest
1 teaspoon pure vanilla extract
⅓ teaspoon liquid stevia
2 cups heavy (whipping) cream
1 cup whipped coconut cream

1. In a medium bowl, whisk together the yolks, lemon juice and zest, vanilla, and liquid stevia.
2. Whisk in the heavy cream and divide the mixture between 4 ramekins.
3. Place a rack at the bottom of the insert of the slow cooker and place the ramekins on it.
4. Pour in enough water to reach halfway up the sides of the ramekins.
5. Cover and cook on low for 3 hours.
6. Remove the ramekins from the insert and cool to room temperature.
7. Chill the ramekins completely in the refrigerator and serve topped with whipped coconut cream.

Per Serving
calories: 319 | fat: 30g | protein: 7g
carbs: 3g | net carbs: 3g | fiber: 0g

Almond-Peanut Butter Cheesecake

Prep time: 15 minutes | Cook time: 5 to 6 hours | Serves 10

¼ cup butter, melted, divided
1 cup ground almonds
2 tablespoons cocoa powder
1 cup granulated erythritol, divided
12 ounces (340 g) cream cheese, room temperature
½ cup natural peanut butter
2 eggs, room temperature
1 teaspoon pure vanilla extract

1. Lightly grease a 7-inch springform pan with 1 tablespoon butter.
2. In a small bowl, stir together the almonds, cocoa powder, and ¼ cup erythritol until blended. Add the remaining 3 tablespoons of the butter and stir until coarse crumbs form.
3. Press the crust mixture into the springform pan along the bottom and about 2 inches up the sides.
4. In a large bowl, using a handheld mixer, beat together the cream cheese and peanut butter until smooth. Beat in the remaining ¾ cup of the erythritol, eggs, and vanilla.
5. Spoon the batter into the springform pan and smooth out the top.
6. Place a wire rack in the insert of slow cooker and place the springform pan on the wire rack.
7. Cover and cook on low for 5 to 6 hours, or until the cheesecake doesn't jiggle when shaken.
8. Cool completely before removing from pan.
9. Chill the cheesecake completely before serving, and store leftovers in the refrigerator.

Per Serving
calories: 311 | fat: 28g | protein: 11g
carbs: 5g | net carbs: 3g | fiber: 2g

Strawberry Mousse

Prep time: 10 minutes | Cook time: 0 minutes | Serves 6

8 ounces (227 g) strawberries, sliced
¼ cup granulated erythritol–monk fruit blend; less sweet: 2 tablespoons
½ ounce (14 g) full-fat cream cheese, at room temperature
1 cup heavy whipping cream, divided
⅛ teaspoon vanilla extract
⅛ teaspoon salt

1. Put the large metal bowl in the freezer to chill for at least 5 minutes.
2. In a blender or food processor, purée the strawberries and erythritol–monk fruit blend. Set aside.
3. In the chilled large bowl, using an electric mixer on medium high, beat the cream cheese and ¼ cup of heavy cream until well combined, stopping and scraping the bowl once or twice, as needed. Add the vanilla and salt and mix to combine. Add the remaining ¾ cup of heavy cream and beat on high for 1 to 3 minutes, until very stiff peaks form.
4. Gently fold the purée into the whipped cream. Refrigerate for at least 1 hour and up to overnight before serving.
5. Serve in short glasses or small mason jars.
6. Store leftovers in an airtight container for up to 5 days in the refrigerator.

Per Serving
calories: 160 | fat: 15.9g | protein: 0.9g
carbs: 4.0g | net carbs: 3.0g | fiber: 1.0g

Creamy Chocolate Mousse

Prep time: 10 minutes | Cook time: 0 minutes | Serves 2

1½ tablespoons heavy (whipping) cream
4 tablespoons butter, at room temperature
1 tablespoon unsweetened cocoa powder
4 tablespoons cream cheese, at room temperature
1 tablespoon Swerve natural sweetener

1. In a medium chilled bowl, use a whisk or fork to whip the cream. Refrigerate to keep cold.
2. In a separate medium bowl, use a hand mixer to beat the butter, cocoa powder, cream cheese, and sweetener until thoroughly combined.
3. Take the whipped cream out of the refrigerator. Gently fold the whipped cream into the chocolate mixture with a rubber scraper.
4. Divide the pudding between two dessert bowls.

Cover and chill for 1 hour before serving.

Per Serving
calories: 460 | fat: 50g | protein: 4g
carbs: 10g | net carbs: 4g | fiber: 6g

Chocolate Chip Ice Cream with Mint

Prep time: 10 minutes | Cook time: 30 minutes | Serves 2

½ tablespoon butter
1 tablespoon Swerve natural sweetener
10 tablespoons heavy (whipping) cream, divided
¼ teaspoon peppermint extract
2 tablespoons sugar-free chocolate chips

1. Put a medium metal bowl and your hand-mixer beaters in the freezer to chill.
2. In a small, heavy saucepan over medium heat, melt the butter. Whisk in the sweetener and 5 tablespoons of cream.
3. Turn the heat up to medium-high and bring the mixture to a boil, stirring constantly. Turn the heat down to low and simmer, stirring occasionally, for about 30 minutes. You want the mixture to be thick, so it sticks to the back of a spoon.
4. Stir in the peppermint extract.
5. Pour the thickened mixture into a medium bowl and refrigerate to cool.
6. Remove the metal bowl and the mixer beaters from the freezer. Pour the remaining 5 tablespoons of cream into the bowl. With the electric beater, whip the cream until it is thick and fluffy and forms peaks. Don't overbeat, or the cream will turn to butter. Take the cream mixture out of the refrigerator.
7. Using a rubber scraper, gently fold the whipped cream into the cooled mixture.
8. Transfer the mixture to a small metal container that can go in the freezer.
9. Mix in the chocolate chips, and cover the container with foil or plastic wrap.
10. Freeze the ice cream for 4 to 5 hours before serving, stirring it twice during that time.

Per Serving
calories: 325 | fat: 33g | protein: 3g
carbs: 17g | net carbs: 4g | fiber: 13g

Avocado-Chocolate Pudding

Prep time: 5 minutes | Cook time: 0 minutes | Serves 2

1 ripe medium avocado, cut into chunks	4 tablespoons unsweetened cocoa powder
2 ounces (57 g) cream cheese, at room temperature	¼ teaspoon vanilla extract
1 tablespoon Swerve natural sweetener	Pinch pink Himalayan salt

1. In a food processor (or blender), combine the avocado with the cream cheese, sweetener, cocoa powder, vanilla, and pink Himalayan salt. Blend until completely smooth.
2. Pour into two small dessert bowls, and chill for 30 minutes before serving.

Per Serving
calories: 281 | fat: 27g | protein: 8g
carbs: 27g | net carbs: 12g | fiber: 15g

Ginger-Pumpkin Pudding

Prep time: 5 minutes | Cook time: 3 to 4 hours | Serves 8

1 tablespoon coconut oil	1 tablespoon grated fresh ginger
2 cups pumpkin purée	¾ teaspoon liquid stevia
1½ cups coconut milk	Pinch ground cloves
2 eggs	1 cup whipped coconut cream
½ cup almond flour	
1 ounce (28 g) protein powder	

1. Lightly grease the insert of the slow cooker with coconut oil.
2. In a large bowl, stir together pumpkin, coconut milk, eggs, almond flour, protein powder, ginger, liquid stevia, and cloves.
3. Transfer the mixture to the insert.
4. Cover and cook on low 3 to 4 hours.
5. Serve warm with whipped coconut cream.

Per Serving
calories: 217 | fat: 19g | protein: 8g
carbs: 7g | net carbs: 3g | fiber: 4g

Pumpkin Compote with Mix Berries

Prep time: 10 minutes | Cook time: 3 to 4 hours | Serves 10

1 tablespoon coconut oil	½ cup coconut milk
2 cups diced pumpkin	1 teaspoon ground cinnamon
1 cup cranberries	½ teaspoon ground allspice
1 cup blueberries	¼ teaspoon ground nutmeg
½ cup granulated erythritol	1 cup whipped cream
Juice and zest of 1 lemon	

1. Lightly grease the insert of the slow cooker with the coconut oil.
2. Place the pumpkin, cranberries, blueberries, erythritol, lemon juice and zest, coconut milk, cinnamon, allspice, and nutmeg in the insert.
3. Cover and cook on low for 3 to 4 hours.
4. Let the compote cool for 1 hour and serve warm with a generous scoop of whipped cream.

Per Serving
calories: 113 | fat: 9g | protein: 4g
carbs: 7g | net carbs: 4g | fiber: 3g

Blueberry-Pecan Crisp

Prep time: 10 minutes | Cook time: 3 to 4 hours | Serves 8

5 tablespoons coconut oil, melted, divided	1 teaspoon baking soda
4 cups blueberries	½ teaspoon ground cinnamon
¾ cup plus 2 tablespoons granulated erythritol	2 tablespoons coconut milk
1 cup ground pecans	1 egg

1. Lightly grease a 4-quart slow cooker with 1 tablespoon of the coconut oil.
2. Add the blueberries and 2 tablespoons of erythritol to the insert.
3. In a large bowl, stir together the remaining ¾ cup of the erythritol, ground pecans, baking soda, and cinnamon until well mixed.
4. Add the coconut milk, egg, and remaining coconut oil, and stir until coarse crumbs form.
5. Top the contents in the insert with the pecan mixture.
6. Cover and cook on low for 3 to 4 hours.
7. Serve warm.

Per Serving
calories: 222 | fat: 19g | protein: 9g
carbs: 9g | net carbs: 5g | fiber: 4g

Flaxseed Coconut Bread Pudding

Prep time: 20 minutes | Cook time: 2 hours | Serves 12

Unsalted butter, for greasing
6 tablespoons coconut flour
4 ounces (113 g) full-fat cream cheese, at room temperature
½ cup golden flaxseed meal, re-ground in a clean coffee grinder
2 large eggs
1 tablespoon granulated erythritol–monk fruit blend
1 teaspoon baking powder
⅛ teaspoon salt
6 tablespoons heavy whipping cream
¼ cup water
2 tablespoons unsalted butter, at room temperature, plus more for greasing
¾ cup heavy whipping cream
2 tablespoons water
2 large eggs
¼ cup granulated erythritol–monk fruit blend
½ teaspoon vanilla extract
⅛ teaspoon salt
2 tablespoons unsalted butter, at room temperature
6 tablespoons allulose
¼ cup heavy whipping cream
¼ teaspoon salt
½ tablespoon dark rum or ¼ teaspoon rum extract

1. Preheat the oven to 350°F (180°C). Grease the baking sheet with butter and set aside.
2. In a large bowl, using an electric mixer on high, mix the coconut flour, cream cheese, flaxseed meal, eggs, erythritol–monk fruit blend, baking powder, and salt until just combined, stopping and scraping the bowl once or twice, as needed. Slowly add the heavy cream and water to the batter and mix until thoroughly combined.
3. Pour the batter into the prepared baking sheet and bake for 30 to 35 minutes, or until lightly browned. Allow the bread to fully cool, 15 to 20 minutes, and cut into 1-inch squares. Put the cubed bread in another large mixing bowl. Leave the oven on.
4. Grease another baking sheet generously with butter and set aside.
5. In the medium saucepan, bring the heavy cream and water almost to a boil, then reduce the heat and add the 2 tablespoons of butter.
6. In the medium bowl, whisk the eggs, erythritol–monk fruit blend, vanilla, and salt. Temper the egg mixture by adding 3 tablespoons of the hot cream mixture to it and mixing well. Stir the remaining cream mixture into the egg mixture.
7. Pour the cream and egg mixture over the cubed bread in the large mixing bowl, toss to coat, and pour everything into the buttered baking sheet. Using a spoon, press down the bread to ensure the liquid covers it.
8. Bake for 40 to 45 minutes at 350°F (180°C) or until the egg mixture has set and the top is lightly browned. Cool for 5 minutes.
9. Store leftovers in an airtight container in the refrigerator for up to 3 days.
10. In the small saucepan, brown the butter over medium-low heat, stirring constantly. The butter will begin to foam and bubble, and after 2 to 4 minutes, you should begin to see browned bits on the bottom of the pan. At this point, remove the pan from the heat and continue to stir until the butter begins to lightly brown to a golden amber color.
11. Add the allulose, heavy cream, and salt to the browned butter and stir until well combined. Simmer over low heat for 15 minutes. Resist the urge to stir. At the 15-minute mark, turn off the stove and add the rum. Note that the sauce will foam up when you add the rum. Stir and turn the heat to low and allow the sauce to cook for another 10 minutes without stirring. This will thicken the sauce and cook down the alcohol.
12. To serve, cut the bread pudding into 12 slices and pour the rum sauce over each slice.
13. Store leftover sauce in an airtight container in the refrigerator for up to 3 days.

Per Serving
calories: 325 | fat: 32.0g | protein: 5.0g | carbs: 7.1g | net carbs: 2.9g | fiber: 4.2g

Blueberry, Strawberry, and Raspberry Parfaits

Prep time: 10 minutes | Cook time: 10 minutes | Serves 4

2 cups heavy whipping cream
1 teaspoon vanilla extract
6 large egg yolks
¼ cup granulated erythritol–monk fruit blend
1 tablespoon unsalted butter, at room temperature
1 cup blueberries

5 strawberries, thinly sliced
1 cup raspberries
¼ cup freshly squeezed lemon juice
1 tablespoon granulated erythritol–monk fruit blend
½ cup slivered almonds, for topping

1. In the medium saucepan, heat the heavy cream over low heat until hot. Stir in the vanilla, then set aside to cool.
2. In a medium bowl, whisk the egg yolks, erythritol–monk fruit blend, and butter for about 2 minutes, until the mixture is a pale yellow.
3. Once the cream has cooled to the touch, pour one-quarter of the heavy cream mixture into the egg mixture and whisk until well combined. Add the remainder of the cream mixture and mix well.
4. Pour the cream and egg mixture back into the saucepan and cook over low heat, stirring continuously for about 5 minutes, or until the mixture begins to thicken. You'll know the pudding is thick enough when it coats the back of the spoon without dripping.
5. Pour the pudding through the sieve into another medium bowl. Put a sheet of plastic wrap directly onto the surface of the pudding to prevent a skin from forming. Move the pudding to the refrigerator for 1 to 2 hours to cool completely.
6. While the pudding cools, in the small bowl, combine the blueberries, strawberries, raspberries, lemon juice, and erythritol–monk fruit blend and mix.
7. Once the pudding has cooled, completely assemble the parfaits. In a mason jar or any 8-ounce (227-g) glass container, add ⅓ cup of pudding and top with the berry mixture, repeating the layers until the glass is full, ending with berries. Top with slivered almonds before serving.
8. Store leftovers in an airtight container for up to 5 days in the refrigerator.

Per Serving
calories: 646 | fat: 60.8g | protein: 10.0g | carbs: 18.9g | net carbs: 14.2g | fiber: 4.7g

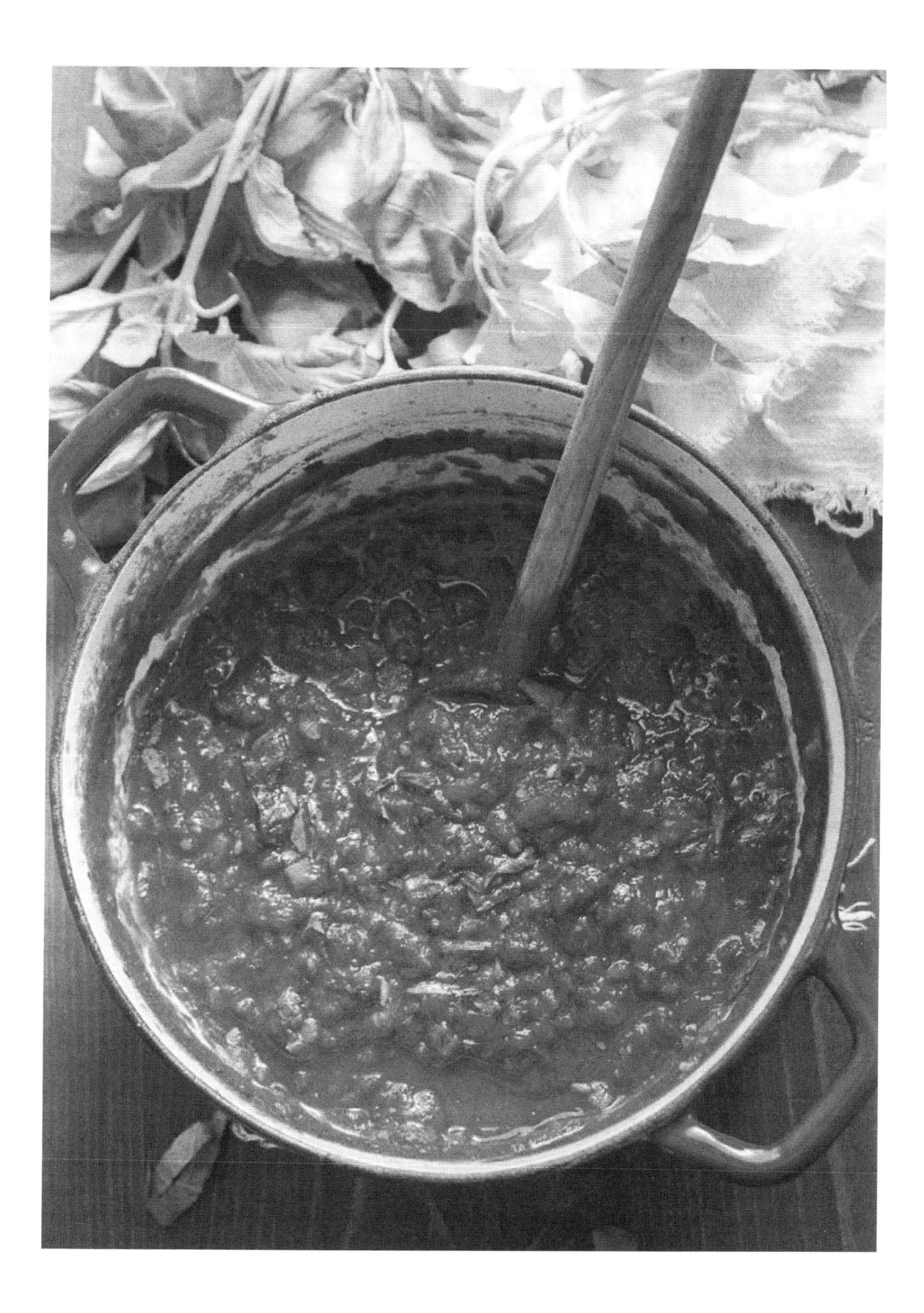

Chapter 12 Sauces and Dressings

Sriracha Sauce

Prep time: 5 minutes | Cook time: 0 minutes | Makes ¾ cup

½ cup sugar-free mayonnaise
1½ tablespoons lime juice
1½ tablespoons Sriracha sauce
1 tablespoon granulated erythritol

1. Place all of the ingredients in a small bowl and stir well until combined. Store in an airtight container in the refrigerator for up to 1 week.

Per Serving
calories: 140 | fat: 15.8g | protein: 0g
carbs: 1.0g | net carbs: 1.0g | fiber: 0g

Fettuccine Alfredo

Prep time: 5 minutes | Cook time: 10 minutes | Serves 2

4 tablespoons butter
2 ounces (57-g) cream cheese
1 cup heavy (whipping) cream
½ cup grated Parmesan cheese
1 garlic clove, finely minced
1 teaspoon dried Italian seasoning
Pink Himalayan salt, to taste
Freshly ground black pepper, to taste

1. In a heavy medium saucepan over medium heat, combine the butter, cream cheese, and heavy cream. Whisk slowly and constantly until the butter and cream cheese melt.
2. Add the Parmesan, garlic, and Italian seasoning. Continue to whisk until everything is well blended. Turn the heat to medium-low and simmer, stirring occasionally, for 5 to 8 minutes to allow the sauce to blend and thicken.
3. Season with pink Himalayan salt and pepper, and stir to combine.
4. Toss with your favorite hot, precooked, keto-friendly noodles and serve.
5. Keep this sauce in a sealed glass container in the refrigerator for up to 4 days.

Per Serving
calories: 294 | fat: 30g | protein: 5g
carbs: 2g | net carbs: 2g | fiber: 0g

BBQ Sauce

Prep time: 8 minutes | Cook time: 0 minutes | Makes ¾ cup

½ cup reduced-sugar ketchup, store-bought or homemade
2 tablespoons apple cider vinegar
2 tablespoons granulated erythritol
1 tablespoon filtered water
1½ teaspoons ground allspice
1½ teaspoons ground mustard powder
1 teaspoon blackstrap molasses (optional; see note)
½ teaspoon liquid smoke
½ teaspoon onion powder
½ teaspoon Worcestershire sauce
¼ teaspoon ground cloves
¼ teaspoon xanthan gum (optional, to thicken)

1. Place all of the ingredients in a medium-sized bowl and whisk together. Store in an airtight container in the refrigerator for up to 2 weeks.

Per Serving
calories: 15 | fat: 0g | protein: 0g
carbs: 2.8g | net carbs: 2.8g | fiber: 0g

Orange Chili Sauce

Prep time: 5 minutes | Cook time: 0 minutes | Makes 1¼ cup

1 cup sugar-free orange marmalade
1 tablespoon filtered water
1 tablespoon fish sauce (no sugar added)
1 tablespoon lime juice
1 teaspoon granulated erythritol
1 teaspoon red pepper flakes
1 teaspoon toasted sesame oil

1. Place all of the ingredients in a small bowl and mix well. Store in an airtight container in the refrigerator for up to 2 weeks.

Per Serving
calories: 21 | fat: 0g | protein: 0g
carbs: 5.9g | net carbs: 4.9g | fiber: 1.0g

Cheesy Hot Crab Sauce

Prep time: 10 minutes | Cook time: 5 to 6 hours | Makes 4 cups

8 ounces (227-g) cream cheese	1 tablespoon granulated erythritol
8 ounces (227-g) goat cheese	2 teaspoons minced garlic
1 cup sour cream	12 ounces (340-g) crabmeat, flaked
½ cup grated Asiago cheese	1 scallion, white and green parts, chopped
1 sweet onion, finely chopped	

1. In a large bowl, stir together the cream cheese, goat cheese, sour cream, Asiago cheese, onion, erythritol, garlic, crabmeat, and scallion until well mixed.
2. Transfer the mixture to an 8-by-4-inch loaf pan and place the pan in the insert of the slow cooker.
3. Cover and cook on low for 5 to 6 hours.
4. Serve warm.

Per Serving (½ cup)
calories: 361 | fat: 28g | protein: 17g
carbs: 10g | net carbs: 8g | fiber: 2g

Scallion Ginger Dressing

Prep time: 8 minutes | Cook time: 0 minutes | Makes ¾ cup

¼ cup chopped scallions	granulated erythritol
3 tablespoons avocado oil or other light-tasting oil	1 tablespoon lime juice
2 tablespoons filtered water	1 tablespoon white vinegar
2 tablespoons fish sauce (no sugar added)	1 tablespoon peeled and minced fresh ginger
2 tablespoons	1 teaspoon toasted sesame oil

1. Place all of the ingredients in a small blender and blend until mostly smooth. Store in an airtight container in the refrigerator for up to 1 week.

Per Serving
calories: 76 | fat: 8.0g | protein: 1.0g
carbs: 1.0g | net carbs: 1.0g | fiber: 0g

Marinara

Prep time: 5 minutes | Cook time: 0 minutes | Makes 4 cups

1 (28-ounce / 794-g) can peeled whole San Marzano tomatoes	1 teaspoon dried parsley leaves
¼ cup extra-virgin olive oil	1 teaspoon garlic powder
2 tablespoons red wine vinegar	1 teaspoon kosher salt
1 teaspoon dried basil leaves	1 teaspoon onion powder
1 teaspoon dried oregano leaves	½ teaspoon red pepper flakes
	¼ teaspoon ground black pepper

1. Place the tomatoes and olive oil in a blender and blend for 30 seconds, or until the desired consistency is reached. If you prefer a chunkier sauce, pulse instead of blending for about 15 seconds. Stir in the remaining ingredients.
2. Store in an airtight container for up to 1 week in the refrigerator or 6 months in the freezer.

Per Serving
calories: 85 | fat: 6.8g | protein: 1.0g
carbs: 5.0g | net carbs: 3.0g | fiber: 2.0g

Parmesan Basil Vinaigrette

Prep time: 5 minutes | Cook time: 0 minutes | Makes ¾ cup

¼ cup fresh basil leaves	1 tablespoon lemon juice
¼ cup sugar-free mayonnaise	1 tablespoon granulated erythritol
2 tablespoons extra-virgin olive oil	1 tablespoon grated Parmesan cheese
2 tablespoons full-fat sour cream	½ teaspoon kosher salt
1 tablespoon apple cider vinegar	¼ teaspoon ground black pepper

1. Place all of the ingredients in a small blender and blend until mostly smooth. Store in an airtight container in the refrigerator for up to 1 week.

Per Serving
calories: 124 | fat: 14.0g | protein: 0g
carbs: 0g | net carbs: 0g | fiber: 0g

Tzatziki Sauce

Prep time: 10 minutes | Cook time: 0 minutes | Serves 4

½ large English cucumber, unpeeled
1½ cups Greek yogurt (I use Fage)
2 tablespoons olive oil
Large pinch pink Himalayan salt
Large pinch freshly ground black pepper
Juice of ½ lemon
2 garlic cloves, finely minced
1 tablespoon fresh dill

1. Halve the cucumber lengthwise, and use a spoon to scoop out and discard the seeds.
2. Grate the cucumber with a zester or grater onto a large plate lined with a few layers of paper towels. Close the paper towels around the grated cucumber, and squeeze as much water out of it as you can. (This can take a while and can require multiple paper towels. You can also allow it to drain overnight in a strainer or wrapped in a few layers of cheesecloth in the fridge if you have the time.)
3. In a food processor (or blender), blend the yogurt, olive oil, pink Himalayan salt, pepper, lemon juice, and garlic until fully combined.
4. Transfer the mixture to a medium bowl, and mix in the fresh dill and grated cucumber.
5. I like to chill this sauce for at least 30 minutes before serving. Keep in a sealed glass container in the refrigerator for up to 1 week.

Per Serving
calories: 149 | fat: 11g | protein: 8g
carbs: 5g | net carbs: 4g | fiber: 1g

Garlic Aioli Sauce

Prep time: 5 minutes | Cook time: 0 minutes | Serves 4

½ cup mayonnaise
2 garlic cloves, minced
Juice of 1 lemon
1 tablespoon chopped fresh flat-leaf Italian parsley
1 teaspoon chopped chives
Pink Himalayan salt, to taste
Freshly ground black pepper, to taste

1. In a food processor (or blender), combine the mayonnaise, garlic, lemon juice, parsley, and chives, and season with pink Himalayan salt and pepper. Blend until fully combined.

2. Pour into a sealed glass container and chill in the refrigerator for at least 30 minutes before serving. (This sauce will keep in the fridge for up to 1 week.)

Per Serving
calories: 204 | fat: 22g | protein: 1g
carbs: 3g | net carbs: 2g | fiber: 1g

Tomato and Bacon Dressing

Prep time: 8 minutes | Cook time: 0 minutes | Makes ¾ cup

¼ cup sugar-free mayonnaise
5 cherry tomatoes
3 slices bacon, cooked and chopped
1 clove garlic, peeled
2 tablespoons chopped fresh parsley
½ teaspoon granulated erythritol
¼ teaspoon kosher salt
⅛ teaspoon ground black pepper

1. Place all of the ingredients in a small blender and blend until mostly smooth. Store in an airtight container in the refrigerator for up to 1 week.

Per Serving
calories: 95 | fat: 10.0g | protein: 2.0g
carbs: 1.0g | net carbs: 1.0g | fiber: 0g

Creamy Caesar Dressing

Prep time: 5 minutes | Cook time: 0 minutes | Serves 4

½ cup mayonnaise
1 tablespoon Dijon mustard
Juice of ½ lemon
½ teaspoon Worcestershire sauce
Pinch pink Himalayan salt
Pinch freshly ground black pepper
¼ cup grated Parmesan cheese

1. In a medium bowl, whisk together the mayonnaise, mustard, lemon juice, Worcestershire sauce, pink Himalayan salt, and pepper until fully combined.
2. Add the Parmesan cheese, and whisk until creamy and well blended.
3. Keep in a sealed glass container in the refrigerator for up to 1 week.

Per Serving
calories: 222 | fat: 23g | protein: 2g
carbs: 2g | net carbs: 2g | fiber: 0g

Blue Cheese Dressing

Prep time: 5 minutes | Cook time: 0 minutes | Makes 1 cup

⅓ cup sugar-free mayonnaise
¼ cup crumbled blue cheese
1 ounce (28 g) cream cheese (2 tablespoons), softened
2 tablespoons heavy whipping cream
1 teaspoon lemon juice

1. Place all of the ingredients in a small blender and blend for 30 seconds, until creamy and nearly entirely smooth. Store in an airtight container in the refrigerator for up to 1 week.

Per Serving
calories: 101 | fat: 10.2g | protein: 1.0g
carbs: 0.5g | net carbs: 0.5g | fiber: 0g

Asian Peanut Sauce

Prep time: 5 minutes | Cook time: 0 minutes | Serves 4

½ cup creamy peanut butter (I use Justin's)
2 tablespoons coconut aminos
1 teaspoon Sriracha sauce
1 teaspoon toasted sesame oil
1 teaspoon garlic powder

1. In a food processor (or blender), blend the peanut butter, coconut aminos, Sriracha sauce, sesame oil, and garlic powder until thoroughly mixed.
2. Pour into an airtight glass container and keep in the refrigerator for up to 1 week.

Per Serving
calories: 185 | fat: 15g | protein: 7g
carbs: 8g | net carbs: 6g | fiber: 2g

Ketchup

Prep time: 5 minutes | Cook time: 1 hour | Makes 2 cups

1 (28-ounce / 794-g) can tomato purée
⅓ cup granulated erythritol
¼ teaspoon cayenne pepper
½ cup white vinegar
1½ teaspoons dehydrated onions
½ teaspoon celery salt
½ teaspoon whole cloves
1 (1-inch) piece of cinnamon stick, broken

1. Combine the tomato purée, sweetener, and cayenne pepper in a medium-sized saucepan and bring to a boil over medium heat, then reduce the heat to low. Simmer until it reduces by half, about 30 minutes, stirring occasionally.
2. Meanwhile, in another small saucepan, combine the vinegar, onions, celery salt, cloves, and cinnamon stick pieces. Bring to a boil, then remove from the heat. Strain out the solids.
3. Add the flavored vinegar to the tomato mixture. Simmer for another 20 minutes, or until the ketchup reaches the desired consistency. Remove from the heat and let cool.
4. Blend the cooled ketchup with an immersion blender or in a small blender until smooth. Store in a clean jar with an airtight lid for up to 1 month in the refrigerator.

Per Serving
calories: 15 | fat: 0g | protein: 0g
carbs: 3.8g | net carbs: 2.8g | fiber: 1.0g

Strawberry Vinaigrette

Prep time: 5 minutes | Cook time: 0 minutes | Makes ½ cup

¼ cup chopped fresh strawberries
2 tablespoons avocado oil or other light-tasting oil
1 tablespoon chopped fresh basil
1 tablespoon filtered water
2 teaspoons red wine vinegar
½ teaspoon granulated erythritol
⅛ teaspoon kosher salt
⅛ teaspoon ground black pepper

1. Place all of the ingredients in a small blender and blend until mostly smooth. Store in an airtight container in the refrigerator for up to 1 week.

Per Serving
calories: 66 | fat: 7.0g | protein: 0g
carbs: 1.0g | net carbs: 1.0g | fiber: 0g

Appendix 1 Measurement Conversion Chart

VOLUME EQUIVALENTS(DRY)

US STANDARD	METRIC (APPROXIMATE)
1/8 teaspoon	0.5 mL
1/4 teaspoon	1 mL
1/2 teaspoon	2 mL
3/4 teaspoon	4 mL
1 teaspoon	5 mL
1 tablespoon	15 mL
1/4 cup	59 mL
1/2 cup	118 mL
3/4 cup	177 mL
1 cup	235 mL
2 cups	475 mL
3 cups	700 mL
4 cups	1 L

VOLUME EQUIVALENTS(LIQUID)

US STANDARD	US STANDARD (OUNCES)	METRIC (APPROXIMATE)
2 tablespoons	1 fl.oz.	30 mL
1/4 cup	2 fl.oz.	60 mL
1/2 cup	4 fl.oz.	120 mL
1 cup	8 fl.oz.	240 mL
1 1/2 cup	12 fl.oz.	355 mL
2 cups or 1 pint	16 fl.oz.	475 mL
4 cups or 1 quart	32 fl.oz.	1 L
1 gallon	128 fl.oz.	4 L

TEMPERATURES EQUIVALENTS

FAHRENHEIT(F)	CELSIUS(C) (APPROXIMATE)
225 °F	107 °C
250 °F	120 °C
275 °F	135 °C
300 °F	150 °C
325 °F	160 °C
350 °F	180 °C
375 °F	190 °C
400 °F	205 °C
425 °F	220 °C
450 °F	235 °C
475 °F	245 °C
500 °F	260 °C

WEIGHT EQUIVALENTS

US STANDARD	METRIC (APPROXIMATE)
1 ounce	28 g
2 ounces	57 g
5 ounces	142 g
10 ounces	284 g
15 ounces	425 g
16 ounces (1 pound)	455 g
1.5 pounds	680 g
2 pounds	907 g

Appendix 2 Recipe Index

A
Alaskan Cod Fillet   84
Almond and Rind Crusted Zucchini Fritters   47
Almond Breaded Hoki   80
Almond Fat Bombs with Chocolate Chips   148
Almond-Peanut Butter Cheesecake   154
Almond-Sour Cream Cheesecake   153
Anchovies and Veggies Wraps   76
Anchovies with Caesar Dressing   69
Anchovy Fat Bombs   18
Arugula and Avocado Salad   25
Asiago Drumsticks with Spinach   89
Asian Peanut Sauce   163
Asian Scallop and Vegetable   78
Asian Turkey and Bird's Eye Soup   88
Asian-Flavored Beef and Broccoli   133
Asparagus and Trout Foil Packets   80
Avocado and Berry Smoothie   1
Avocado and Ham Stuffed Eggs   18
Avocado Crostini Nori with Walnuts   60
Avocado Sausage Stacks   5
Avocado-Bacon Sushi   20
Avocado-Chocolate Pudding   156

B
Bacon and Beef Stew   133
Bacon and Jalapeño Egg Muffins   2
Bacon and Pork Omelet   111
Bacon Fudge   147
Bacon Green Soup   41
Bacon-Wrapped Chicken with Asparagus   104
Bacon-Wrapped Enoki Mushrooms   21
Bacon-Wrapped Poblano Poppers   16
Bacon, Avocado, and Veggies Salad   25
Baked Cheesecake Bites   152
Baked Cheesy Chicken and Spinach   104
Baked Cheesy Pork and Veggies   121
Baked Chicken in Tomato Purée   101
Baked Cocktail Franks   14
Baked Tilapia with Black Olives   75
Balsamic Brussels Sprouts Cheese Salad   32
Balsamic Glazed Brussels Sprouts   50
Balsamic Glazed Meatloaf   131
Balsamic Mushroom Beef Meatloaf   125
Basil Feta Flank Steak Pinwheels   137
BBQ Grilled Pork Spare Ribs   109
BBQ Pork Ribs   113
BBQ Sauce   160
Beef and Broccoli Casserole   125
Beef and Cauliflower Rice Casserole   139
Beef and Fennel Provençal   141
Beef and Mushroom Cheeseburgers   130
Beef and Mushroom Soup   43
Beef and Onion Stuffed Zucchinis   127
Beef and Pimiento in Zucchini Boats   128
Beef and Spinach Salad   26
Beef and Veggie Stuffed Butternut Squash   125
Beef Brisket with Red Wine   137
Beef Casserole with Cauliflower   138
Beef Chuck Roast with Mushrooms   132
Beef Chuck Roast with Veggies   138
Beef Hamburger Soup   35
Beef Lasagna with Zucchinis   138
Beef Meatloaf with Balsamic Glaze   130
Beef Ragout with Green Beans   132
Beef Sausage Casserole with Okra   135
Beef Steaks with Mushrooms and Bacon   131
Beef Stew with Black Olives   135
Beef Tripe with Onions and Tomatoes   140
Beef-Stuffed Peppers   21
Beef, Pancetta, and Mushroom Bourguignon 127
Bell Pepper and Tomato Sataraš   49
Bell Pepper Turkey Casserole   90
Blackberry Cobbler with Almonds   152
BLT Cups   16
Blue Cheese Dressing   163
Blueberry-Pecan Crisp   156
Blueberry, Strawberry, and Raspberry Parfaits   158
Boiled Stuffed Eggs   47
Bolognese Pork Zoodles   108
Braised Chicken and Veggies   103
Braised Cream Kale   51
Broccoli and Cauliflower Mash   51
Broccoli and Ham Egg Bake   4
Broccoli Cheese   56
Broccoli Soup   42
Buttered Broccoli   58
Butternut Squash and Beef Stew   136

C
Caesar Salad with Salmon and Egg   29
Cajun Tilapia Fish Burgers   72
Caprese Salad   27
Caprese Sticks   15
Caramel-Cream Chocolate Crepes   10
Caribbean Baked Wings   13
Caribbean Beef with Peppers   135

Catalan Shrimp   71
Catfish Flakes and Cauliflower Casserole   85
Cauliflower and Celery Soup   62
Cauliflower and Lamb Soup   34
Cauliflower and Tomato Beef Curry   134
Cauliflower Bites   19
Cauliflower Chowder with Fresh Dill   64
Cauliflower Egg Bake   49
Cauliflower Soup   44
Cauliflower Soup with Sausage   45
Cheddar Anchovies Fat Bombs   21
Cheddar Bacon and Egg Frittata   3
Cheddar Bacon Stuffed Chicken Fillets   97
Cheddar Buffalo Chicken Bake   50
Cheddar Cauliflower Soup   38
Cheese and Egg Spinach Nests   8
Cheese and Shrimp Stuffed Celery   14
Cheese Bites with Pickle   14
Cheese Stuffed Spaghetti Squash   53
Cheesecake Fat Bomb with Berries   146
Cheesy Egg and Bacon Quesadillas   7
Cheesy Ham and Chicken Bites   20
Cheesy Ham-Egg Cups   15
Cheesy Hot Crab Sauce   161
Cheesy Lemonade Fat Bomb   151
Cheesy Prosciutto Balls   20
Cheesy Shrimp Stuffed Mushrooms   83
Chicken and Bell Pepper Kabobs   91
Chicken and Cabbage Soup   35
Chicken and Spinach Meatballs   17
Chicken and Tomato Packets   93
Chicken Breast Fritters with Dill Dip   58
Chicken Drumsticks in Capocollo   92
Chicken Mélange   91
Chicken Paella and Chorizo   98
Chicken Thigh and Kale Stew   90
Chicken Thigh Green Salad   27
Chicken Wings in Spicy Tomato Sauce   13
Chicken with Cream of Mushroom Soup   103
Chicken with Mayo-Avocado Sauce   102
Chicken-Stuffed Cucumber Bites   53
Chicken, Pepper, and Tomato Bake   95
Chili Con Carne   113
Chinese Cauliflower Rice with Eggs   48
Chinese Flavor Chicken Legs   99
Chipotle Beef Spare Ribs   124
Chipotle Tomato and Pumpkin Chicken Chili   90
Chive-Sauced Chili Cod   73
Chocolate Almond Bark   145
Chocolate Chip Ice Cream with Mint   155
Chocolate Fudge   146
Chocolate Pecan-Berry Mascarpone Bowl   152
Chocolate Truffles   145

Chocolate-Coconut Shake   144
Chorizo, Kale, and Avocado Eggs   3
Cinnamon Crusted Almonds   149
Cinnamon-Cream-Cheese Almond Waffles   6
Cioppino   40
Citrus Asparagus and Cherry Tomato Salad   64
Classic Devilled Eggs with Sriracha Mayo   50
Classic Flan   147
Classic Greek Salad   27
Classic Jerk Chicken   96
Cocktail Meatballs   18
Coconut and Pecorino Fried Shrimp   81
Coconut and Seed Bagels   1
Coconut Carrot Soup   36
Coconut Milk and Pumpkin Soup   37
Coconut Mussel Curry   82
Coconut Pumpkin Soup   40
Coconut Shrimp Stew   70
Coconut Turkey Breast   94
Cod Patties with Creamed Horseradish   85
Coffee-Coconut Ice Pops   151
Colby Bacon-Wrapped Jalapeño Peppers   52
Colby Broccoli Bake   67
Colden Gazpacho Soup   44
Cottage Kale Stir-Fry   48
Cream Cheese Almond Muffins   9
Cream Cheese Fat Bombs   150
Cream Cheese Stuffed Mushrooms   17
Cream of Broccoli Soup   41
Cream of Onion Pork Cutlets   107
Creamy Cabbage and Cauliflower   63
Creamy Caesar Dressing   162
Creamy Cashew Lemon Smoothie   1
Creamy Chocolate Mousse   155
Creamy Dijon Pork Filet Mignon   111
Creamy Pepper Loin Steaks   115
Creamy Reuben Soup with Sauerkraut   137
Creamy Ricotta Almond Cloud Pancakes   11
Creamy Spinach   49
Creamy Strawberry Shake   144
Creamy-Lemony Chicken Thighs   93
Creole Beef Tripe Stew with Onions   134
Crispy Chorizo with Parsley   52
Crispy Five Seed Crackers   19
Crispy Strawberry Chocolate Bark   153
Cumin Green Cabbage Stir-Fry   54
Curry Green Beans and Shrimp Soup   45
Curry White Fish Fillet   81

D–E

Dijon Crab Cakes   70
Dijon-Tarragon Salmon   73
Dill-Cream-Cheese Salmon Rolls   1
Double Cheese Kale Bake   67

Double-Cheese Ranch Chicken   100
Duo-Cheese Broccoli Croquettes   57
Duo-Cheese Lettuce Rolls   57
Duo-Cheese Pork and Turkey Patties   111
Easy Chicken and Onion Soup   36
Easy Peanut Butter Smoothie   3
Egg and Chicken Salad in Lettuce Cups   30
Egg and Ham Muffins   10
Egg-Stuffed Avocados   63

F
Fajita Spareribs   17
Fennel and Trout Parcels   83
Feta Cucumber Salad   28
Feta Zucchini and Pepper Gratin   59
Fettuccine Alfredo   160
Flank Steak and Kale Roll   136
Flaxseed Coconut Bread Pudding   157
French Scrambled Eggs   2
Fresh Strawberry Cheesecake Mousse   145

G
Gambas al Ajillo   74
Garlic Aioli Sauce   162
Garlicky Chicken Salad   32
Garlicky Coconut Milk and Tomato Soup   36
Garlicky Mackerel Fillet   75
Garlicky Sweet Chicken Skewers   103
Ginger-Pumpkin Pudding   156
Goan Sole Fillet Stew   77
Greek Aubergine-Egg Casserole   66
Greek Caper Salad   25
Greek Drumettes with Olives   89
Greek Tilapia with Tomatoes and Olives   69
Green Minestrone Soup   34
Grilled Beef Skewers with Fresh Salad   142
Grilled Lemony Chicken Wings   87
Grilled Prosciutto-Chicken Wraps   47
Grilled Ribeye Steaks with Green Beans   134
Grilled Rosemary Wings with Leeks   88
Grilled Salmon Steak   76
Ground Beef and Cauliflower Curry   123
Gruyere and Mushroom Lettuce Wraps   11

H
Haddock with Mediterranean Sauce   70
Halibut Tacos with Cabbage Slaw   71
Halloumi Asparagus Frittata   66
Ham, Cheese and Egg Cups   7
Hazelnut Haddock Bake   79
Hearty Chicken Soup   39
Hearty Pork Stew Meat   116
Herbed Balsamic Turkey   97
Herbed Beef and Zucchini Soup   35
Herbed Beef Soup   37
Herbed Eggplant   53

Herbed Eggplant and Kale Bake   55
Herbed Pork and Turkey Meatloaf   112
Herbed Pork Chops with Cranberry Sauce   118
Herbed Provolone Cheese Chips   19
Herbed Turkey with Cucumber Salsa   89
Herbed Veggie and Beef Stew   141
Homemade Poulet en Papillote   101
Hot Spare Ribs   22
Hungarian Chicken Thighs   102

I-J
Indian White Cabbage Stew   48
Italian Asiago and Pepper Stuffed Turkey   95
Italian Bacon Omelet   2
Italian Broccoli and Spinach Soup   65
Italian Haddock Fillet   73
Italian Sausage and Okra Stew   127
Italian Tomato and Cheese Stuffed Peppers   56
Italian Tomato Soup   41
Italian Turkey Meatballs with Leeks   87
Italian Veal Cutlets with Pecorino   142
Itanlian Chicken Cacciatore   99
Jalapeño Pepper Cream Cheese Omelet   9
Juicy Beef Meatballs with Parsley   139
Juicy Beef with Thyme and Rosemary   129

K-L
Kale and Smoked Salmon Salad   29
Kale Chips   16
Ketchup   163
Keto Peanut Butter Cookies   153
King Size Beef Burgers   123
Lamb and Cheddar Taco Soup   36
Lamb Chops with Fennel and Zucchini   131
Lamb Curry   126
Leek and Pumpkin Turkey Stew   92
Leek and Turkey Soup   43
Lemon Custard   154
Lemony Beef Rib Roast   126
Lemony Chicken and Chive Soup   34
Lemony Chicken Skewers   105
Lemony Cucumber-Avocado Salad   62
Lemony Ginger Pancakes   8
Lemony Mustard Pork Roast   107
Lemony Prawn and Arugula Salad   31
Lemony Rosemary Chicken Thighs   89
Lime and Coconut Panna Cotta   150
Lobster and Cauliflower Salad Rolls   74

M-N
Mackerel and Green Bean Salad   31
Marinara   161
Marinated Chicken with Peanut Sauce   96
Marinated Pork and Veg Salad   26
Mascarpone Beef Balls with Cilantro   128

Mascarpone Turkey Pastrami Pinwheels 57
Mashed Cauliflower with Bacon and Chives 52
Meaty Jalapeños 23
Mediterranean Aïoli 4
Mediterranean Halibut Fillet 77
Mediterranean Roasted Chicken Drumettes 96
Mediterranean Spiced Pork Roast 107
Mediterranean Tomato and Avocado Salad 28
Meringues 149
Mexican Beef and Tomato Chili 126
Mexican-Flavored Stuffed Peppers 65
Mini Bacon and Kale Muffins 23
Mozzarella Beef Gratin 134
Mozzarella Prosciutto Wraps with Basil 58
Mushroom and Bell Pepper Omelet 63
Mushroom and Broccoli Quiche 6
Mushroom and Kale Tofu Scramble 8
Mushroom and Zucchini Stew 62
Mushroom Stroganoff 50
Mustard Pork Meatballs 109
Nacho Soup 43

O
Old Bay Sea Bass Fillet 82
Olla Podrida 112
Olla Tapada 93
Onion Sauced Beef Meatballs 136
Orange Chili Sauce 160
Oregano Chicken Breast 105

P
Pancetta Veg Salad with Kale Frittata 5
Panna Cotta 148
Paprika Chicken Wings 105
Paprika Pork Loin Shoulder 114
Paprika Riced Cauliflower 47
Paprika Veggie Bites 19
Parma Ham-Wrapped Stuffed Chicken 100
Parmesan Bacon-Stuffed Pork Roll 119
Parmesan Basil Vinaigrette 161
Parmesan Cauliflower Fritters 59
Parmesan Chicken Wings with Yogurt Sauce 104
Parmesan Spinach Stuffed Chicken 101
Parmesan Veggie Fritters 65
Parsley-Lemon Salmon 77
Peanut Butter and Chocolate Fat Bombs 151
Pecan Pralines 148
Pecorino Cauli Bake with Mayo 57
Pecorino Mushroom Burgers 59
Peppery Omelet with Cheddar Cheese 66
Pesto Bacon and Avocado Mug Cakes 9
Pickle and Ham Stuffed Pork 113
Pinwheel Beef and Spinach Steaks 130
Pistachio Nut Salmon with Shallot Sauce 69
Pork and Beef Meatballs 110

Pork and Butternut Squash Stew 118
Pork and Mashed Cauliflower Crust 121
Pork and Mustard Green Soup 38
Pork and Vegetable Soup 40
Pork and Veggies Burgers 120
Pork and Yellow Squash Traybake 114
Pork Chops and Bacon 110
Pork Chops and Brussel Sprouts 116
Pork Chops with Greek Salsa 116
Pork Chops with Veggies 119
Pork Cutlets with Juniper Berries 108
Pork Kofte with Cauliflower Mash 120
Pork Lettuce Wraps 109
Pork Medallions 118
Pork Paprikash 107
Pork Ragout 115
Pork Rind Crusted Beef Meatballs 133
Pork Skewers with Greek Dipping Sauce 22
Pork Soup 35
Pork Steaks with Chimichurri Sauce 111
Pork with Raspberry Sauce 110
Posset 150
Power Green Soup 42
Prosciutto-Wrapped Piquillo Peppers 60
Provençal Lemony Fish Stew 79
Pulled Boston Butt 117
Pumpkin and Cauliflower Curry 49
Pumpkin Cheesecake Bites 152
Pumpkin Compote with Mix Berries 156

R
Raspberry and Kale Smoothie 4
Red Snapper Fillet and Salad 79
Reuben Beef Soup 42
Riced Cauliflower Stuffed Bell Peppers 55
Rich Taco Soup 44
Rind and Cheese Crusted Chicken 91
Ritzy Baked Chicken with Vegetable 100
Roasted Asparagus 58
Roasted Cauliflower with Serrano Ham 52
Roasted Chicken Breasts with Capers 99
Roasted Pork Shoulder 115
Roasted Stuffed Pork Loin Steak 119
Romano and Asiago Cheese Crisps 15
Romano Cheese Meatballs 13
Romano Zucchini Cups 48
Russian Beef and Dill Pickle Gratin 140

S
Saffron Coconut Shrimp Soup 39
Salmon and Cucumber Panzanella 83
Salmon Fillet and Spinach Cobb Salad 29
Salmon Fillets with Broccoli 73
Salmon with Radish and Arugula Salad 74
Salsa Verde Chicken Soup 39

Salted Vanilla Caramels   146
Sardine Burgers   82
Sardine Pepper Boats   18
Sardines with Zoodles   72
Sausage Quiche   4
Scallion Ginger Dressing   161
Seafood Chowder   81
Seared Pork Medallions   108
Seared Scallops with Sausage   75
Shirataki Mushroom Ramen   64
Shirataki Noodles with Grilled Tuna   80
Shrimp and Pork Rind Stuffed Zucchini   78
Shrimp and Vegetable Bowl   78
Shrimp Jambalaya   84
Shrimp Salad with Lemony Mayonnaise   28
Simple Beef Burgers   123
Simple Peanut Butter Fat Bomb   151
Simple White Wine Drumettes   87
Skirt Steak with Green Beans   140
Skirt Steak, Veggies, and Pecan Salad   30
Slow Cooked Chicken Cacciatore   94
Slow Cooked Faux Lasagna Soup   37
Slow Cooker Chocolate Pot De Crème   154
Smoked Haddock Burgers   85
Smoked Salmon and Avocado Omelet   70
Spanish Chicken and Pepper Salad   26
Spanish Cod à La Nage   77
Spiced Cauliflower Cheese Bake   54
Spiced Duck Goulash   95
Spicy Beef Brisket Roast   129
Spicy Chicken Drumettes   20
Spicy Pork and Capers with Olives   109
Spicy Pork and Spanish Onion   110
Spicy Pork Meatballs with Seeds   117
Spinach and Bacon Salad   28
Spinach Cheese Balls   51
Spinach-Cucumber Smoothie   3
Sriracha Sauce   160
St. Louis Ribs   112
Stir-Fried Chicken, Broccoli and Cashew   102
Strawberries Coated with Chocolate Chips   149
Strawberry Mousse   155
Strawberry Vinaigrette   163
Summer Stew with Chives   63
Super Cheesy Bacon-Cauliflower Soup   37
Swedish Herring and Spinach Salad   75
Swiss Chard, Sausage, and Squash Omelet   7
Swiss Cheese Broccoli   62
Swiss Zucchini Gratin   67

T

Tangy Pork Rib Roast   117
Tangy-Garlicky Pork Chops   114
Teriyaki Turkey with Peppers   92

Texas Chili   124
Texas Pulled Boston Butt   121
Thai Beef Steak with Mushrooms   129
Thai Tuna Fillet   84
Thyme Roasted Drumsticks   88
Tiger Shrimp with Chimichurri   76
Tikka Masala   87
Tilapia and Riced Cauliflower Cabbage Tortillas   71
Tilapia Tacos with Cabbage Slaw   71
Tomato and Bacon Cups   2
Tomato and Bacon Dressing   162
Tomato purée Pork Chops   120
Tomato Soup   42
Traditional Walnut Fat Bombs   15
Tuna Cheese Caprese Salad   25
Tuna Fillet Salade Niçoise   69
Tuna Omelet Wraps   74
Tuna Salad with Olives and Lettuce   27
Tuna Shirataki Pad Thai   72
Tuna-Mayo Topped Dill Pickles   53
Tuna, Ham and Avocado Wraps   76
Turkey and Avocado Roll-Ups   21
Turkey and Canadian Bacon Pizza   88
Turkey and Pumpkin Ragout   94
Turkey Stuffed Mini Peppers   14
Turkey Taco Soup   34
Turkey Wing Curry   98
Turkish Chicken Thigh Kebabs   98
Tuscan Chicken Breast Sauté   97
Tzatziki Sauce   162

V

Vanilla Chocolate Pudding   144
Vanilla Mascarpone Cups   5
Veal, Mushroom, and Green Bean Stew   132
Vegetable Mix   55
Veggie Cauliflower Rice with Beef Steak   128

W-Z

Whiskey-Glazed Chicken Wings   16
White Chowder   72
White Wine Pork with Cabbage   108
Wrapped Asparagus with Prosciutto   17
Yellow Cheddar Pork Patties Salad   30

Z

Zoodles with Beef Bolognese Sauce   123
Zucchini and Beef Lasagna   124
Zucchini and Carrot Coconut Bread   6
Zucchini and Celery Soup   38
Zucchini Casserole   54
Zucchini Chips   13
Zucchini Fritters   51
Zucchini Sticks with Garlic Aioli   56

Printed in Great Britain
by Amazon